HEART CELL COMMUNICATION IN HEALTH AND DISEASE

Developments in Cardiovascular Medicine

R.J. Siegel (ed.): *Ultrasound Angioplasty.* 1995   ISBN 0-7923-3722-0
D.M. Yellon and G.J. Gross (eds.): *Myocardial Protection and the Katp Channel.* 1995
                                        ISBN 0-7923-3791-3
A.V.G. Bruschke. J.H.C. Reiber. K.I. Lie and H.J.J. Wellens (eds.): *Lipid Lowering
Therapy and Progression of Coronary Atherosclerosis.* 1996 ISBN 0-7923-3807-3
A.S.A. Abd-Elfattah and A.S. Wechsler (eds.): *Purines and Myocardial Protection.* 1995
                                        ISBN 0-7923-3831-6
M. Morad, S. Ebashi, W. Trautwein and Y. Kurachi (eds.): *Molecular Physiology and
Pharmacology of Cardiac Ion Channels and Transporters.* 1996 ISBN 0-7923-3913-4
A.M. Oto (ed.): *Practice and Progress in Cardiac Pacing and Electrophysiology.* 1996
                                        ISBN 0-7923-3950-9
W.H. Birkenhager (ed.): *Practical Management of Hypertension. Second Edition.* 1996
                                        ISBN 0-7923-3952-5
J.C. Chatham, J.R. Forder and J.H. McNeill(eds.):*The Heart In Diabetes.* 1996
                                        ISBN 0-7923-4052-3
M. Kroll, M. Lehmann (eds.): *Implantable Cardioverter Defibrillator Therapy: The
Engineering-Clinical Interface.* 1996   ISBN 0-7923-4300-X
Lloyd Klein (ed.): *Coronary Stenosis Morphology: Analysis and Implication.*
1996   ISBN 0-7923-9867-X
Johan H.C. Reiber, Ernst E. Van der Wall (eds.): *Cardiovascular Imaging.*
1996   ISBN 0-7923-4109-0
A.-M. Salmasi, A. Strano (eds.): *Angiology in Practice.*   ISBN 0-7923-4143-0
Julio E. Perez, Roberto M. Lang, (eds.): *Echocardiography and Cardiovascular
Function: Tools for the Next Decade.* 1996   ISBN 0-7923-9884-X
Keith L. March (ed.): *Gene Transfer in the Cardiovascular System: Experimental
Approaches and Therapeutic Implications.* 1997 ISBN 0-7923-9859-9
Anne A. Knowlton (ed.): *Heat Shock Proteins and the Cardiovascular System.*
1997   ISBN 0-7923-9910-2
Richard C. Becker (ed.): *The Textbook of Coronary Thrombosis and Thrombolysis.* 1997
                                        ISBN 0-7923-9923-4
Robert M. Mentzer, Jr., Masafumi Kitakaze, James M. Downey, Masatsugu Hori, (eds):
Adenosine, Cardioprotection and its Clinical Application
                                        ISBN 0-7923-9954-4
Ian Graham, Helga Refsum, Irwin H. Rosenberg, Per Magne Ueland (eds.):
Homocysteine Metabolism: From Basic Science to Clinical Medicine
                                        ISBN 0-7923-9983-8
Antoine Lafont, Eric Topol (eds.): *Arterial Remodeling: A Critical Factor in
Restenosis.*   1997   ISBN 0-7923-8008-8
Michele Mercuri, David D. McPherson, Hisham Bassiouny, Seymour Glagov (eds.):
Non-Invasive Imaging of Atherosclerosis   ISBN 0-7923-8036-3
Walmor C. DeMello, Michiel J. Janse(eds.): *Heart Cell Communication in Health
and Disease*   ISBN 0-7923-8052-5

HEART CELL COMMUNICATION

IN HEALTH AND DISEASE

Edited by

Walmor C. De Mello
and
Michiel J. Janse

Kluwer Academic Publishers
Boston/Dordrecht/London

Distributors for North America:
Kluwer Academic Publishers
101 Philip Drive
Assinippi Park
Norwell, Massachusetts 02061 USA

Distributors for all other countries:
Kluwer Academic Publishers Group
Distribution Centre
Post Office Box 322
NL-3300 AH Dordrecht, THE NETHERLANDS

Library of Congress Cataloging-in-Publication Data

Heart cell communication in health and disease / edited by Walmor C.
De Mello and Michiel J. Janse.
      p. cm. -- (Developments in cardiovascular medicine ; v. 200)
      Includes bibliographical references and index.
      ISBN 0-7923-8052-5 (alk. paper)
      1. Heart cells. 2. Gap junctions (Cell biology) 3. Cell
Interaction. I. De Mello, Walmor C. II. Janse, Michiel Johannes.
III. Series
      [DNLM: 1. Heart--physiology. 2. Heart--physiopathology. 3. Gap
Junctions--physiology. 4. Cell Communication--physiology. W1
DE997VME v.200 1998 / WG 202 H4363 1998]
QP114.C44H42   1998
612.1'7--dc21
DNLM/DLC
for Library of Congress   97-40862
                                               CIP

Printed on acid-free paper.
Printed in the United States of America

CONTENTS

Contributing Authors vii
Preface ix
Dedication xi

Contributing Authors

Arnsdorf, Morton F.
Section of Cardiology
Department of Medicine,
Pritzker Medical School,
University of Chicago,
Chicago, IL, USA

De Mello, Walmor C.
Department of Pharmacology,
School of Medicine,
Medical Sciences Campus,
University of Puerto Rico,
San Juan, PR, USA

Dudley, Samuel C.
Section of Cardiology,
Department of Medicine,
Pritzker Medical School,
University of Chicago,
Chicago, IL, USA

Eisenberg, Leonard M.
Department of Cell Biology
and Anatomy,
Medical University
of South Carolina,
Charleston, SC, USA

Kléber, André G.
Department of Physiology,
University of Bern,
Bern, Switzerland

Litchenberg, Wanda H.
Department of Cell Biology
and Anatomy,
Medical University of South Carolina
Charleston, SC, USA

Beyer, Eric
Department of Pediatrics
Washington University,
School of Medicine,
Saint Louis, MO, USA

Dekker, Lukas R.C.
Laboratory of Experimental
Cardiology,
Academic Medical Center,
University of Amsterdam,
Amsterdam, The Netherlands

Janse, Michiel J.
Laboratory of Experimental
Cardiology,
Academic Medical Center,
University of Amsterdam,
Amsterdam, The Netherlands

Gourdie, Robert G.
Department of Cell Biology
and Anatomy,
Medical University
of South Carolina,
Charleston, SC, USA

Larson, David
Mallory Institute of Pathology,
Boston University,
School of Medicine,
Boston, MA, USA

Rudy, Yoram
Department of Cardiac
Bioelectricity,
Case Western Reserve University
Cleveland, OH, USA

Seul, Kyung Hwan
Department of Pediatrics,
Washington University,
School of Medicine,
Saint Louis, MO, USA

Shaw, Robin
Department of Cardiac
Bioelectricity,
Case Western Reserve
University,
Cleveland, OH, USA

Veenstra, Richard D.
Department of Pharmacology,
Medical College,
SUNY, at Syracuse
Syracuse, NY, USA

Severs, Nicholas J.
Imperial College of Medicine,
at the National Heart and
Lung Institute,
London, England

Tan, Hanno H.
Laboratory of Experimental
Cardiology,
Academic Medical Center,
University of Amsterdam,
Amsterdam, The Netherlands

Wang, Hong-Zhan
Department of Pharmacology,
College of Medicine,
SUNY, at Syracuse
Syracuse, NY, USA

Preface

This volume presents an extensive review of different aspects of heart cell communication. It starts with the fundamental concept that cardiac cells are communicated, and then goes to the role of gap junction in heart development, the molecular biology of gap junctions, the biophysics of the intercellular channels, the control of junctional conductance and the influence of gap junctions on impulse propagation.

For the first time, the intricacies of cell communication in the normal heart as well as under different pathological conditions, are presented in a single volume. Gap junction communication in heart failure, coronary artery disease, myocardial ischemia and cardiac arrhythmias is presented by different authors, each an expert in his own field. The process of cell communication is then analyzed at different levels of complexity, providing the reader with a broad view of this field and its relevance to cardiology.

We are grateful for the collaboration of our distinguished colleagues who participated in this important publication, and thank Kluwer Academic Publishers for their advice and professionalism.

Walmor C. De Mello
Michiel J. Janse

DEDICATION

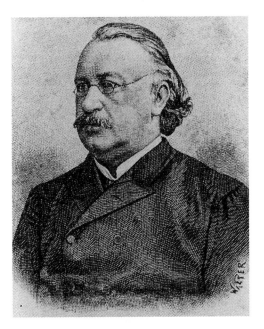

Theodor Wilhelm Engelmann
(1843-1909)

Theodore Wilhelm Engelmann started his career in Utrecht. In 1897 he was appointed to the Chair of Physiology in Berlin after the retirement of du Bois Raymond. His contribution to muscle and particularly to cardiac physiology is recognized as of fundamental importance for the ulterior development of this field. In several articles published in Pflugers Archiv he emphasized the notion that the "death of a heart cell does not necessarily lead to the death of neighboring myocytes." Because of the relevant role of Engelmann's work in our knowledge of heart cell communication, we would like to dedicate this volume in his memory.

Walmor C. De Mello
Michiel Janse

HEART CELL COMMUNICATION
IN HEALTH AND DISEASE

1 ON THE SYNCYTIAL NATURE OF CARDIAC MUSCLE

Walmor C. De Mello

Department of Pharmacology, Medical Science Campus, UPR

The heart muscle was initially conceptualized as an anatomical syncytium. Indeed, at the beginning of the century, intercalated discs were interpreted as sarcomere differentiation or even as contraction artefacts (1,2,3). In morphological studies performed by Heidenhain he mentioned Godlewisky's observations emphasizing the absence of cell boundaries. Quoting his original words:

> "... einen Tangentialschnitt durch the Herzwand eines drei-tagigen Entenembryos vorstellt. Nun ist allerdings richtig, dass sich damals trotz genauer Untersuchungen keine Zellengrenzen fanden".

These findings confirmed previous results of Fredericq (4) using embryonic heart muscle. He concluded: "Examiné a un grossissement 500 il se montré composé de mêmes elements que les muscles volontaires: une masse granuleuse protoplasmique dans lequelle se trouvant plonges des nombreaux noyau. Ici egalement les cellules embryonaires paraissent s'être fusioneés".

To avoid the concept of isolated cell Purkinje fibers were initially described as composed of grains (Körnchen) with a "Zwichensubstanz" between the Körnchen (5). Although the studies of Werner (6) recognized that the heart muscle consists of "territories with clear boundaries" the cellular nature of cardiac muscle was only accepted with the development of electronmicroscopy and the work of Sjostrand and Andersson, (7). These authors showed that heart cells are enveloped by a membrane what demonstrated that the cardiac muscle is composed of isolated cells.

This finding certainly represented a serious problem for the explanation of how the electrical impulse propagates throughout the heart. The same question was a central point of controversy in neurophysiology with the neuronal theory of Ramon y Cajal (8) because the nervous system was classically visualized as a net-like structure which is the reticular theory of Gerlach (9). With the work of Loewi (10), Dale (11) and Katz (12) the possibility of electrical synaptic transmission was discarded. As emphasized by Katz (13) the impedance of nerve endings and the skeletal muscle fiber are mismatched, indicating that the electrical mechanism of synaptic transmission is not correct. Indeed, the end-plate potential was due to the removal of charge from the postsynaptic membrane which was found to be thousands of time larger than any removal process caused by presynaptic action current alone (14).

It was then conceivable that the release of some chemical transmitter by the myocyte might induce the depolarization of the neighboring cell. Contrary to the neurons, however, a chemical machinery necessary for the synthesis and the storage of transmitters into synaptic vesicles does not exist in cardiac muscle.

The classical observations of van Bremen (15), Moore and Ruska, (16), Poche and Lindner (17) and Sjostrand and Andersson (7), however, indicated that the plasma cell membrane is modified at the intercellular region showing junctional specializations like macula adherents (demosomes), fasciae adherents and nexuses (see Fig. 1). In desmosome the apposing plasma cell membranes are separated by a gap of 250-300 A while at the nexus the cell membranes are in intimate contact (Fig. 1). Using the electron opaque lanthanum hydroxide to mark the extracellular space Revel and Karnovsky (18) showed, however, that at the nexus or "gap junction" there is gap of 2 nm between the two plasma cell membranes (see also Fig. 1). In addition, these observations suggested that gap junctions are composed of membrane particles organized like a plaque.

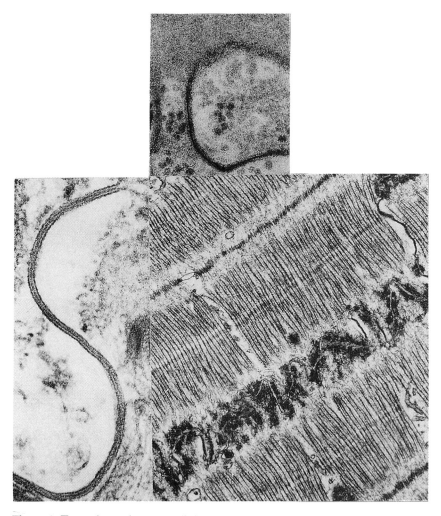

Figure 1. Top - shows the extracellular space in gap junction marked with electron opaque lanthanum hydroxide. Bottom-Right - Thin section electronmicrograph of gap junction showing internal structure. Left - electronmicroscopy of heart muscle showing intercalated disc. Kindly provided by Dr. JR Sommer, with permission.

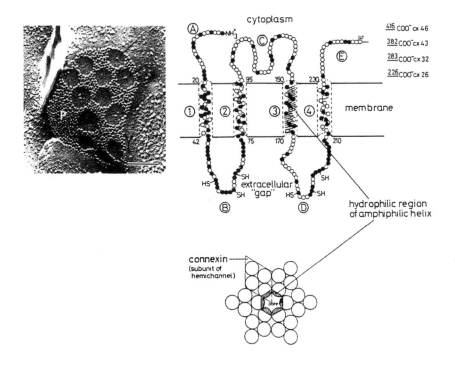

Figure 2. Left - vertebrate gap junction from calf heart showing closely packed particles in hexagonal array kindly provided by Dr. C Peracchia. Right - hypothetical topological model of connexins based on evaluation of hydropathy. In lower part of the figure hypothetical structure of hemichannel viewed perpendicularly to the plane of the membrane. From reference 61, with permission.

An important information about the organization of cytoplasmic and external surfaces of gap junctions was achieved by using freeze -fracture- etch methods (19) (see Fig. 2). These and posterior studies indicated that each cell contributes to a hemi-channel or connexon (20) and that each connexon is composed of six protein subunits surrounding an aqueous pore (Figs. 2 and 3).

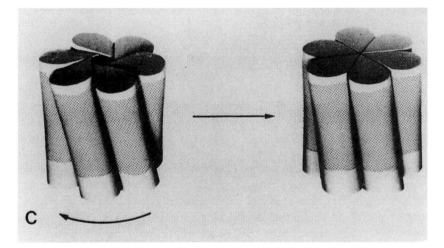

Figure 3. Models of gap junctions derived from tri-dimensional maps. The hemichannel is oriented with the cytoplasmic domain to the top. The hemichannel consists of six subunits that enclose the small hydrophilic cavity. The conformation changes that open and closes the channel consists of a cooperative change in the angle of inclination of the subunits. From reference 24, with permission.

Subsequent physiological and biophysical observations demonstrated that hydrophilic channels located at the center of nexus subunits, connect the interior of adjacent cardiac cells (21) (see chapters 3 and 4). Recently, observations of Veenstra et al., (22) are consistent with the view that the conventional simple aqueous pore model of a gap junction channel must be replaced by a new model for channel conductance and permeability based on electrostatic interaction (see Chapter 4).

The first model describing conformational changes which are responsible for channel gating was presented by Mackowiski et al., (23) and represented the combination of chemical data, of low-angle-X-ray diffraction studies and electron microscopic information. In this model the gate was located in the external subunit of the channel and the change in channel conductance was visualized as a displacement of mass into the lumen (for more details on other models see 24). An alternative mechanism of channel gating involves a coordinate rearrangement of the entire channel due to tilting or sliding of the individual subunits along their lines of contact (see Fig. 3 and 20, 24).

1. Cell communication assayed by electrical methods

The first evidence that heart fibers present cable properties was presented by Weidmann (25). Applying one dimensional cable theory to cardiac Purkinje fibers he demonstrated that the data is well described by the cable theory. Indeed, when current is injected into a Purkinje cell appreciable changes in membrane potential can be seen in adjacent cell. These studies demonstrated that the core resistivity is quite low and the space constant (1.9 mm) is larger than the length of a single heart cell (125 um). Moreover, Draper and Weidmann (26) showed that the conduction velocity of the action potential in these fibers is 3-4 m/sec what means that a single myocyte is traversed in 30 us. Since the action potential upstroke uses 0.3-0.5 ms it is possible to conclude that 10-15 cells participate simultaneously in the upstroke. As emphasized by Fozzard (27) these observations support the view that the cells are electrically coupled because transmission through chemical synapses require longer times.

Using a method similar to that of Osthout and Hill (28) Barr et al., (29) showed that the impulse conduction in atrial muscle is blocked by increasing the extracellular resistance in the central portion of a thin bundle (see Fig. 4). The blockade of the action potential was, however, reversed by connecting an appropriate resistance between both sides of the central gap (Fig. 4) what implies that low extracellular and intracellular resistances are required for the propagation of the action potential.

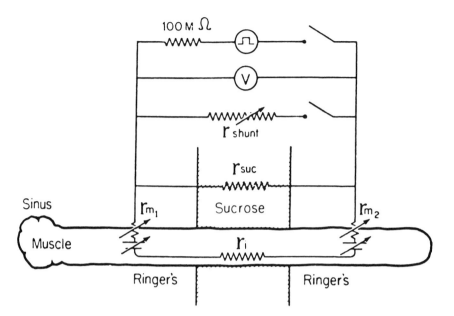

Figure 4. Diagram showing the experimental procedure followed by Barr et al., to demonstrate the electrical coupling in frog atrial muscle. The central area of the bundle was perfused with isotonic sucrose solution while the two peripheral regions were bathed with Ringer's solution and separated from the central zone by a partition. From reference 29, with permission.

The remaining question was whether intercellular junctions were necessary for the propagation of the impulse or was the electrical signal able to jump the gap between two apposing cells.

It is known since the work of Hodgkin (30) that electrotonic potentials can jump across a short inexitable zone. If the amplitude of the signal is not decreased to less than 1/5 across the inexitable zone the threshold will be reached in the cell beyond the block and consequently a propagated action potential will be generated. As the terminal membrane impedance falls with the inverse square of the fiber diameter it is easy to understand that in some preparations like the septate axon the attenuation of the electrical impulse across the septa is about 1/10 what means that the longitudinal propagation of the impulse will be "almost" possible even if we assume the absence of gap junctions (31).

For cardiac fibers with a small diameter the situation is quite different since the attenuation factor here is extremely large and the possibility that the electrical impulse cross the gap is impossible.

This means that the hypothesis of impulse propagation across intercellular gaps can be discarded and the presence of intercellular channels is then required for the intercellular spread of current. Indeed, experiments performed on cultured heart cells indicated that the coupling resistance is high (> 100 MΩ) at the moment of cell contact but starts falling immediately after reaching values of 20 MΩ at the moment electrical synchronization is achieved (32). Assuming a resistance of 10^{-10} Ω for a single hydrophilic channel the rate of channel synthesis was found to be one channel per cell per minute (32). Furthermore, during the establishment of the gap junction the conductance is increased by quantal steps suggesting a gradual increment in number of channels (33). When neonatal heart cells are pushed together and one of the cells is stimulated, an action potential is recorded in the stimulated cell but no response is detected in the other cell (34). In about 5-15 min, however, the non-stimulated cell starts showing subthreshold depolarization and finally total cell communication is established (Fig. 5).

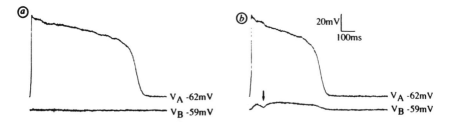

Figure 5. Membrane potentials recorded from two heart cells in the process of coupling under current clamp conditions. A: just after the cells have been pushed together, B: 7 min later. From reference 34, with permission.

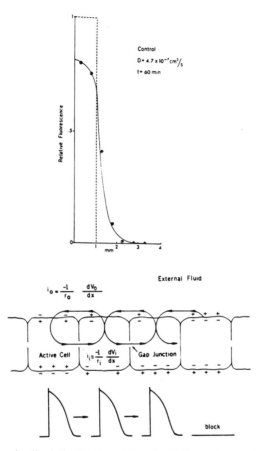

Figure 6. Top - longitudinal distribution of Lucifer Yellow along trabecula dissected from the right atrium of dog's heart. D = diffusion coefficient. From reference 56, with permission. Bottom - diagram illustrating the flow of local current in a cardiac fiber and the role of gap junctions in the spread of propagated activity,. From reference 57, with permission.

These and other findings lead us to conclude that the mechanism of impulse propagation in the heart is through local current flow what means that current flows the active areas along the myoplasm and gap junctions, outward through the resting adjacent cell membrane, back along the extracellular fluid and inward through the active region, so completing the local circuit (see Fig. 6). The potential change across the non-junctional membrane (V_m) is given by the difference between the potential on the inside (V_i) and the potential on the outside (V_o): $V_m = (V_i - V_o)$. The current flowing along the outside of the membrane is $i_o = (1/ro)(dVo/dx)$, where dVo/dx is the extracellular potential gradient and r_o the resistance per unit length of the extracellular fluid. The current flowing along the core of the cardiac fiber is given by $i_i = (-1/ri)(dVi/dx)$ where dVi/dx is the intracellular gradient and r_i the intracellular resistance per unit length, which represents the myoplasmic and the junctional resistance. Contrary to nerve cells the cardiac myocytes have a highly structured intracellular medium in which the sarcoplasmic reticulum occupies a quite large proportion of this space. Despite of this the cytoplasm of the heart and other muscle fibers has a specific resistance similar to that of the extracellular fluid (14, 35).

The complex geometry of the myocardium has a great influence on the spread of current. In the rat atrium, for instance, the depolarization of one cell causes an appreciable change in the membrane potential of adjacent cells (36) but a steep decline of the electrotonic potentials was found (λ = 130 um) when an intracellular electrode was used to polarize the cell. The enormous decrement of the electrotonic potentials was due to the three - dimensional characteristics of the rat trabecula and was not related to a high intracellular or extracellular resistance or to a low non-junctional membrane resistance. The decay of the electrotonic potential in this case is better fitted by a Bessel function (36).

It is essential to recognize that the coupling coefficient (Cc) between two isopotential cells is given by the following ratio:

$$Cc = gj/gj + gjn$$

where gj is the junctional conductance and gjn the conductance of the surface cell membrane. This means that an increase in gjn will result in a smaller coupling coefficient.

In specialized fibers of the A-V node as well as in the sinoatrial node, for instance, acetylcholine causes a decline in the electrical coupling mainly through an increase in surface cell membrane conductance (37, 38).

In both tissues the spread of electrical current is limited by a small space constant (465 um for the sinoatrial node (39) and 430 um for the A-V node (37).

Gap junctions have been identified between pacemaker cells (40) but their mean area is smaller than those found in the myocardium. In the sinoatrial node, for instance, the nexuses represent 0.2% of cell surface area which is about 10 times less than in working myocardial cells. In the A-V node, a high intracellular resistance contributes to the small conduction velocity (37) and makes the cell-to-cell propagation greatly dependent on changes in non-junctional membrane resistance. Although it is known that a slower depolarizing mechanism in the A-V node cell is also responsible for slow conduction there is evidence that in atrial muscle appreciable amounts of conexin43, connexin40 and connexin45 can be found while the A-V node and sinoatrial node are devoid of connexin43 (41). These observations highly suggest that the different expression of the connexins influences the junctional conductance and consequently the conduction velocity.

Since the membrane potential of sinoatrial fibers is about -60 to -65 mV compared to -85 to -90 mV in the atrium the obvious question is how the pacemaker cells that are electrically coupled with atrial cells are not hyperpolarized by the atrium. A reasonable explanation is the establishment of a gradient in coupling between the pacemaker and the atrium (42).

Because gj is dependent upon Cai (43) the question of whether the junctional conductance is constant or changes during the cardiac cycle merits serious consideration. Measurements of intracellular resistance and space constant performed during diastolic depolarization in isolated Purkinje fibers indicated that the electrical coupling is gradually increased during diastole (44). The increment in electrical coupling is due to both a fall in the intracellular resistance (r_i) and an increase in non-junctional membrane resistance (r_m). According to these findings the firing of the action potential coincides with the moment a maximal degree of cell coupling is achieved. Although the mechanism by which r_i falls during diastole remains to be determined, it is known that epinephrine increases the electrical coupling during diastole depolarization (44) suggesting that this phenomenon is enhanced by cAMP and consequent phosphorylation of gap junction proteins.

A major advance in the study of heart cell communication came through the development of patch clamp technique (45). The double whole-cell recording technique was initially used in measurements of junctional conductance in chick embryonic heart cell pairs (46,48) and subsequently in neonatal heart cells (34,49) or adult rat ventricular cell pairs (50,51,52). A full description of this technique including its limitation was presented by Giaume (53).

2. Cell-to-cell coupling assayed by fluorescent probes

Further evidence that heart cells are intercommunicated was provided by studies of ion or dye-coupling. In 1966 Weidmann (54) demonstrated that potassium ions diffuse through the gap junctions of sheep and calf ventricular muscle.

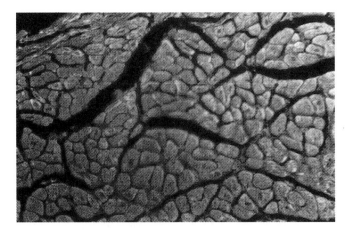

Figure 7. Spread of Lucifer Yellow along cardiac fibers. Note the absence of the dye in the extracellular space. From De Mello, unpublished.

Subsequent studies showed that Lucifer Yellow CH - a non-toxic substituted naphtalimide with two sulfonated groups, diffuses through the cytoplasm and gap junctions in heart fibers and has the advantage that does not cross the surface cell membrane (55). As shown in Fig. 6 the introduction of Lucifer yellow CH into dog trabeculae with the cut-end method was followed by its redistribution over distances larger than the length of a single cell. Considering that the permeability of the surface cell membrane to the dye is negligible the results represent a strong evidence that the cardiac cells are connected by permeable channels (56). The diffusion coefficient (D_j) can be quantitatively evaluated by fitting the experimental results to theoretical points estimated using the Crank's equation for the diffusion in a cylinder assuming no loss of tracer through the surface cell membrane. Fluorescence microscopy showed indeed, Lucifer Yellow CH located exclusively inside the heart fibers (see Fig. 7).

The average value of D_j for the dog trabeculae estimated by an interactive computer program for non-linear regression was $4\pm0.63x$ 10^{-7} cm^2/s (56). For Lucifer Yellow CH the value of D_j is smaller than the diffusion coefficient of the dye in the sarcoplasm ($D_s=2x10^{-6}$ cm^2/s) indicating that there is a restrictive diffusion at the gap junctions.   Indeed, studies performed with other compounds not only supported this view but also indicated that the junctional permeability (P_{nexus}), which has the physical dimension of velocity (cm/s), is inversely proportional to the molecular weight of the compounds (57).   For Lucifer Yellow CH (mol.wt.473) $P_{nexus}=3x10^{-4}$ cm/s (54) for TEA (mol wt.130) was 1.27 x 10^{-3} cm/s (58) for cAMP (mol.wt. 328) was 1.33 x 10^{-6} cm/s (59) and for K was 7.68 x 10^{-3} cm/s (54). The diameter of the pore connecting two apposing cells was found to be 1-1.5 nm while Procion Yellow (mol.wt. 697) - an elongated structure measuring 0.5 x 1 x 2.7 nm, is the largest molecule to pass the channel (60). It is important to add that the terms "ionic permeability" and "ionic conductance" are not interchangeable because permeability $P=(uB/d)(RT/F)$ where u is electrical mobility, B is the partition coefficient between solution and membrane and d is thickness of the membrane. The two properties are, however, in intimate relation.

The studies of dye coupling were extremely valuable in studies of intercellular communication in different systems and helped to demonstrate that the junctional permeability is not constant but it can be modulated. Certainly, the combination of different techniques and preparations is extremely useful and permits a more penetrating insight into the dynamics of the process of intercellular communication whose biological importance in the heart is not solely related to the control of electrical and molecular coupling but also proved to be an important protective mechanism in case of heart injury (healing-over).

References

1. Ebner V (1900). Ueber die Kittlinien der Herzmuskelfasern. Sitzungsber. Wien Akad Math Nat Kl, 109, 3.
2. Heidenhain M (1991). Ueber die Structur des menschlichen Herzmuskels. Anat Anz 20:33.
3. Godlewisky E (1902). Die Entwicklung des Skelet-und Herzmuskelgewebes der Saugthiere. Arch Mikros Anat 60:111.
4. Fredericq L (1875). Génération et structure du tissu musculaire. Bruxelles.
5. Purkinje JE (1845). Mikroskopisch-neurologische Beobachtungen. Arch Anat Physiol Leipzig, 281.
6. Werner M (1910). Besteht die Herzmuskulatur der Saugethiere aus allseitz scharf begrentzen Zellen oder nicht? Arch Mikrosk Anat 71:101.
7. Sjöstrand FS and Andersson KE (1954). Electron microscopy of the intercalated disks of cardiac muscle tissue. Experientia, 10, 369-371.
8. Ramon y Cajal S (1895). Les nouvelles idées sur la structure du systéme nerveux chez l'homme et chez les vertebrés. Reinwald, Paris.
9. Gerlach J (1877) Von dem Ruckenmarke. In: Handbuch der Lehre von den Geweben. Bd 2, (S Stricker, ed).
10. Loewi O (1921). Uber humorale Ubertragbarkeit der Herznervenwirkung. Pflüg. Arch. ges. Physiol. 189:239-242.
11. Dale HH (1935). Pharmacology and nerve endings. Proc R Soc Med 28; 319-332.
12. Katz B (1935). The transmission of impulses from nerve to muscle and the subcellular unit of synaptic action. Proc Roy Soc (London) Ser B 155:455-477.
13. Katz B (1966). Nerve, muscle, and synapse. McGraw-Hill Inc.
14. Fatt P and Katz B (1951). An analysis of the end-plate potential recorded with an intracellular microelectrode. J Physiol (London) 115: 320-370.
15. van Bremen VL (1953). Intercalated discs in heart muscle studied with the electron microscope. Anat Rec 117; 49-54.
16. Moore D and Ruska H (1957). Electron microscope study of mammalian cardiac muscle cells. J Biophys Biochem Cytol 3:261-269.
17. Poche R and Lindner E (1955). Untersuchungen zur Frage der Glanzstreifen des Herzmuskelgewebes beim Warmblutter und beim Kaltblutter. Z. Zellforch Mikrosk Anat 43:104-108.
18. Revel JP and Karnovsky MJ (1967). Hexagonal arrays of subunits in intercellular junctions of the mouse heart and liver. J Cell Biol 33:C7-C12.
19. Goodenough DA and Gilula NB (1974). The splitting of hepatocyte gap junctions and zonnulae occludents with hypertonic solution. J Cell Biol 61:575-590.
20. Unwin PNT and Zampihi G (1980). Structure of junctions between communicating cells. Nature 283:545-549.

21. McNutt NS and Weinstein RS (1970). The ultrastructure of the nexus. A correlated thin section and freeze cleave study. J Cell Biol 47:666-673.

22. Veenstra RD, Wang HZ, Beblo DA, Chilton MG, Harris AL, Beyer EG and Brink PR (1995). Selectivity of connexin-specific gap junctions does not correlate with channel conductance. Circ Res 77:1156-1165.

23. Makowsky L, Caspar DLD, Phillips WC and Goodenough DA (1977). Gap junction structures II. Analysis of the X-ray diffraction data. J Cell Biol 74: 629-645.

24. Zampighi G (1987). Gap junction structure. In: Cell-to-cell communication (De Mello, WC, ed) pp 4-28, Plenum Press, New York.

25. Weidmann S (1952). The electrical constants of Purkinje fibers. J Physiol (London), 118:348-360.

26. Draper MH and Weidmann S (1951). Cardiac resting and action potentials recorded with an intracellular electrode. J Physiol (London), 115:74-94.

27. Fozzard H (1979). Conduction of the action potential. In Handbook of Physiology, Section 2 Vol 1 pp 335-358 (Berne RM , Sperelakis N and Geiger SR, eds) American Physiological Society, Washington.

28. Osterhout WJV and Hill SE (1930). Salt bridges and negative variations. J Gen Physiol 13, 547-553.

29. Barr L, Dewey MM and Berger W (1965). Propagation of action potentials and the structure of the nexus in cardiac muscle. J Gen Physiol, 48:797-823.

30. Hodgkin A (1937). Evidence for electrical transmission in nerve. J Physiol (London) 90:183-232.

31. Katz B (1939). Electric excitation of nerve. Oxford University, Press, London.

32. Clapham DE, Shrier A and DeHaan RL (1980). Junctional resistance and action potential delay between embryonic heart cell aggregates. J Gen Physiol 75:633-654.

33. Loewenstein WR, Kanno Y and Socolar SJ (1978). Quantum jumps of conductance during formation of membrane channels at cell-cell junction. Nature, London, 274:133-136.

34. Rook MB, Jongsma HY and Van Ginnecken ACG (1988). Properties of single gap junctional channels between isolated neonatal rat heart cells. Am J Physiol 255:H770-H782.

35. Falk G and Fatt P (1964). Linear electrical properties of striated fibres observed with intracellular electrodes. Proc Roy Soc London Ser B 160:69-123.

36. Woodbury YW and Crill WE (1961). On the problem of impulse conduction in the atrium. In: Nervous Inhibition (Florey, L ed) Plenum, pp 24-35, New York.

37. De Mello WC (1977). Passive electrical properties of the atrioventricular node. Pflugers Arch Ges Physiol 371:135-139.

38. De Mello WC (1980). Intercellular communication and junctional permeability In: Membrane Structure and Function (EE Bittar, ed) Vol 3, pp 128-164, Wiley, New York.

39. Bonke EIM (1973). Electrotonic spread in the sinoatrial node of the rabbit heart. Pflugers Arch 339:17-24.
40. Masson-Pevet M, Bleeker WK, Besselsen E, Mackaay JC, Jongsma HJ and Bouman LN. On the ultrastructural identification of pacemaker cell types within the sinus node. In: Cardiac rate and Rhythm. (Bouman LN and Jongsma HJ, eds) pp 19-34, Martinus Nijhoff Publishers, 1982, Boston.
41. Davis LM, Kanter Kanter HL, Beyer EG and Saffitz JE (1994). Distinct gap junction protein phenotypes in cardiac tissues with disparate conduction properties. J Am Cell Cardiol 24:1124-1132.
42. Joyner RW and Van Capelle FJL (1986). Propagation through electrically coupled cells - how a small SA node drives a large atrium. Biophys J 50:1157-1164.
43. De Mello WC (1975). Effect of intracellular injection of calcium and strontium on cell communication in heart. J Physiol (London) 250:231-245.
44. De Mello WC (1986). Increased spread of electrotonic potentials during diastolic depolarization in cardiac muscle. J Mol Cell Cardiol 18:23-29.
45. Hamill OR, Marty P, Neher A, Sakmann B and Sigworth EJ (1981). Improved patch-clamp techniques for high resolution current recording from cells and cell-free membrane patches. Pflugers Arch 39: 85-100.
46. Ayer RK, DeHaan RL and Fischmeister R (1983). Measurement of membrane patch and seal resistance with two patch electrodes in chick embryo cardiac cells. J Physiol (London) 345, 29P.
47. Fischmeister R, Ayer RK and DeHaan RL (1984). Some limitations of the cell attached patch-clamp technique: a two electrode analysis. Pflugers Arch 406:73-76.
48. Veenstra RD and DeHaan RL (1986). Measurements of single channel currents from cardiac gap junctions. Science, 233, 972.
49. Burt JM and Spray DC (1988). Single channel events and gating behavior of the cardiac gap junction channel. Proc Natl Acad Sci, USA, 85:3431.
50. White RL, Spray DC, Campos de Carvalho A,m Wittenberg BA and Bennett MVL (1985). Some electrical and pharmacological properties of gap junctions between adult ventricular myocytes. Am J Physiol 18, C447-C551.
51. Weingart R (1986). Electrical properties of the nexal membrane studied in rat ventricular cell pairs. J Physiol 370:267-284.
52. De Mello WC (1988). Increase in junctional conductance caused by isoproterenol in heart cell pairs is suppressed by cAMP-dependent protein-kinase inhibitor. Biochem Biophys Res Comm 154:509-514
53. Giaume C (1991). Aplication of the patch-clamp technique to the study of junctional conductance. In: Biophysics of Gap Junction Channels (C. Peracchia, ed) pp 176-188, CRC Press, Boca Raton.
54. Weidmann S (1966). The diffusion of radiopotassium across intercalated discs of mammalian cardiac muscle. J. Physiol (London) 187:323-342.

55. De Mello WC, González Castillo M and van Loon, P (1983). Intercellular diffusion of Lucifer Yellow CH in mammalian cardiac fibers. J Mol Cell Cardiol 15:637-643.
56. De Mello WC and van Loon P (1987). Further studies on the influence of cyclic nucleotides on junctional permeability in heart. J Mol Cell Cardiol 19:763-771.
57. De Mello WC (1987). Modulation of Junctional Permeability. In: Cell-to-Cell Communication (De Mello, WC, ed) 29-64, Plenum Press, New York.
58. Weingart R (1974). The permeability to tetraethylammonium ions of the surface membrane and the intercalated disks of the sheep and calf myocardium. J Physiol (London) 240:741-762.
59. Tsien R and Weingart R (1976). Inotropic effect of cyclic AMP in calf ventricular muscle studied by a cut-end-method. J Physiol (London) 260:117-141.
60. Imanaga I (1974). Cell-to-cell diffusion of procion yellow in sheep and calf Purkinje fibers. J Memb Biol 16:381-388.
61. Willecke K and Traub O (1990). Molecular biology of mammalian gap junctions. In Cell Intercommunication (WC De Mello, ed) pp 22-33, CRC Press Boca Raton.

2 GAP JUNCTIONS AND HEART DEVELOPMENT

Robert G. Gourdie, Wanda H. Litchenberg and Leonard M. Eisenberg

Department of Cell Biology and Anatomy, MUSC

The function of gap junctions in propagation of the cardiac action potential is one of the best characterized roles for intercellular communication. Comprehending the part played by cell-to-cell dialogue in embryological processes, including development of the heart, has proven to be a more complex problem. Nonetheless, research at the conjunction of cardiac development and gap junctions is a diverse and fast-moving arena. Significant recent advances have resulted from mutational analysis or transgenic alterations of the genes encoding the subunits which comprise the gap junction channel--the connexin proteins (1-3). Such work has directly linked proper gap junction gene function to normal cardiac organogenesis and also implicated altered intercellular communication in certain congenital abnormalities of the heart. Of further interest is the suggestion that alteration to coupling patterns in the diseased mature heart may result from pathological reiteration of developmental processes involved in the cellular organization of gap junctions (4,5). Such insight may be clinically relevant, as disruptions to myocyte coupling patterns have been implicated in the genesis of arrhythmias and other disturbances of cardiac conduction (see chapter 8).

The intent of this chapter is to provide an overview of the field, updating the reader with information on current progress and trends. In the first section, we survey developmental variation in gene expression patterns for cardiac connexins. The next section deals largely with structural aspects of gap junctions in differentiating cardiac tissues. Here, particular emphasis is placed on postnatal development and how progressive changes to myocyte coupling patterns within the heart may influence the maturation of essential electrophysiological properties. Finally, we consider genetic and transgenic studies of gap junction function in heart development. For those interested in broadening their reading beyond the scope of this text, several general reviews of intercellular communication in developmental processes and control of growth are available (6-10).

1. CONNEXIN GENE EXPRESSION DURING CARDIAC DEVELOPMENT

Gap junctions are aggregates of transmembrane channels (connexons) which provide sieve-like points of direct, but regulated coupling between the cytoplasm of adjoining cells. The connexin proteins that comprise gap junctional channels are encoded by a family of related genes of which more than 12 have been identified in mammalian cells, with several homologues isolated from non-mammalian species, including chick, *Xenopus* and skate (11-16). The embryonic heart undergoes profound and dynamic alterations in size, structure and function as development proceeds. Accordingly, intercellular communication in this developing organ is likely to be adapted for a variety of roles including cellular electrical connectivity, metabolic coupling, homeostatic interchange of ions and other small cytoplasmic molecules and the passage of signaling molecules potentially involved in developmental processes. Consistent with such diversity of function, there is evidence for complex patterns of expression of a number of distinct connexin isoforms in cardiac tissues (see chapter 3 for in-depth coverage of cardiac gap junction molecular biology). To some extent, the pace of discovery on gap junctions and connexins in the developing and mature heart has outpaced our ability to interpret the morphogenetic and physiological implications of the data. Perplexing variations in expression have been reported both within and between muscular and non-muscular cells of the heart, including those comprising the valvular tissues and coronary vascular bed. Multiple connexin isoforms may be present in certain cardiac cells--e.g. recent data indicate that the terminal Purkinje fiber cells of the mammalian conduction system may express three different connexin isoforms. The picture is further complicated by species differences and variations in the detection methodologies employed by various laboratories. Nonetheless, it seems we have reached an interesting juncture as certain pieces of the puzzle are beginning to fall into place.

1.1   Connexin43 in developing mammalian heart

Connexin43, the first connexin identified in the heart (17-18) was subsequently confirmed to be the main gap junctional isoform found in working atrial and ventricular myocytes in developing mammals (19-29).

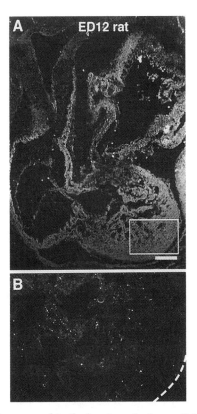

Figure 1. *Connexin43 is expressed in the looping tube heart of the rat embryo.* A) Low magnification survey of a looping tube heart from an ED 12 rat embryo. The boxed region in the primitive left ventricle indicates the tissue location shown in detail below. B) Detail of a gradient of connexin43 immunolabeling in ventricular myocardium. Punctate connexin43 signal is seen mainly within the inner trabeculated muscle. Near the epicardial (dotted line) outer surface of the heart, connexin43 immunolabeling is much lower. Reproduced from Anatomy and Embryology (24) by permission of Springer-Verlag Berlin Heidelberg. Scale bar 100 μm.

This protein has also been reported to be present in myocardial conduction tissues (24) and coronary and aortic smooth muscle cells (19,30). Immunofluorescence studies of mouse (23,26) and rat (20,24) demonstrated initial localization of connexin43 at probable gap junctions in ventricular myocardium between the 10th (ED 10) and 12th (ED 12) days of embryonic development (Figure 1). At these stages, rodent hearts are relatively primitive structures, resembling a looped tube. The appearance of connexin43 protein in mouse ventricle coincides well with reports of the initial detection of connexin43 transcript on ED 10 by in situ hybridization (25) and on ED 11 by Northern blotting (19). The timing of this detection occurs subsequent to the initiation of coordinate pulsatile activity by the myocardial rudiment (ED 8-9), although appearance of connexin43 coincides somewhat with the differentiation of ultrastructurally identifiable gap junctions in the primitive murine heart on ED 9-10 (31-33).

Detailed analyses of the spatial and temporal distributions of mRNA (29) and protein immunolocalization (22,24) have revealed a striking regionalization of connexin43 within the developing rat heart. From ED 13, high levels of connexin43 transcript were detected within atrial and ventricular myocardium (29), coinciding with marked increases in the densities of immunoreactive connexin43-puncta in these tissues (22,24). Connexin43 signal was found to be particularly abundant within the inner trabeculated muscle of the ventricles, but was absent or negligible at the subepicardial myocardium, the crest of the interventricular septum, the atrioventricular junction, and the outflow and inflow regions of the embryonic heart (20,22,24,29). There is some debate as to whether connexin43 is actually expressed at all in the atrioventricular junction of the rat. However, whether absent or present at low levels, this region is characterized by a relative paucity of connexin43 throughout development, a feature which persists into probable tissue derivatives comprising the atrioventricular node and proximal bundles of the mature rat conduction system. Interestingly, connexin43 occurs at high levels in Purkinje fiber cells in rats and other mammals, where it is co-expressed with connexin40 (34-36). Studies using *Xenopus* oocyte expression systems suggest that connexin40 and connexin43 half-channels are incompatible, being unable to form functional intercellular channels (37). Consequently, it has been proposed that segmented patterns of expression and co-expression of connexin43 and connexin40, by different myocardial compartments, may play an important role in electrical integration of the conduction system and correct patterns of linkage between Purkinje fiber cells and working myocytes (34,38).

Quantitative analyses of the relative abundance of connexin43 mRNA and immunoblotted protein have been undertaken in cardiac tissues from the developing mouse (19) and rat (21). These studies revealed that levels of connexin43 transcript rose sharply over the fetal and perinatal period before peaking 5 to 7 days after birth. The relative abundance of connexin43 protein also showed pronounced increases during the fetal and perinatal period; although curiously, protein maxima lagged some 10 to 14 days behind that of mRNA. The reason for this dissociation in the variation of connexin43 mRNA and its translation product remain unclear. During later postnatal growth, the abundance of both protein and transcript fall. These maturational declines in connexin43 gene products are consistent with reported sharp decreases in the level of ultrastructurally definable junctions in mammalian ventricle following birth (39,40). It is important to note that these quantitative studies relate only to overall gap junctional or connexin43 content within ventricular tissue samples. As such, interpretation of these indices will be confounded by factors such as cellular hypertrophy and heterogeneity of cell types in developing cardiac tissues. At present, virtually nothing is known about temporal variation in levels of connexin43 (or any other connexin) gene products within individual myocytes during postnatal growth. This data will likely be important for gaining insight into the differentiation of myocyte coupling patterns. As discussed subsequently in section 2, the precise configuring of such patterns is thought to be one of the key processes in maturation of normal electrophysiological function in the mammalian heart.

1.2 Other connexins in developing mammalian heart

Two further connexin isoforms, connexin40 and connexin45, have been reported to be expressed by developing and mature myocardial tissues in mammals, including humans (28,29,34,35,38,41-50). Currently, only limited information is available regarding connexin45 in developing heart. Quantitative Northern analyses of heart tissues from mouse (28) indicated an initially low and steadily declining abundance of connexin45 transcript from ED 14 (i.e. relative to levels of cardiac connexin43 mRNA). This variation accords with a time course described for levels of connexin45 mRNA in developing chick heart (51). However, in the adult mouse heart, the connexin45 transcript was reported as undetectable (28). This result from mouse is perplexing, as earlier studies of adult heart from other mammals suggest that connexin45 mRNA and protein are ubiquitously expressed at low to moderate levels in both working and conducting myocardium (44,46-50,52). There is presently no explanation for this interesting discrepancy. However, the pronounced decline of connexin45 mRNA levels observed over mouse embryogenesis would be consistent with restriction of expression into more specialized cardiac lineages. There is considerably more information on connexin40, the third myocardial-associated isoform found in mammals. Northern blotting indicated the presence of connexin40 in mouse embryos on ED 11, the stage at which immunofluorescence also reveals the presence of connexin40 within atrial and ventricular myocardium (28). With the progression of development, atrial connexin40 levels were found to be maintained. However, in ventricles, the pattern became more restricted. Immunopositive signal decreased in ventricular trabeculations from ED 14 onwards, with connexin40 eventually becoming preferentially expressed at relatively high levels in ventricular conduction cells (i.e. Purkinje fiber cells). Consistent with this maturational coalescence of connexin40 into conductile lineages, quantitative Northern blotting suggested connexin40 transcript levels declined over development and growth of the mouse heart. A similar pattern of spatial and temporal variation for connexin40 mRNA has been described from in situ hybridization studies in developing rat (29). In this latter study, an interesting asymmetric variation in connexin40 mRNA levels over time was described between the embryonic left and right ventricles, suggesting an independent maturational progression of gap junction-mediated communication in these two cardiac chambers.

While myocytes are the major constituent cell type in the developing heart, a heterogeneous mix of other cell types is also present in this organ. Current developmental data on connexins in non-myocardial cardiac tissues in mammals is fragmentary and mainly relates to expression by different vascular cell types (28,29). In addition to preferential expression by atrial and conduction cells, it has been determined that connexin40 is expressed at high levels in vascular endothelium of forming and mature coronary blood vessels (28,35,46,53). Expression of connexin37 mRNA has been reported to occur at low levels in the developing mouse heart (28). The precise cell type expressing connexin37 is uncertain, although it seems unlikely to be myocardial. In adult mouse, connexin37 has been reported to be present in endocardial endothelium and vascular smooth muscle tissues of coronary arteries and the aorta (54). An antibody against connexin50 has been immunolocalized to junction-like puncta in valve tissues from rat postnates (24). Interestingly, connexin50 is abundant in the lens and corneal epithelium of the eye (55). Like heart valves, neither of these two ocular tissues are supplied with blood vessels--an observation that has led to speculation that connexin50 may form channels specialized for functioning in avascular tissues.

1.3   Connexins in the non-mammalian heart

To date, knowledge on connexins in non-mammalian heart has come largely from studies of chick embryos (51,56-60). These data suggest certain similarities to mammals, but also some striking differences. The most surprising of which is an apparent absence of connexin43 in mature avian myocardial tissues. An important starting point for our knowledge of cardiac connexin diversity in bird, and for that matter in mammals, was the isolation and sequencing of genes encoding chick connexin45 and connexin42 (51).

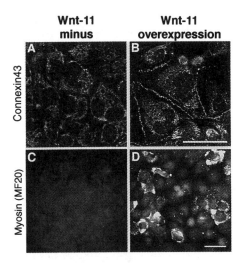

Figure 2. *WNT-11 regulates expression of connexin43 and differentiation of myocardial lineage.* A and C) Connexin43 and MF20 (a marker of myosin within cells of myocardial lineage) are poorly expressed in WNT-11 minus QCE6 cells--a mesodermal cell line derived from quail in which WNT-11 expression has been downregulated. B and D) High levels of connexin43 and MF20 are observed in QCE6 cells in which WNT-11 has been overexpressed. Reproduced from Development (61) by permission of the Company of Biologists. Scale bars A and B 17 μm and C and D 40 μm.

At the time, these represented two novel proteins, although mammalian cognates (connexin45 and connexin40, respectively) were soon described (41-44). Northern blot analyses indicated the expression of connexin43, connexin42 and connexin45 mRNAs in chick heart, though levels of connexin45 transcript declined sharply over development (51). As with embryonic mammals, the tissue specificity of connexin45 in the developing chick embryo remains uncharacterized. High levels of connexin42 have been reported to be immunolocalized in ventricular conduction tissues in the developing chick (from ED 10) and adult bird (56,58), with lower levels present in working myocardium (57,58). Immunofluorescence studies suggest that connexin43 is localized in the vessel walls of the outflow tract (57) and smooth muscle cells of prominent coronary arteries, but not veins (56). While absent between myocardial cells in bird, connexin43-coupling may be significant for specification of myocyte progenitors at the very earliest stages of avian cardiac differentiation (61). WNT-11-mediated changes in connexin43 expression in a quail mesodermal cell line (QCE6) were associated with altered potential of this cell line to undergo differentiation into cardiomyocyte-like cells (Figure 2). In ongoing work, it is being assessed whether this modulation of phenotypic potential by WNT-11, a gene expressed during the initial coalescence of the cardiogenic mesoderm (61), is directly correlated with alterations in levels of gap junctional coupling between cells.

The spatiotemporal variation of connexin42 in the avian heart has provided some important and unexpected insights into the developmental origin and maturation of cardiac conduction tissues (Figure 3 and references 56,58,59,62,63). From embryonic day 9 (ED 9), vascular endothelial cells of presumptive coronary arteries express relatively high levels of connexin42. At this stage, the gross morphogenesis of the chick heart is nearly complete, although the level of differentiation of accessory and specialized cardiac structures, such as nerves, blood vessels and the conduction system remains limited. During subsequent embryonic development, increasing levels of connexin42 were localized in definitive Purkinje fiber cells surrounding the already connexin42-positive arterial vessels. The correlated pattern of connexin42 expression by these two disparate tissues has led to cell lineage studies using replication-defective retroviruses (38,58,63). Data from these experiments suggest that cells comprising the developing vascular bed induce differentiation of embryonic myocytes into specialized lineages such as periarterial Purkinje fibers. Interestingly, the fascicular components of the ventricular conduction system, including the atrioventricular bundle and bundle branches, were found to have low connexin42 content until after hatching (56). Subsequently, a distal to proximal (i.e. relative to the atrioventricular node) gradient of connexin42 immunoreactivity differentiated along these conduction fascicles. A comparable spatial variation in connexin40 content has also been identified along the mature atrioventricular conduction system of mammalian heart (29, 34-36). At present, the functional implications of these peripheral to central gradients in connexin40 (the mammalian homologue of connexin42) have not been explored. However, consideration of the succession of differentiation in bird suggests that emergence of mature gap junctional communication patterns occur centripetally, from the most peripheral elements of the conduction system inward (i.e. Purkinje fibers toward atrioventricular bundle). This developmental sequence is counter-intuitive, as it opposes the direction of anterograde propagation and consequently raises interesting questions as to the integration of different elements of the conduction system during development. Indeed, the implication is that linkage of different compartments of the conduction system in the chick embryo may be an unexpectedly discontinuous process. These data also point to the potential for important changes in cardiac gap junction organization and function in the period following hatching in birds or birth in mammals, a theme that will be explored further in the subsequent section.

2. DIFFERENTIATION OF MYOCYTE COUPLING PATTERNS AND MATURATION OF CARDIAC ELECTROPHYSIOLOGICAL FUNCTION

2.1 Cardiac muscle is a discontinuous anisotropic media

The classical description of the heart as an electrical syncytium has provided a useful model for conceptualizing conduction of impulses in cardiac tissue. However, in the last decade new information has led to a significant conceptual shift. The work of Madison Spach and others has laid to rest the idea that action potential propagates smoothly through compartments of cardiac muscle as if in a continuous media (64-71). Propagation of electrical excitation in myocardium is discontinuous and stochastic. At the microscopic level, an electrical impulse stutters as it moves along paths determined by non-uniformly distributed points of coupling between muscle cells. In adult mammalian ventricle, this non-uniformity takes the form of polarized distributions of gap junctions at sites of end to-end abutment between myocytes--termed intercalated disks. Although, no direct correlation of structure and function has yet been made, the preferential concentrations of electrical connections at ventricular myocyte termini/disks has been speculated to account for the anisotropic or directional nature of impulse propagation found in mature myocardial tissues, in which impulse velocity along the myocyte long axis exceeds that transverse to this cellular axis (52,70,72,73). Uniform discontinuous anisotropic conduction of action potential is an important component of stable electromechanical function in heart. However, a decrease in transverse propagation velocity (and hence increased anisotropy) due to losses of gap junctions at domains of lateral contact between aging myocytes has been proposed to be a (and possibly **the**) substrate for micro-reentry and arrhythmia (69,74,75). It is therefore an important task to investigate the mechanisms underpinning the generation of cellular non-uniformities in cardiac gap junction distribution. This point is further emphasized by recent data indicating that the Kv1.5 potassium channel (76) and the rH1 sodium channel (77) both co-distribute with gap junctions at intercalated disks in adult mammalian ventricle.

2.2 Patterning of gap junctional coupling in the postnatal ventricle

Although the morphogenesis of the heart is nearly complete at birth (in a number of mammalian species, including humans), the physiology and the differentiation state of myocytes remains immature (78,79). During postnatal development, myocytes undergo profound changes in size, morphology and molecular phenotype. Several workers have now also confirmed that a striking re-organization of electrical connectivity occurs between working muscle cells in the mammalian ventricle during the maturational period following birth (5,20,23,24,72,76,80). This sequence was first and best characterized in rodent hearts (5,20,23,24). In the neonatal rat ventricle, gap junctions have relatively uniform distributions, being dispersed more or less randomly across the membranes of myocytes. During postnatal growth, concomitant with the loss of lateral interconnections, there is a progressive accumulation of gap junctions into polarized distributions at intercalated disks. This process continues over a relatively extended time

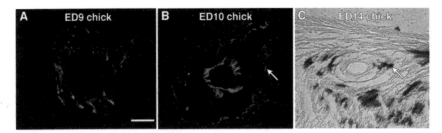

Figure 3. *Connexin42 expression and retroviral lineage tracing of cardiac Purkinje fibers.* A) Connexin42 immunolabeling of endothelial cells surrounding the lumen of a coronary vessel in an ED 9 chick embryo. B) Connexin42 labeling of endothelial cells and presumptive Purkinje fibers (arrowed) around a coronary artery at ED 10. The changing pattern of connexin42 expression (A and B) may be explained by a direct contribution of coronary vasculogenic cells to cardiac conduction tissues or an inductive relationship between forming blood vessels and adjacent embryonic myocardial cells. To determine which hypothesis accounted for the observed expression pattern, retroviral cell lineage studies were undertaken (58). C) A virally-infected clone of β -galactosidase-expressing cells (blue) around a coronary artery in an ED 14 chick heart. Both perivascular Purkinje fibers (arrowed) and working myocytes are contained within this clone, indicating that Purkinje fibers have a common cellular origin with working myocytes. Reproduced from Development (58) by permission of the Company of Biologists. Scale bar 10 μm.

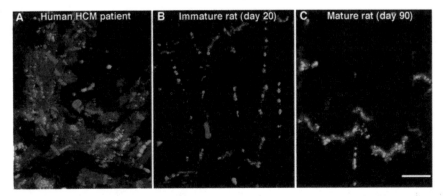

Figure 4. *Common patterns of association between gap junctions and cell adhesion junctions in diseased and differentiating myocardium.* A) Region of ventricular myofiber disarray in a hypertrophic cardiomyopathy patient doubled-labeled for connexin43 (green) and desmosomal desmoplakin (red). Punctate connexin43 signal is dispersed from desmoplakin which is localized mainly at disks. B) Dissociated patterning of putative gap junctions (green) and cell adhesion junctions (red) in ventricle of a 20 day rat. Gap junctions are largely not associated with disks, but dispersed along myocyte sides. C) In the ventricle of a 90 day rat, gap and adhesion junctions co-localize mainly at disks. Reproduced from Circulation Research (61) by permission of the American Heart Association. Scale bar 10 μm.

course and does not culminate until the animal is past sexual maturity (40 postnatal days). Comparable results indicating a prolonged phase of re-organization of cardiac intercellular junctions have been reported for humans in early childhood (72,76,80). As alluded to previously, this progressive change in the geometry of connectivity between mycoytes has been proposed as one of the main factors underlying changes in the rate and anisotropy of conduction during postnatal development (70,72).

2.3 A role for cell adhesion in gap junctional patterning?

Recent studies may have provided further clues as to potential mechanisms governing the generation of non-uniform distributions of cardiac gap junctions. Early reports, based on studies of human ventricular tissues, suggested that gap junctions co-distributed with cell adhesion junctions during postnatal development (72). However, more detailed quantitative studies of rat ventricle have characterized the emergence of a striking, but transient dissociation in the distribution of gap junctions and adhesive junctions during early postnatal life (5). While gap junctions show steady accumulation to myocyte termini during maturational growth of the heart, desmosomal and fascia adherentes junctions quickly differentiate into definitive intercalated discs in the days following birth (Figure 4). One explanation proposed to account for the observed developmental changes in electrical contact between myocytes relates to variation in the relative stability of different domains of myocyte sarcolemma (5). This hypothesis suggests that gap junctions proximal to high concentrations of cell adhesion junctions (e.g. at disks) will be preserved over those positioned distal from regions of dense mechanical coupling (e.g. myocyte sides). Conceivably, small variations in gap junction degradation rates at different domains of the cell membrane generated by this, or some other mechanism, could, over postnatal growth, give rise to the patterns of electromechanical coupling observed in mature ventricular myocardium. At present, there is no direct support of this hypothesis. Indeed other processes, such as active promotion of gap junctional assembly at disks, may account wholly or in part for the observed data. Nonetheless, indirect evidence for the potential importance of degradative processes to the generation of myocyte coupling patterns comes from several studies which have reported conspicuous increases in endocytotic-like gap junctional figures in ventricular myocytes from neonates in various mammalian species (72,81-83).

2.4 Clinical implications

Pursuit of the mechanism(s) involved in differentiation of myocardial cell coupling patterns is important to clinicians for several reasons. First, disruption to the normal organization of myocyte connectivity in diseases such as ischemic heart disease and hypertrophic cardiomyopathy have been strongly implicated as anatomical substrates for reentry, arrhythmia and other pathological disturbances of conduction (see chapters 8 and 9). Information on the processes governing gap junctional patterning during development could provide insight into the breakdown of electrical connectivity in diseases of the heart characterized by electromechanical dysfunction. Pertinently, recent data suggest that gap junctions in regions of myofiber disarray from patients with hypertrophic cardiomyopathy are dispersed from cell adhesion junctions (Figure 4 and reference 4). This histopathology is reminiscent of the maturational changes described by Angst and co-workers (5) and suggests that one consequence of cardiomyopathy may be a reiteration of more immature patterns of association between electrical and mechanical intercellular junctions in tissue exhibiting myofiber disarray. A second area of medical pertinence concerns the plasticity and remodeling of myocardium in response to surgery. It has been shown that corrective surgery of congenital cardiac malformations is more effective, in terms of reduction of postoperative arrhythmias and cardiac function, when performed earlier in infant life (84-87). These improved outcomes have been suggested to be related to an increased ability of the ventricle to electromechanically remodel when surgery is undertaken earlier in postnatal life (72,88). Finally, recent studies have indicated the possibility of transplantational repair of diseased myocardium by undifferentiated cardiac cells (89-92). The effectiveness of this approach may hinge on ensuring the homogeneous integration of cellular coupling at the donor-recipient interface and differentiation of normal patterns of association between gap junctions and cell adhesion junctions within the grafted tissue.

3. GENETIC AND TRANSGENIC STUDIES

The potential of intercellular communication to influence development was recognized almost as soon as the existence of low resistance pathways between cells was characterized (93-96). An obstacle to subsequent progress has been that gap junction coupled networks, such as those found in developing embryos, represent complex, non-linear systems.

As such, they are difficult to probe experimentally and consequently problematic to model. Recently, a promising route has been provided by molecular biology and the so-called "reverse genetic approach . Specific disruptions to connexin genes have been shown to have significant developmental consequences, in effect, providing a top-down perspective into the enigmatic role played by gap junctions. An initial breakthrough came with the recognition that point mutations in the human connexin32 gene were associated with peripheral nerve degeneration and the X-linked form of Charcot-Marie-Tooth syndrome (97,98). Subsequent work also implicated disrupted connexin gene function in cardiac disease. An inherited conduction system defect and dilated cardiomyopathy were mapped to a chromosomal locus suggestive of involvement of the connexin40 gene (99). In this case, connexins were excluded as the cause of malady; however, other studies have provided evidence indicative of a direct role for gap junctions in congenital abnormalities of the heart. Britz-Cunningham and co-workers (2), identified specific mutations in the connexin43 gene that were correlated with the occurrence of visceroatrial heterotaxia--a spectrum of profound anomalies distinguished by laterality defects to a number of organs, including the heart. The mutations were characterized as substitutions at serine or threonine residues which are potential phosphorylation sites in the C-terminal domain of the connexin43 protein. These mutations were shown to have direct functional consequences on coupling between cultured cells. The work of others have indicated that the particular (set of) mutations in the study of Britz-Cunningham et al. may be confined to a distinct cohort of individuals with the heterotaxia syndrome (100, 101). A fuller account of this interesting topic is provided in chapter 10.

A second arm of the "reverse genetic approach has been provided by direct manipulation of connexin genes using mouse transgenesis. Reaume and co-workers (1) reported a null mutant mouse in which virtually all coding sequence of the connexin43 gene had been deleted. Connexin43 is expressed early in mouse development and is thought to be involved in normal compaction of the preimplantation embryo (102, 103). It was unexpected then that some embryos homozygous for the deletion mutation survived to term. However, all such "knockout mice died shortly after birth from breathing difficulties. The observed postnatal mortality was attributed to abnormalities in the pulmonary outflow region of the heart, including a tissue blockage at the base of the pulmonary outflow tract which apparently compromised blood flow to the lungs of newborn null mutants once separated from the maternal circulation. These results suggest that connexin43 is not essential for cardiac function, at least not until partuition. As connexin40 is widely expressed in embryonic and fetal heart, it may be that this isoform fulfills a compensatory role. A germane, but not widely appreciated part of this story, is that while connexin43 is strongly expressed in normal embryonic rodent heart, as detailed in section 1.1, the pattern is far from uniform. Indeed, the outflow pole of the rat embryo (i.e. the main apparent site of defect in the mouse null mutant) has been shown have an extreme paucity of connexin43 expression (22,24). This poses an interesting quandary as to how the observed cardiac phenotype arises in the connexin43 knockout mouse. Further clues regarding the role of connexin43 in cardiac development came from work carried out by the group of Lo and her collaborators (3,104). In these studies, transgenic mice were constructed which overexpressed the connexin43 gene under control of a cytomegaloviral promoter. In such CMV43 animals, overexpression of the transgene was not targeted to myocardial tissues, but to the dorsal neural tube and to neural crest derivatives emigrating from the tube. Significantly, CMV43 mice also exhibited congenital heart defects, with involvement of a similar region affected in Cx43 knockout transgenics--the outflow pole of the right ventricle. However, unlike connexin43 null mutants, connexin43-overexpressors did not die at birth and detailed study revealed that their heart defects were also functionally and structurally unique. Other anomalies included defects in the cardiac conduction system and in the deployment of coronary vessels. Ultrasound of CMV43 embryos demonstrated the presence of unstable heart rhythms and also evidence of a reduction in the outflow of blood from the aorta and pulmonary artery. More detailed examinations of living fetal hearts by magnetic resonance imaging showed a narrowing of the ductus arteriosus, a blood vessel often attenuated in human fetuses with heart defects. Perhaps of most pertinence, breeding of the CMV43 transgene into the connexin43 knockout mouse, extended postnatal viability of mice homozygous for the null allele, implying that overexpression of connexin43 in neural lineages somehow resulted in partial rescue of newborns afflicted with connexin43 deletion. An explanation, posed by the authors, was that the cardiac neural-crest, a well-characterized player in the proper formation of the cardiac outflow tract (105), was being targeted via disrupted connexin43 function in both the CMV43 and connexin43 knockout transgenic constructs. A mechanism that could mediate such a process remains to be demonstrated. One conclusion that might be drawn from this work is that in order to gain insight into the role of intercellular communication in cardiac organogenesis, we may have to understand the part played by gap junctions in differentiation of extracardiac lineages migrating into the developing heart.

4. CONCLUSIONS AND THE FUTURE

The evidence that gap junctions have important roles in the normal differentiation of the heart is compelling. The work highlighted in this review indicates that research in this area is diverse and currently moving at a rapid pace. Findings such as those suggesting the potential effects of gap junctions in the migratory neural crest on heart development and the potential interplay between cell adhesion junctions and gap junctions in maturation of function in the ventricular myocardium are leading the field in unexpected and exciting new directions. There are some gaps in our present knowledge for which future progress will probably be straightforward. The status of connexin45 is unresolved. This is particularly the case in relation to the tissue specificity and function of connexin45 during early development, the period in which this isoform is most highly expressed in heart. Structural, molecular, and physiological aspects of cellular connectivity within the mature and developing atrioventricular node remain poorly characterized. Future studies of gap junctions and connexins in this structure could usefully incorporate our growing understanding of the morphogenesis of the central conduction axis, including concepts such as the primary conduction ring, identified from studies of developing hearts from humans (106) and birds (107). Progress in certain other important areas will likely require patience and persistence. It is interesting to speculate on the distant prospect of transposing principals learned from conduction of impulse within the myocardium, such as Spachs concepts of discontinuous signal propagation and stochastic coupling, to future modeling of the function of gap junctions in developing systems. Research on the cardiac gap junction has often led the way in establishing general notions on intercellular communication, applicable to both excitable and non-excitable tissues. Consistent with this historical role, ongoing work in the heart will continue to assist us in unraveling the complexities of intercellular communication in developmental processes.

5. ACKNOWLEDGMENTS

The authors wish to thank Drs Madison Spach and Andy Wessels for their critical reading of this manuscript. Dr Gourdie's laboratory is supported by the NIH/NHLBI, American Heart Association (SC Affiliate) and the March of Dimes Birth Defects Foundation (Basil OConnor Scholarship).

REFERENCES

1. Reaume AG, de Sousa PA, Kulkarni S, Langille BL, Zhu D, Davies TC, Juneja SC, Kidder GM and Rossant J (1995). Cardiac malformation in neonatal mice lacking connexin43. Science 267:1831-1834.
2. Britz-Cunningham SH, Shah MM, Zuppan CW and Fletcher WH (1995). Mutations in the connexin43 gap-junction gene in patients with heart malformations and defects of laterality. N Engl J Med 332:1323-1329.
3. Ewart JL, Cohen MF, Meyer RA, Huang GY, Wessels A, Gourdie RG, Chin AJ, Park SMG, Lazatin BO, Villabon S and Lo CW (1997). Heart and neural tube defects in transgenic mice overexpressing the Cx43 gap junction gene. Development 124:1281-1292.
4. Sepp R, Severs NJ and Gourdie RG (1996). Altered patterns of cardiac intercellular junction distribution in hypertrophic cardiomyopathy. Heart 76:412-417.
5. Angst BD, Khan LUR, Severs NJ, Whitely K, Rothery S, Thompson RP, Magee AI and Gourdie RG (1997). Dissociated spatial patterning of gap junctions and cell adhesion junctions during postnatal differentiation of ventricular myocardium. Circ Res 80:88-94.
6. Green CR (1988). Evidence mounts for the role of gap junctions during development. Bioessays 8:7-10.
7. Warner A (1992). Gap junctions in development—a perspective. Sem in Cell Biol 3:81-91.
8. Paul DL (1995). New functions for gap junctions. Curr Opin Cell Biol 7:665-672.
9. Lo CW (1996). The role of gap junction membrane channels in development. J Bioenerg Biomembr 28:379-385.
10. Yamasaki H and Naus CC (1996). Role of connexin genes in growth control. Carcinogenesis 17:1199-1213.
11. Beyer EC (1993). Gap junctions. Int Rev Cytol 137C:1-37.
12. Bennett MV, Zheng X and Sogin ML (1994). The connexins and their family tree. Soc Gen Physiol Ser 49:223-233.

13.   Bruzzone R, White TW and Paul DL (1996). Connections with connexins:
       the molecular basis of direct intercellular signaling. Eur J Biochem 238:1-27.
14.   Goodenough DA, Goliger JA, Paul DL (1996). Connexins, connexons, and
       intercellular communication. Ann Rev Biochem 65:475-502.
15.   Kumar NM and Gilula NB (1996). The gap junction communication channel.
       Cell. 84:381-388.
16.   Willecke K and Haubrich S (1996). Connexin expression systems: to what
       extent do they reflect the situation in the animal? J Bioenerg Biomembr
       28:319-326.
17.   Beyer EC, Paul DL and Goodenough DA (1987). Connexin43: a protein
       from rat heart homologous to a gap junction protein from liver. J Cell Biol
       105:2621-2629.
18.   Beyer EC, Kistler J, Paul DL and Goodenough DA (1989). Antisera directed
       against connexin43 peptides react with a 43-kD protein localized to gap
       junctions in myocardium and other tissues. J Cell Biol 108:595-605.
19.   Fromaget C, el Aoumari A, Dupont E, Briand JP and Gros D (1990).
       Changes in the expression of connexin 43, a cardiac gap junctional protein,
       during mouse heart development. J Mol Cell Cardiol 22:1245-1258.
20.   Gourdie RG, Green CR, Severs NJ and Thompson RP (1990).
       Three-dimensional reconstruction of gap junction arrangement in developing
       and adult rat hearts. Trans R Microscop Soc 1:417-420.
21.   Fishman GI, Hertzberg EL, Spray DC and Leinwand LA (1991). Expression
       of connexin43 in the developing rat heart. Circ Res 68:782-787.
22.   van Kempen MJ, Fromaget C, Gros D, Moorman AF and Lamers WH
       (1991). Spatial distribution of connexin43, the major cardiac gap junction
       protein, in the developing and adult rat heart. Circ Res 68:1638-1651.
23.   Fromaget C, el Aoumari A and Gros D (1992). Distribution pattern of
       connexin 43, a gap junctional protein, during the differentiation of mouse
       heart myocytes. Differentiation 51:9-20.
24.   Gourdie RG, Green CR, Severs NJ and Thompson RP (1992).
       Immunolabelling patterns of gap junction connexins in the developing and
       mature rat heart. Anat Embryol 185:363-378.
25.   Ruangvoravat CP and Lo CW (1992). Connexin43 expression in the mouse
       embryo: localization of transcripts within developmentally significant domains.
       Dev Dyn 194:261-281.
26.   Yancey SB, Biswal S and Revel JP (1992). Spatial and temporal patterns of
       distribution of the gap junction protein connexin43 during mouse gastrulation
       and organogenesis. Development 114:203-212.
27.   Dahl E, Winterhager E, Traub O and Willecke K (1995). Expression of gap
       junction genes, connexin40 and connexin43, during fetal mouse development.
       Anat Embryol 191:267-278.

28. Delorme B, Dahl E, Jarry-Guichard T, Marics I, Briand J-P, Willecke K, Gros D and Théveniau-Ruissy M (1995). Developmental regulation of connexin 40 gene expression in mouse heart correlates with the differentiation of the conduction system. Dev Dyn 204:358-371.

29. van Kempen MJA, Vermeulen JLM, Moorman AFM, Gros D, Paul DL and Lamers WH (1996). Developmental changes of connexin40 and connexin43 mRNA distribution patterns in the rat heart. Cardiovasc Res 32:886-900.

30. Blackburn JP, Peters NS, Yeh HI, Rothery S, Green CR and Severs NJ (1995). Upregulation of connexin43 gap junctions during early stages of human coronary atherosclerosis. Arterioscler Thromb Vasc Biol 15:1219-1228.

31. Gros D and Challice CE (1976). Early development of gap junctions between the mouse embryonic myocardial cells. A freeze-etching study. Experientia 32:996-998.

32. Gros D, Mocquard JP, Challice CE and Schrevel J (1978). Formation and growth of gap junctions in mouse myocardium during ontogenesis: a freeze-cleave study. J Cell Sci 30:45-61.

33. Navaratnam V, Kaufman MH, Skepper JN, Barton S and Guttridge KM (1986). Differentiation of the myocardial rudiment of mouse embryos: an ultrastructural study including freeze-fracture replication. J Anat 146:65-85.

34. Gourdie RG, Severs NJ, Green CR, Rothery S, Germroth P and Thompson RP (1993).The spatial distribution and relative abundance of gap-junctional connexin40 and connexin43 correlate to functional properties of components of the cardiac atrioventricular conduction system. J Cell Sci 105:985-991.

35. Gros D, Jarry-Guichard T, ten Velde I, de Maziere A, van Kempen MJA, Davoust J, Briand JP, Moorman AFM and Jongsma HJ (1994). Restricted distribution of connexin40, a gap junctional protein, in mammalian heart. Circ Res 74:839-851.

36. van Kempen MJA, ten Velde I, Wessels A, Oosthoek PW, Gros D, Jongsma HJ, Moorman AFM and Lamers WH (1995). Differential connexin distribution accommodates cardiac function in different species. Microsc Res Tech 31:420-436.

37. White TW and Bruzzone R (1996). Multiple connexin proteins in single intercellular channels: connexin compatibility and functional consequences. J Bioenerg Biomembr 28: 339-350.

38. Gourdie RG (1995). A map of the heart: gap junctions, connexin diversity, and retroviral studies of conduction myocyte lineage. Clin Sci 88:257-262.

39. Stewart JM and Page E (1978). Improved stereological techniques for studying myocardial cell growth: application to external sarcolemma, T system, and intercalated disks of rabbit and rat hearts. J Ultrastruct Res 65:119-134.

40. Shibata Y, Nakata K and Page E (1980). Ultrastructural changes during development of gap junctions in rabbit left ventricular myocardial cells. J Ultrastruct Res 71:258-271.

41. Beyer EC, Reed KE, Westphale EM, Kanter HL and Larson DM (1992). Molecular cloning and expression of rat connexin40, a gap junction protein expressed in vascular smooth muscle. J Membr Biol 127:69-76.

42. Haefliger JA, Bruzzone R, Jenkins NA, Gilbert DJ, Copeland NG and Paul DL (1992). Four novel members of the connexin family of gap junction proteins. Molecular cloning, expression and chromosome mapping. J Biol Chem 267:2057-2064.

43. Hennenmann H, Suchyna T, Lichtenberg-Frate H, Jungbluth S, Dahl E, Schwarz J, Nicholson BJ and Willecke K. Molecular cloning and functional expression of mouse connexin40, a second gap junction gene preferentially expressed in lung. J Cell Biol 117:1299-1310.

44. Kanter HL, Saffitz JE and Beyer EC (1992). Cardiac myocytes express multiple gap junction proteins. Circ Res 70:438-444.

45. Bastide B, Neyses L, Ganten D, Paul M, Willecke K and Traub O (1993). Gap junction protein connexin40 is preferentially expressed in vascular endothelium and conductive bundles of rat myocardium and is increased under hypertensive conditions. Circ Res 73:1138-1149.

46. Kanter HL, Laing JG, Beau SL, Beyer EC and Saffitz JE (1993). Distinct patterns of connexin expression in canine Purkinje fibers and ventricular muscle. Circ Res 72:1124-1131.

47. Chen SC, Davis LM, Westphale EM, Beyer EC and Saffitz JE (1994). Expression of multiple gap junction proteins in human fetal and infant hearts. Pediatr Res 36:561-566.

48. Davis LM, Kanter HL, Beyer EC and Saffitz JE (1994). Distinct gap junction protein phenotypes in cardiac tissues with disparate conduction properties. J Am Coll Cardiol 24:1124-1132.

49. Davis LM, Rodefeld ME, Green K, Beyer EC and Saffitz JE (1995). Gap junction protein phenotypes of the human heart and conduction system. J Cardiovasc Electrophysiol 6:813-822.

50. Verheule S, van Kempen MJA, te Welscher PHJA, Kwak BR and Jongsma HJ (1997). Characterization of gap junction channels in adult rabbit atrial and ventricular myocardium. Circ Res 80:673-681.

51. Beyer EC (1990). Molecular cloning and developmental expression of two chick embryo gap junction proteins. J Biol Chem 265:14439-14443.

52. Saffitz JE, Kanter HL, Green KG, Tolley TK and Beyer EC (1994). Tissue-specific determinants of anisotropic conduction velocity in canine atrial and ventricular myocardium. Circ Res 74:1065-1070.

53. Bruzzone R, Haefliger J-3, Gimlich RL and Paul DL (1993). Connexin40, a component of gap junctions in vascular endothelium, is restricted in its ability to interact with other connexins. Mol Biol Cell 4:7-20.

54. Gros DB and Jongsma HJ (1996). Connexins in mammalian heart function. Bioessays 18:719-730.

55. Kistler J, Evans C, Donaldson P, Bullivant S, Bond J, Eastwood S, Roos M, Dong Y, Gruijters T and Engel A (1995). Ocular lens gap junctions: protein expression, assembly, and structure-function analysis. Microsc Res Tech 31:347-356.

56. Gourdie RG, Green CR, Severs NJ, Anderson RH and Thompson RP (1993). Evidence for a distinct gap-junctional phenotype in ventricular conduction tissues of developing and mature avian heart. Circ Res 72:278-289.

57. Minkoff R, Rundus VR, Parker SB, Beyer EC and Hertzberg EL (1993). Connexin expression in the developing avian cardiovascular system. Circ Res 73:71-78.

58. Gourdie RG, Mima T, Thompson RP and Mikawa T (1995). Terminal diversification of the myocyte lineage generates Purkinje fibers of the cardiac conduction system. Development 121:1423-1431.

59. McCabe CF, Gourdie RG, Thompson RP and Cole GJ (1995). Developmentally regulated neural protein EAP-300 is expressed by myocardium and cardiac neural crest during chick embryogenesis. Dev Dyn 203:51-60.

60. Wiens D, Jensen L, Jasper J and Becker J (1995). Developmental expression of connexins in the chick embryo myocardium and other tissues. Anat Rec 241:541-553.

61. Eisenberg CA, Gourdie RG and Eisenberg LM (1997). *Wnt-11* is expressed in early avian mesoderm and required for the differentiation of the quail mesoderm cell line QCE-6. Development 124:525-536.

62. Mikawa T and Gourdie RG (1996). Pericardial mesoderm generates a population of coronary smooth muscle cells migrating into the heart along with ingrowth of the epicardial organ. Dev Biol 174: 221-232.

63. Mikawa T, Hyer J, Itoh N and Wei Y (1996). Retroviral vectors to study cardiovascular development. Trends Cardiovasc Med 6:679-686.

64. Spach MS, Miller WT 3rd, Miller-Jones E, Warren RB and Barr RC (1979). Extracellular potentials related to intracellular action potentials during impulse conduction in anisotropic canine cardiac muscle. Circ Res 45:188-204.

65. Spach MS, Miller WT 3rd, Geselowitz DB, Barr RC, Kootsey JM and Johnson EA (1981). The discontinuous nature of propagation in normal canine cardiac muscle. Evidence for recurrent discontinuities of intracellular resistance that affect the membrane currents. Circ Res 48:39-54.

66. Spach MS, Miller WT 3rd., Dolber PC, Kootsey JM, Sommer JR, Mosher CE, Jr. (1982). The functional role of structural complexities in the propagation of deploarization in the atrium of the dog. Cardiac conduction disturbances due to discontinuities of effective axial resistivity. Circ Res 50:175-191.

67. Spach MS (1983). The discontinuous nature of electrical propagation in cardiac muscle. Consideration of a quantitative model incorporating the membrane ionic properties and structural complexities. The ALZA distinguished lecture. Ann Biomed Eng 11:209-261.

68. Spach MS, Dolber PC and Sommer JR (1985). Discontinuous propagation: an hypothesis based on known cardiac structural complexities. Int J Cardiol 7:167-174.

69. Spach MS (1991). Anisotropic structural complexities in the genesis of reentrant arrhythmias. Circulation 84:1447-1450.

70. Spach MS (1994). Changes in the topology of gap junctions as an adaptive structural response of the myocardium. Circulation 90:1103-1106.

71. Spach MS and Heidlage JF (1995). The stochastic nature of cardiac propagation at a microscopic level. Electrical description of myocardial architecture and its application to conduction. Circ Res 76:366-80.

72. Peters NS, Severs NJ, Rothery SM, Lincoln C, Yacoub MH and Green CR (1994). Spatiotemporal relation between gap junctions and fascia adherens junctions during postnatal development of human ventricular myocardium. Circulation 90:713-725.

73. Saffitz JE, Davis LM, Darrow BJ, Kanter HL, Laing JG and Beyer EC (1995). The molecular basis of anisotropy: role of gap junctions. J Cardiovasc Electrophysiol 6:498-510.

74. Spach MS and Dolber PC (1986). Relating extracellular potentials and their derivatives to anisotropic propagation at a microscopic level in human cardiac muscle. Evidence for electrical uncoupling of side-to-side fiber connections with increasing age. Circ Res 58:356-371.

75. Spach MS and Josephson ME (1994). Initiating reentry: the role of nonuniform anisotropy in small circuits. J Cardiovasc Electrophysiol 5:182-209.

76. Mays DJ, Foose JM, Philipson LH and Tamkun MM (1995). Localization of the Kv1.5 K+ channel protein in explanted cardiac tissue. J Clin Invest 96:282-292.

77. Cohen SA (1996). Immunocytochemical localization of rH1 sodium channel in adult rat heart atria and ventricle. Presence in terminal intercalated disks. Circulation 94:3083-3086.

78. Hirakow R, Gotoh T and Watanabe T (1980). Quantitative studies on the ultrastructural differentiation and growth of mammalian cardiac muscle cells. I. The atria and ventricles of the rat. Acta Anat 108:144-152.

79. Hirakow R and Gotoh T (1980). Quantitative studies on the ultrastructural differentiation and growth of mammalian cardiac muscle cells. II. The atria and ventricles of the guinea pig. Acta Anat 108:230-237.

80. Oosthoek PW, van Kempen MJA, Wessels A, Lamers WH, Moorman AFM Distribution of the cardiac gap junction protein connexin43 in the neonatal and adult human heart. In Marchal G and Carraro U (eds) Muscle and Motility, Vol 2. Proceedings of the XIXth European Conference in Brussels. Andover: Intercept Ltd., 1993.

81. Legato MJ (1979). Cellular mechanisms of normal growth in the mammalian heart. II. A quantitative and qualitative comparison between the right and left ventricular myocytes in the dog from birth to five months of age. Circ Res 44:263-279.

82. Chen L, Goings GE, Upshaw-Earley J and Page E (1989). Cardiac gap junctions and gap junction-associated vesicle: ultrastructural comparison of in situ negative staining with conventional positive staining. Circ Res 64:501-514.

83. Page E. Cardiac gap junctions. In Fozzard HA, Haber E, Jennings RB, Katz AM, Morgan H and Morgan E (eds.): The Heart and Cardiovascular System, 2nd ed. New York, New York: Raven Press, 1992, pp 1003-1047.

84. Kirklin JK, Blackstone EH, Kirklin JW, Pacifico AD and Bargeron LM Jr (1986). The Fontan operation. Ventricular hypertrophy, age, and date of operation as risk factors. J Thorac Cardiovasc Surg 92:1049-1064.

85. Colan SD, Trowitzsch E, Wernovsky G, Sholler GF, Sanders SP and Castaneda AR (1988). Myocardial performance after arterial switch operation for transposition of the great arteries with intact ventricular septum. Circulation 78:132-141.

86. Gustafson RA, Murray GF, Warden HE, Hill RC and Rozar GE Jr (1988). Early primary repair of tetralogy of Fallot. Ann Thorac Surg 45:235-241.

87. Losay J, Touchot-Kone A, Bruniaux J, Serraf A, Lacour-Gayet F, Planche C and Binet JP (1992). Immediate and mid-term results of surgery of aortic valve stenosis in the newborn infant. Arch Mal Coeur Vaiss 85:567-571.

88. Severs NJ, Dupont E, Kaprielian RR, Yeh H-I and Rothery S. Gap junctions and connexins in the cardiovascular system. In Yacoub MH, Carpentier A, Pepper J and Fabiani J-N (eds.): Annual of Cardiac Surgery, 9th ed., London, England: Rapid Science Publishers, 1996, pp 31-44.

89. Soonpaa MH, Koh GY, Klug MG and Field LJ (1994). Formation of nascent intercalated disks between grafted fetal cardiomyocytes and host myocardium. Science 264:98-101.

90. Koh GY, Soonpaa MH, Klug MG, Pride HP, Cooper BJ, Zipes DP, Field LJ (1995). Stable fetal cardiomyocyte grafts in the hearts of dystrophic mice and dogs. J Clin Invest 96:2034-2042.

91. Van Meter CH Jr, Claycomb WC, Delcarpio JB, Smith DM, deGruiter H, Smart F and Ochsner JL (1995). Myoblast transplantation in the porcine model: a potential technique for myocardial repair. J Thorac Cardiovasc Surg 110:1442-1448.

92.   Connold AL, Frischknecht R, Dimitrakos M and Vrbova G (1997). The survival of embryonic cardiomyocytes transplanted into damaged host rat myocardium. J Muscle Res Cell Mot 18:63-70.

93.   Sheridan JD (1966). Electrophysiological study of special connections between cells in the early chick embryo. J Cell Biol 31:C1-5.

94.   Furshpan EJ and Potter DD (1968). Low-resistance junctions between cells in embryos and tissue culture. Curr Top Dev Biol 3:95-127.

95.   Ito S and Loewenstein WR (1969). Ionic communication between early embryonic cells. Dev Biol 19:228-243.

96.   Bennett MV and Trinkaus JP (1970). Electrical coupling between embryonic cells by way of extracellular space and specialized junctions. J Cell Biol 44:592-610.

97.   Bergoffen J, Scherer SS, Wang S, Scott MO, Bone LJ, Paul DL, Chen K, Lensch MW, Chance PF and Fischbeck KH (1993). Connexin mutations in X-linked Charcot-Marie-Tooth disease. Science 262:2039-2042.

98.   Bruzzone R, White TW, Scherer SS, Fischbeck KH and Paul DL (1994). Null mutations of connexin32 in patients with X-linked Charcot-Marie-Tooth disease. Neuron 13:1253-1260.

99.   Kass S, MacRae C, Graber HL, Sparks EA, McNamara D, Boudoulas H, Basson CT, Baker PB III, Cody RJ and Fishman MC, Cox N, Kong A, Wooley CF, Seidman JG and Seidman CE (1994). A gene defect that causes conduction system disease and dilated cardiomyopathy maps to chromosome 1p1-1q1. Nat Genet 7:546-551.

100.   Gebbia M, Towbin JA and Casey B (1996). Failure to detect connexin43 mutations in 38 cases of sporadic and familial heterotaxy. Circulation 94:1909-1912.

101.   Splitt MP, Burn J, Goodship J (1996). Connexin43 mutations in sporadic and familial defects of laterality. N Engl J Med 332:1323-1329.

102.   De Sousa PA, Valdimarsson G, Nicholson BJ, Kidder GM (1993). Connexin trafficking and the control of gap junction assembly in mouse preimplantation embryos. Development.117:1355-1367.

103.   Becker DL and Davies CS (1995). Role of gap junctions in the development of the preimplantation mouse embryo. Microsc Res Tech 31:364-74.

104.   Ewart JL, Cohen MF, Wessels A, Gourdie RG, Chin AJ, Park SMJ, Lazatin S, Villabon S, Lo CW (1997). Heart and neural tube defects in transgenic mice overexpressing the Cx43 gap junction gene. Mol Biol Cell 7: 462a.

105.   Kirby ML and Waldo KL (1995). Neural crest and cardiovascular patterning. Circ Res 77:211-215.

106.   Wessels A, Vermeulen JL, Verbeek FJ, Viragh S, Kalman F, Lamers WH and Moorman AF (1992). Spatial distribution of "tissue-specific" antigens in the developing human heart and skeletal muscle. III. An immunohistochemical analysis of the distribution of the neural tissue antigen G1N2 in the embryonic heart; implications for the development of the atrioventricular conduction system. Anat Rec 232:97-111.

107.   Chan-Thomas PS, Thompson RP, Robert B, Yacoub MH and Barton PJ (1993). Expression of homeobox genes Msx-1 (Hox-7) and Msx-2 (Hox-8) during cardiac development in the chick. Dev Dyn 197: 203-16.

3 CARDIOVASCULAR GAP JUNCTION PROTEINS: MOLECULAR CHARACTERIZATION AND BIOCHEMICAL REGULATION

Eric C. Beyer[1], Kyung Hwan Seul[1], and David M. Larson[2]

[1]Department of Pediatrics, Washington University School of Medicine, St. Louis, MO, and
[2]Mallory Institute of Pathology, Boston University School of Medicine, Boston, MA

Gap junctions are plasma membrane specializations containing channels which permit the intercellular exchange of ions and small molecules. Gap junction channels are of central importance in electrically excitable tissues such as myocardium where cell-to-cell passage of ions allows propagation of action potentials. Gap junctions are also present in many non-excitable cells (for example endothelial cells) where they may facilitate intercellular exchange of nutrients, metabolites, and signaling molecules as well as ions. The present review will focus on molecular biological and biochemical studies that have enhanced our understanding of the molecular composition of cardiac and vascular gap junction channels and the regulation of the subunit proteins that form them.

Electrical coupling of cardiac cells through such low resistance intercellular pathways was first proposed by Weidmann (1) who applied linear cable theory to the spread of electrotonic potentials in cardiac Purkinje fibers. Barr *et al.* (2) subsequently demonstrated that closely apposed regions of adjacent plasma membranes, termed the nexus or gap junction, were the functional site of electrical contact between heart cells; they showed that disruption of these structures by hypertonic solutions also blocked action potential conduction. In thin-section electron micrographs, the gap junction appeared as a pair of parallel membranes separated by a narrow 20 angstrom extracellular gap which was spanned by hexagonally arranged protein subunits (3,4). Each protein bridge was postulated to consist of a pair of hemichannels (or connexons), one from each cell, which traverses (5). Micrographs of cardiovascular gap junctions are shown in figure 1.

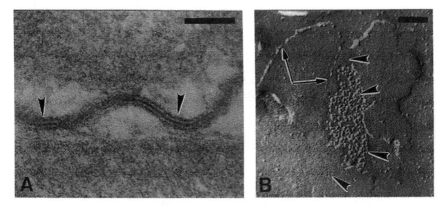

Figure 1 Electron micrographs showing gap junctions between cultured cells. (A) Thin-section view of gap junction (arrowheads) between two rat ventricular myocytes, cultured as in Eid *et al.* (6). Bar = 0.1 μm. (B) Freeze-fracture replica of gap (arrowheads) and tight (arrows) junctions between two bovine brain microvascular endothelial cells, cultured as in Larson *et al.* (7). Note P-face particles and E-face pits in gap junction. Bar = 0.1 μm.

1. Gap junction structure

In the 1970's, procedures were developed for the isolation of gap junctions from liver (8,9). These isolated gap junctions were studied by x-ray diffraction and electron microscopy to develop a low resolution (25 Å) structural model (Figure 2)

(10-12). The model shows that a gap junction plaque is composed of from tens to thousands of channels. Each channel is composed of a hexameric structure (connexon) composed of six integral membrane subunits (connexins) which surround a central pore. The connexon joins in mirror symmetry with a connexon in the plasma membrane of the adjacent cell. While they have been studied less, cardiac gap junctions are believed to have a generally similar structure except for larger cytoplasmic domains (13,14). Recent studies by Unger *et al.* (15) examining expressed gap junctions derived from cloned material have supported and refined this model.

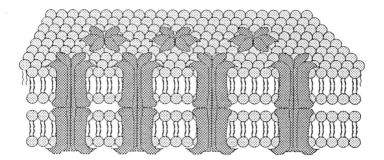

Figure 2. Model of the structure of a gap junction, based on structural analysis of isolated hepatic and cardiac gap junctions (10-13).

In addition to the liver junctions, methods were developed for the isolation of myocardial gap junctions (13,16) and of lens fiber plasma membranes which contain 5-10% gap junction profiles (17-19). SDS-PAGE of these preparations showed that the isolated liver gap junctions are composed primarily of a 27 kDa polypeptide, accompanied by proteolysis fragments, aggregates, and a 21 kDa polypeptide (20). Isolated myocardial gap junctions contain a 43-47 kDa polypeptide, cleaved by endogenous proteases to 34, 32, and 29 kDa bands (16,21,22). Isolated bovine and ovine lens fiber plasma membranes contain a number of polypeptides including one of 70 kDa (MP70) (23). N-terminal sequencing of these proteins by Edman degradation has demonstrated that the liver 27 kDa and 21 kDa proteins, the heart 43-47 kDa protein and its degradation products (24-26), and the lens 70 kDa protein (27) are homologous proteins.

2. Connexin cloning and diversity

Availability of isolated gap junction proteins, development of antibodies, and acquisition of some sequence information allowed the molecular cloning of sequences encoding gap junction proteins. Paul (28) cloned a cDNA for the rat liver 27 kDa protein by antibody screening of a bacteriophage expression library, and Kumar and Gilula (29) cloned a cDNA for its human counterpart by hybridization screening with an amino-terminal oligonucleotide. Both cDNAs encode a polypeptide of 32 kDa. Paul (28) demonstrated by RNA blotting that mRNA hybridizing to this cDNA was expressed in rat liver, brain, stomach, and kidney, but was not detectable in heart or lens.

Beyer *et al.* (30) isolated a related sequence from a rat heart cDNA library by screening with the rat liver cDNA at reduced stringency. The rat heart cDNA codes for a polypeptide of 43 kDa which contains 43% identical amino acids to the protein cloned from rat liver. The amino terminal sequence predicted from the heart clone matches that determined by Edman degradation of the major protein in isolated rat heart gap junctions (25,26). Morphological and functional proof that this protein forms cardiac gap junctional channels was provided by immunocytochemistry using specific anti-peptide antisera (31,32) and by expression of channels produced from the cloned cDNA in *Xenopus* oocytes (33,34).

Cloning of this second gap junction protein confirmed previous suggestions that there was a family of related gap junction proteins. Many of these proteins are not uniquely expressed in a single tissue (28,30). The mobilities of these proteins on SDS-PAGE may vary with electrophoresis conditions (35). Therefore, previous descriptions of gap junction proteins based on tissue of origin or electrophoretic mobility were abandoned, and a new operational nomenclature was developed using the generic term connexin (abbreviated as Cx) for the protein family, with an indication of species (as necessary) and a numeric suffix designating the molecular mass in kiloDaltons, predicted from the derived polypeptide sequence (30,36,37). Thus, the 27 kDa protein from rat liver is termed rat connexin32 (Cx32), the 43 kDa protein from rat heart is termed rat connexin43 (Cx43).

The amino acid sequences derived from the cloned cDNAs have been used to predict the structures of the connexins. Hydropathy plots of Cx32 and of Cx43 suggest four hydrophobic domains, with a large carboxyl-terminal hydrophilic tail. Three smaller hydrophilic domains separate the hydrophobic regions (28). These data, together with the results of proteolysis studies of isolated junctions, have been used to construct a topology model for the relation of these polypeptides to the junctional plasma membrane, assuming that each hydrophobic domain represents a transmembrane segment of the molecule (30,38). The model has been tested by examining the protease sensitivity of isolated liver gap junctions and by the mapping of site-specific antisera by immunocytochemistry. The controlled proteolytic cleavage has demonstrated that both the N- and C-termini of Cx32 face the cytoplasm, and that an additional cytoplasmically-accessible proteolytic site is located between the second and third transmembrane segments (38,39). Antisera have been raised against synthetic oligopeptides representing various segments of Cx32 and Cx43, and have been used to map the topology in the electron microscope (14,31,32,40,41), unambiguously showing that the amino-terminus, the carboxyl terminus and a loop in the middle of the protein are all located on the cytoplasmic face of the junctional membrane. And, to the degree that the harsh experimental conditions do not alter the protein topology, they also demonstrate that the predicted extracellular connexin domains can be detected on the extracellular surfaces of the junctional membranes.Demonstration that the connexins are a family of proteins containing conserved and unique regions has led to a search for further family members. Two general strategies have been employed: low stringency hybridization screening of cDNA and genomic libraries and use of the polymerase chain reaction with

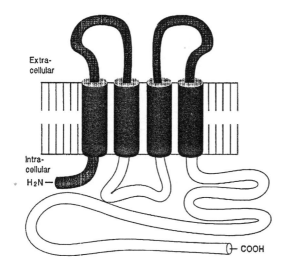

Figure 3. Topology of the connexin protein relative to the junctional plasma membrane. Shaded regions represent sequences within the polypeptide that are conserved among all connexins while unshaded regions are unique.

consensus/degenerate primers derived from the conserved regions (42-47). To date over 13 different connexins have been identified from rodent sources.

Similar strategies have been used to identify orthologues or additional connexin family members in various different vertebrate species. Cx43 orthologues have been cloned from *Xenopus* (48), chicken (49), human (50), mouse (51), and cow (52), as well as rat (30). The sequences are extremely similar: the mammalian Cx43 proteins show >97% amino acid identity; the chick protein has 92% identical amino acids to the rat; the *Xenopus* protein has 87% identical amino acids to the rat. Many of the substitutions are conservative. Some other connexins are also well conserved: human, dog and mouse Cx45 are about 97% identical (46,53,54), while 85% of amino acids in the chicken Cx45 are identical to those in mammals. A zebrafish connexin (Cx43.4) with substantial similarity to mammalian Cx45 has recently been cloned (55). Cx37 is rather well conserved in mouse, rat, and man (44,56,57). But, Cx40 shows substantial divergence between species: rodent Cx40 is 83% identical to dog Cx40; human Cx40 is 89% identical to dog Cx40 (43,44,47,53,54); the closest avian counterpart of mammalian Cx40 is a 42 kDa protein, Cx42, which contains 70% identical amino acids.

The genes have been cloned for several connexins and the gene structure of other connexins has been partially assessed by DNA blotting and by the polymerase chain reaction (58-61). All connexin genes appear to be single copy genes with a first exon containing only 5'-untranslated sequences and a large second exon containing the complete coding region as well as all remaining untranslated sequences. While some of the non-cardiac connexins (Cx26 and Cx32) do not have TATA boxes (58,60) or may start transcription from alternate first exons (62), Cx43 has been shown to have a single start site in proximity to a reasonable TATA box (61,63). While only preliminary analysis of connexin transcription has been performed in cardiovascular cells (64), reporter gene transfections of various cell lines have identified several enhancer or repressor elements within the Cx43 gene implicated in estrogen responsiveness (65), myometrial-specific regulation (63), or regulation by protein kinase C (66). In humans, a Cx43 pseudogene has also been identified (50).

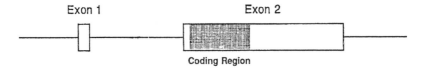

Figure 4. Structure of a connexin gene.

The availability of cloned connexin sequences has made it possible to express the proteins encoded by the different sequences and to examine the properties of the channels produced. Two major strategies have been utilized extensively: injection of *Xenopus* oocytes with *in vitro* transcribed connexin mRNAs (33,34,67) and stable transfection of communication-deficient cell lines with connexin DNAs (68,69). Data derived from some of these studies will be examined in more detail elsewhere (see chapter by Veenstra), but they can be summarized by concluding that each of the connexins forms channels with unique characteristics, including unitary conductance, gating by voltage or pH, and selectivity/permeability (69-74).

3. Connexin distribution in the cardiovascular system

The cloned connexin sequences or protein information derived from them have been used to examine the distribution of different connexins in various organs, tissues, and cell types. Connexin-specific DNA or RNA probes have been used for hybridization to RNA blots prepared from organ or cell culture homogenates or for *in situ* hybridization studies of tissue sections. Antibodies raised against connexin-specific synthetic peptides or bacterially-expressed polypeptides representing the unique cytoplasmic domains have been used for immunoblots and immunohistochemical localization studies.

3.1 *Connexins in the heart.*

By various of these techniques, up to six connexins (Cx37, Cx40, Cx43, Cx45, Cx46, and Cx50=MP70) have been detected in the mammalian heart. RNA blots show hybridization of Cx37, Cx40, Cx43, Cx45, and Cx46 probes to corresponding mRNAs in total RNA prepared from heart homogenates (30,43,44,46,47,53,56,75), but only Cx40, Cx43, and Cx45 have been unambiguously detected in RNA from cardiac myocytes (53). Cx37 was cloned from endothelial cell cDNA (57) (among other sources), and those cells are presumably the source of Cx37 in the heart. The cardiac source of Cx46 expression has not been defined. Cx50 mRNA has not been detected in heart, but Harfst et al. (76) found immunostaining in heart valves using a monoclonal antibody directed against the ovine orthologue of Cx50, MP70.

Table 1. Connexin mRNAs expressed in the heart

Cx37
Cx40
Cx43
Cx45
Cx46

While Cx40, Cx43, and Cx45 have all been detected in cardiac myocytes, immunohistochemistry and *in situ* hybridization studies have shown that these myocyte connexins have different distributions in different cardiac regions. Davis *et al.*(77) have surveyed the distribution of different connexins within different regions of the canine heart. Cx45 is present in all cardiac regions examined. Cx43 is abundant in atrium, ventricle, and in Purkinje fibers, but is not detectable in the canine sinus or atrio-ventricular nodes or the proximal His-Purkinje system. Cx40 is abundant in atrium, bundle branches and Purkinje fibers, present in the sinus and A-V nodes and scarce in ventricular myocardium. The differential distribution of Cx40 and Cx43 is illustrated by the immunofluorescent staining of a frozen section of mouse heart shown in Figure 5. The distribution of Cx40, Cx43, and, in some cases Cx45, have also been examined in other mammalian species including human, mouse, rat, rabbit, and guinea pig (78-82) showing similar patterns of expression. In addition to differences in the patterns of connexins expressed, different cardiac tissues also differ in the size and number of their gap junctions (see Table 2). Changes in levels of connexins during cardiac development are considered in other chapters.

In cardiac cells that contain two or more connexins, those connexins appear to be in the same gap junctions. Double label immunohistochemistry has been performed using a mouse monoclonal antibody to Cx43 and polyclonal antibodies directed against Cx40 or Cx45. Analysis of immunoreactive material in frozen sections or in isolated myocytes with immunofluorescence microscopy and double label immunoelectron microscopy has revealed an identical distribution of both proteins in gap junctions (77,83).

While the patterns of connexin expression appear rather similar in multiple mammalian species, they apparently differ in birds (and perhaps other vertebrates). Chicken cardiac myocytes predominantly contain Cx42 (a connexin most closely related to the mammalian Cx40 sequence) and only little Cx43 (42,84).

Table 2. Gap Junction Structure and Connexin Phenotypes of Cardiac Regions

Cardiac Tissue	Connexin Phenotype			Gap Junction Structure	
	Cx40	Cx43	Cx45	Size	Number
Sinus node	scant	absent	scant	small	few
Right Atrium	abundant	abundant	moderate	large	many
AV Node and Proximal His Bundle	scant	absent	scant	small	few
Distal His Bundle and Proximal BundleBranches	abundant	abundant	moderate	large	moderat
Ventricle	scant	abundant	moderate	moderate	many

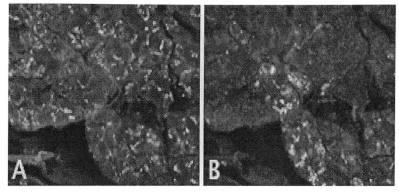

Figure 5. Localization of connexins by confocal immunofluoescence in a frozen section of mouse heart. A. Anti-Cx43 antibodies predominantly label gap junctions between ventricular myocytes. B. Anti-Cx40 antibodies label only sub-endocardial Purkinje fiber cells. There is some overlap of Cx40 and Cx43 immunoreactivity.

3.2 *Connexin distribution in blood vessels*

Several ultrastructural studies have shown gap junctions between endothelial cells or between smooth muscle cells in the vascular wall (reviewed by Larson (85), Dejana, *et al.* (86), and Christ *et al.*, (87)). Heterocellular gap junctions between endothelial cells and pericytes or smooth muscle cells have also been demonstrated (88,89). Recent assessments of dye or electrical transfer *in vivo* have confirmed the presence of functional intercellular communication (90,91).

In 1990, Larson *et al.* (92) surveyed a wide variety of cultured endothelial cells, smooth muscle cells and pericytes from several species and determined that they all expressed Cx43 at the level of transcript. In addition, freshly isolated preparations of bovine aortic endothelium and smooth muscle each contained Cx43 mRNA (92). Subsequently, Beyer *et al.* (43) cloned Cx40 from rat genomic DNA and showed that this connexin was expressed in A7r5 cells (immortalized rat aortic smooth muscle) and cultured bovine aortic smooth muscle cells but not in bovine endothelium. Reed *et al.* (57), cloned human Cx37 from a human umbilical vein endothelial cell library and demonstrated expression in human and bovine endothelial cells including freshly isolated bovine aortic endothelium but not in cultured smooth muscle cells. Subsequent investigations by a variety of groups using DNA or antibody probes to screen for connexins have demonstrated some variability in expression *in vivo* and in culture, depending on vascular bed and species, as shown in Table 3. In general, vessel wall cells all express Cx43, *in vivo* and *in vitro*. *In vivo*, Cx40 mRNA or protein have been demonstrated in large and small vessel endothelium and in smooth muscle from several species but not others. Cx37 has been less extensively studied; however, it has been shown in various endothelia but not in smooth muscle in vivo or in culture. Interestingly, Larson *et al.* (85) have shown that Cx37 is expressed at high levels in confluent endothelial cells (in vivo and in vitro) yet it is barely detectable in subconfluent cultured cells. The relatively small amount of information on vascular pericytes suggests an expression pattern similar to that of smooth muscle cells, as might be expected. An additional connexin, Cx45, has been identified in one smooth muscle line, A7r5 (93).

Table 3: Connexins expressed in vascular wall cells

Cell Type	Source	Species	Cx43	Cx40	Cx37
Endothelium					
in vivo	aorta	bovine	(92), (57)		(57)
		rat	(94)	(94)	
	microvessels	rat	(95)	(95)	
		hamster	(95)	(95)	
	heart vessels	rat		(78)	
	umbilical artery and vein	human	(96)	(96)	(96)
	muscular arteries	rat	Absent (94)	(94)	
culture	aorta	bovine	(92) (57) (85)(97)	Absent (92)	(57) (85)
		porcine	(92) (98)	Absent (98)	(98)
	pulmonary artery	bovine	(99)		
	umbilical vein	human	(92)		(57)
	umbilical artery and vein	human	(96)	(96)	(96)
	corpus cavernosum	human	(92)		
	various microvessels	bovine	(92) (57) (99)		(57)
Smooth muscle					
in vivo	aorta	rat	(92) (94) (97)	Absent (94)	
		dog		(43) (100)	
	coronary	dog		(100)	
	microvessels	rat	(95)	(95)	
		hamster	(95)	(95)	
	corpus cavernosum	human	(101)		
	heart vessels	rat		Absent (78)	
Culture	aorta	bovine	(92) (43)	(43) (100)	
		porcine	(92)		
		rat	(92) (43) (100)	(43) (100)	Absent (57)
		rat (A7r5)	(100)	(43)	Absent (57)
	coronary	human	(102)	(102)	
	mesenteric artery	rat	(92)		
	corpus cavernosum	human	(101)		
Pericytes					
culture	retinal and brain	bovine	(92)		Absent (57)
	glomerular. mesangial	human	(92)		

Citations are listed for reports of the detection of a specific connexin by RNA blotting, immunoblotting, or immunohistochemistry. Studies that examined a tissue for a specific connexin, but were unable to detect it are listed as absent.

3.3 *Connexin distribution in leukocytes*

Circulating leukocytes are usually given as an example of one of the cell types that does not make gap junctions and this is apparently true. Once they stop circulating, however, a few studies have shown the capability of these cells to transfer intercellular tracers or have demonstrated the expression of Cx43. Polacek *et al.* (103) have shown Cx43 expression in macrophage foam cells in human atherosclerotic lesions but not in peripheral mononuclear cells. Beyer and Steinberg have demonstrated expression of Cx43 by macrophage-like cell lines and changes in its expression in response to treatment with cytokines (51,104). Jara *et al.* (105) have found that leukocytes, directly stimulated with lipopolysaccharide, or peritoneal macrophages from lipopolysaccharide-stimulated hamsters express Cx43 *de novo* while untreated cells do not. Other examples, such as the reports of dye transfer by lymphocytes during penetration of endothelial monolayers (106), suggest that functional gap junction expression in leukocytes may be necessary for extravasation or subsequent activities in extravascular tissues. Several reports have indicated that precursor cells have gap junctions, are functionally coupled, or express Cx43 in the bone marrow (107,108).

4. Mixing of connexins

The expression of multiple connexins within an organism and within a single tissue or cell implies that gap junctional plaques may not all be composed only of a homogenous population of channels composed of a single connexin. Rather, connexins may potentially intermingle or mix with each other. The co-expression of multiple connexins in cardiac myocytes and vascular cells suggests that connexin mixing might influence cardiovascular intercellular communication.

There are many examples of co-expression of two connexins within the same cell. This was first documented for Cx26 and Cx32 in hepatocytes (109). In many cases, immunocytochemistry experiments show colocalization to the same gap junction plaques, as we have seen in canine ventricular myocytes and the cell line BWEM (83,93). A few electrophysiologic experiments have shown the presence of multiple different channel sizes in cells which express multiple connexins. As examples, A7r5 cells express Cx40 and Cx43 and show multiple channel sizes (43,100) while SKHep 1 cells, transfected with Cx43 or Cx32, contain channels derived from the introduced connexin as well as 30pS channels which are likely due to endogenous Cx45 (50,110-112).

One kind of mixing of connexins within gap junction channels is the formation of *heterotypic* channels. This would occur if two adjacent cells expressed different connexins and formed junctional channels with each hemi-channel formed homogeneously of a single connexin. The formation of heterotypic channels *in vitro* has been examined extensively by the pairing of *Xenopus* oocytes injected with RNAs for two different connexins (33,34). The two connexins may sometimes form heterotypic channels with complicated, novel gating properties (113,114). Not all connexins are compatible partners for the formation of heterotypic channels (33,34,94,115); the second extracellular loop in the connexin molecules may contribute to the specificity of these interactions (116). Heterotypic gap junctions might allow for the interaction of different cells or tissues in vivo and might contribute to the formation of communication compartments with borders determined by the expression of incompatible connexins. This may have some importance in the heart, since two major cardiac connexins, Cx40 and Cx43, do not form functional heterotypic channels (116,117). Except for a single manuscript analyzing hepatocyte gap junctions (118), heterotypic gap junctions have not yet been definitively demonstrated *in vivo*.

In a cell which co-expressed two connexins, the two proteins might mix within a single hemi-channel, forming *heteromeric* hemi-channels. If two co-expressed connexins are freely capable of mixing and forming heteromeric hemichannels, then in any individual cell there might be 2^6 or 64 possible hemichannels which could result in the formation of 4096 different full channels. If a six-fold symmetry axis is assumed then the predicted number of different hemichannels and complete channels are 14 and 196 respectively. This large number of different heteromeric mixtures might lead to a large variety of channels. Immunocytochemistry experiments do not have the resolution to detect heteromeric channels. Rigorous biochemical or physiological demonstration of heteromeric channels formation by the cardiovascular connexins has not yet been accomplished. However, Stauffer (119) has shown that Cx26 and Cx32 can form heteromeric connexons in an expression system, and Jiang and Goodenough have used biochemical approaches to show the presence of heteromeric connexons in the lens (120). Our own recent data suggest that Cx37 and Cx43 can form heteromeric channels when these connexins are transfected into established cell lines (121).

5. Gap junction synthesis and degradation

The development of specific anti-connexin antibody probes have made possible *in vitro* studies of connexin biosynthesis by metabolic labeling and immunoprecipitation. There have been a few studies of the synthesis and post-translational modification of connexins and the assembly and degradation of gap junctions performed in cardiovascular cells. However, there have been extensive studies of these subjects in other systems (primarily immortalized cell lines expressing Cx43). Those studies, which were recently extensively reviewed by Laird (122), are applicable in many (but not all) ways to cardiac connexins. Only certain highlights will be emphasized here. Detailed discussions of the modification of connexins by phosphorylation have been presented by Lau *et al.* (123) and by Saez *et al.* (124).

5.1. *Serine phosphorylation of Cx43.*

Pulse chase studies have demonstrated that Cx43 is initially synthesized as a 42 kDa polypeptide which subsequently is post-translationally modified to forms with slightly slower mobility on SDS-PAGE by the addition of phosphate to serine residues (49,125,126). There are apparently multiple phosphates added to each mole of Cx43, at least some of this phosphorylation may occur in a serine-rich sequence near the carboxyl-terminus containing multiple potential phosphorylation sites. Other connexins (including Cx37, Cx40, Cx45, and Cx46) contain similar sequences and have also been demonstrated to be phosphoproteins (93,127-129).

The kinase(s) responsible for Cx43 phosphorylation have not all been determined, however, protein kinase C is strongly implicated in at least some of the phosphorylation events since treatment of a number of different cell lines with phorbol esters produces an increase in the phosphorylation of Cx43 and a decrease in intercellular coupling (130-132). Lau and colleagues have demonstrated changes in Cx43 phosphorylation due to mitogen activated kinase or epidermal growth factor stimulation (133,134).

Musil *et al.* (135) have investigated some biological consequences of the serine phosphorylation of Cx43. They demonstrated that Cx43 was present in the non-communicating cell lines L929 and S180, but it was not present in cell surface gap junctional plaques, but rather accumulated intercellularly. The Cx43 was incompletely phosphorylated. However, transfection of the S180 cells with the cell adhesion molecule LCAM (E-cadherin) restored gap junctional communication, full phosphorylation of Cx43, and expression in cell surface gap junctions. These findings suggest a relation between the ability of cells to fully phosphorylate Cx43 and the ability to form communicating junctions. They also suggest a hierarchy of events in the formation of intercellular junctions: a primary cell adhesion event is required prior to formation of gap junctions. Similar observations regarding the requirement of cadherin-mediated cell adhesion for development of gap junctions have also been made in epidermal cells (136). Recently, Fujimoto *et al.* (137) used electron microscopy to show co-localization of connexins with E-cadherin or alpha-catenin during gap junction formation in regenerating liver. Meyer *et al.* (138) have shown that antibodies to extracellular epitopes in Cx43 or A-CAM (N cadherin) will inhibit gap junction formation by Novikoff hepatoma cells. However, Wang and Rose (139) have shown inhibition of communication in L cells transfected with N-cadherin and increases in communication between Morris hepatoma H5123 cells by the same treatment, suggesting that a cell type-specific effect. Musil and Goodenough (140) have extended their original observations in NRK cells by showing the presence of extracellularly accessible Cx43 (in the non-phosphorylated form) and a correlation between phosphorylation of Cx43 and acquisition of insolubility in Triton-X-100, suggesting a role for phosphorylation in gap junction formation.

Based on these studies and many more (reviewed by Laird (122)), a scheme for post-translational processing of Cx43 and its assembly is emerging. Cx43 is synthesized and initially phosphorylated in the endoplasmic reticulum or Golgi apparatus. Formation of hexamers (connexons) occurs in the Golgi or TGN ((141), but see (142)). Connexons are inserted into the cell membrane in a shut configuration, perhaps at regions of cadherin-mediated adhesion or near tight junctions. Formation of plaques of channels requires docking of the connexons with connexons from the adjacent cell and correlates with resistance to solubilization in Triton X-100 and with additional phosphorylation.

5.2. *Tyrosine phosphorylation of Cx43.* A large body of data demonstrating that intercellular communication is abolished in fibroblasts infected with Rous sarcoma virus (RSV) (143,144) has led several investigators to investigate the effects of pp60^{src} on Cx43-expressing cells. Crow *et al.* (125) demonstrated that RSV infection uncoupled vole fibroblasts and lead to the incorporation of phosphate in Cx43 tyrosine residues. Filson *et al.* (126) extended these observations by showing that each molecule of phosphorylated Cx43 contained both phosphoserine and phosphotyrosine and by showing that the ability of *src* variants to abolish cellular communication correlated with tyrosine phosphorylation of Cx43. Swenson *et* (145) showed that in a *Xenopus* oocyte expression system coexpression of pp60^{v-src} with Cx43 reduced cell-cell coupling and lead to tyrosine phosphorylation of Cx43. But, site-directed mutagenesis of Tyr265 in Cx43 eliminated the tyrosine phosphorylation and the depression of communication. More recently, Loo *et al.* (146) have demonstrated that the induced tyrosine phosphorylation is even more complex, resulting in modification of multiple residues. Other oncogenes may have similar effects on intercellular communication and connexin phosphorylation (147,148).

5.3. *Degradation of gap junctions.*   Gap junctions are apparently ephemeral constructs; an early estimate by Fallon and Goodenough (149) of the half-life of metabolically-labeled liver junctions *in vivo* was in the range of 5 hours. The mechanisms of gap junctional degradation are incompletely understood. Electron microscopic studies have implied wholesale endosomal internalization of entire junctions (forming so-called annular gap junctions) followed by degradation in lysosomal, multivesicular body, or autophagosomal compartments (150-155). *In vivo* these structures are found primarily following pathological insults such as ischemia or during tissue remodeling. Cell fractionation and immunoelectron microscopic studies have shown an association of connexins with lysosomes in cultured cells as well (156-158). Recently, Laing and Beyer (159) demonstrated that inhibition of proteasomal degradation extended the half-life of Cx43 in cultured cells, suggesting a role for the ubiquitin-protesomal pathway in connexin proteolysis.

6. Molecular interventional approaches to the study of cardiac intercellular communication

The availability of the cloned connexin sequences has made possible strategies to alter the abundance of the various connexins in cultured cells and in animals to test the involvement of gap junctions in cardiovascular development and physiology. Reaume *et al.* (160) have developed a Cx43 "knock out" mouse, and they have found that homozygous null animals are cyanotic and die soon after birth apparently due to right ventricular outflow tract obstruction. These observations implicate Cx43 in cardiac development. Guerrero *et al.* (161) have recently shown that animals that are heterozygous for the Cx43 null mutation contain only half as much Cx43 protein as wild type littermates and exhibit slowed ventricular conduction. These data directly demonstrate the importance of connexin abundance as a determinant of cardiac conduction. It is likely that in the next few years additional useful data will be derived from these animals and from studies employing other connexin "knock out" or transgenic animals.

REFERENCES

1. Weidmann S. The electrical constants of Purkinje fibres. J Physiol (Lond) 1952;118:348-360.
2. Barr L, Dewey MM., Berger W. Propagation of action potentials and the structur e of th e nexus in cardiac muscle. J Gen Physiol 1965;48:797-823.
3. Robertson JD. The occurrence of a subunit pattern in the unit membranes of club endings in Mauthner cell synapses in goldfish brains. J Cell Biol 1963;19:201-221.
4. Revel JP, Karnovsky MJ. Hexagonal array of subunits in intercellular junctions of the mouse heart and liver. J Cell Biol 1967;33:C7-C12.
5. Loewenstein WR. Permeability of membrane junctions. Ann N Y Acad Sci 6;137:441-472.
6. Eid H, Larson DM, Springhorn JP, Attawia MA, Nayak RC, Smith TW, Kelly A. ...Role of epicardial mesothelial cells in the modification of phenotype and function of adult rat ventricular myocytes in primary coculture. Circ Res 1992;71:40-50.
7. Larson DM, Carson MP, Haudenschild CC. Junctional transfer of small molecules in cultured bovine brain microvascular endothelial cells and pericytes. Microvasc Res 1987;34:184
8. Evans WH, Gurd JW. Preparation and properties of nexuses and lipid enriched vesicles from mouse liver plasma membranes. Biochem J 1972;128:691-700.
9. Goodenough DA, Stoeckenius W. The isolation of mouse hepatocyte gap junctions. Preliminary chemical characterization and x-ray diffraction. J Cell Biol. 1972;54:646-656.
10. Makowski L, Caspar DLD., Phillips WC, Goodenough DA. Gap junction structures. II. Analysis of the X-ray diffraction data. J Cell Biol 1977;74:629-645.
11. Caspar DLD, Goodenough DA, Makowski L, Phillips WP. Gap junction structures. I Correlated electron microscopy and X-ray diffraction. J Cell Biol 1977;74:605-628.
12. Unwin PNT, Zampighi G. Structure of the junction between communicating cells. Nature 1980;283:545-549.
13. Manjunath CK, Goings GE, Page E. Cytoplasmic surface and intramembrane components of rat heart gap junctional proteins. Am J Physiol 1984;246:H865-H875.
14. Yeager M, Gilula NB. Membrane topology and quaternary structure of cardiac gap junction ion channels. J Mol Biol 1992;223:929-948.
15. Unger VM, Kumar NM, Gilula NB, Yeager M. Projectino structure of a gap junction membrane channel at 7A resolution. Nature Structural Biology 1996;
16. Kensler RW, Goodenough DA. Isolation of mouse myocardial gap junctions. J Cell Biol 1980;86:755-764.

17. Bloemendal H., Zweers A, Vermorken F, Dunia I, Benedetti EL. The plasma membrane of eye lens fibers. Biochemical and structural characterization. Cell Differ 1972;1:91-106.

18. Alcala J, Lieska N, Maisel H. Protein composition of bovine lens cortical fiber cell membranes. Exp Eye Res 1975;21:581-589.

19. Goodenough DA. Lens gap junctions: a structural hypothesis for nonregulated low-resistance intercellular pathways.Invest Ophthalmol Vis Sci 1979;18:1104-1122.

20. Hertzberg EL, Gilula NB. Isolation and characterization of gap junctions from rat liver. J Biol Chem 1979;254:2138-2147.

21. Manjunath CK, Goings GE, Page E. Proteolysis of cardiac gap junctions during their isolation from rat hearts. J Membr Biol 1985;85:159-168.

22. Manjunath CK, Goings GE, Page E. Human cardiac gap junctions: isolation, ultrastructure, and protein composition. J Mol Cell Cardiol 1987;19:131-134.

23. Kistler J, Kirkland B, Bullivant S. Identification of a 70,000-D protein in lens membrane junctional domains. J Cell Biol 1985;101:28-35.

24. Gros DB, Nicholson BJ, Revel JP. Comparative analysis of the gap junction protein from rat heart and liver: is there a tissue specificity of gap junctions? Cell 1983;35:539-549.

25. Nicholson BJ, Gros DB, Kent SBH, Hood LE, Revel JP. The Mr 28,000 gap junction proteins from rat heart and liver are different but related. J Biol Chem 1985;260:6514-6517.

26. Manjunath CK, Nicholson BJ, Teplow D, Hood L, Page E, Revel JP. The cardiac gap junction protein (Mr 47,000) has a tissue-specific cytoplasmic domain of Mr 17,000 at its carboxy- terminus. Biochem Biophys Res Commun 1987;142:228-234.

27. Kistler J, Christie D, Bullivant S. Homologies between gap junction proteins in lens, heart and liver. Nature 1988;331:721-723.

28. Paul DL. Molecular cloning of cDNA for rat liver gap junction protein. J Cell Biol 1986;103:123-134.

29. Kumar NM, Gilula NB. Cloning and characterization of human and rat liver cDNAs coding for a gap junction protein. J Cell Biol 1986;103:767-776.

30. Beyer EC, Paul DL, Goodenough DA. Connexin43: a protein from rat heart homologous to a gap junction protein from liver. J Cell Biol 1987;105:2621-2629.

31. Beyer EC, Kistler J, Paul DL, Goodenough DA. Antisera directed against connexin43 peptides react with a 43-kD protein localized to gap junctions in myocardium and other tissues. J Cell Biol 1989;108:595-605.

32. Yancey SB, John SA, Lal R, Austin BJ, Revel JP. The 43 - kD polypeptide of heart gap junctions: immunolocalization, topology, and functional domains. J Cell Biol 1989;108:2241-2254.

33. Swenson KI, Jordan JR, Beyer EC, Paul DL. Formation of gap junctions by expression of connexins in Xenopus oocyte pairs. Cell 1989;57:145-155.

34. Werner R, Levine E, Rabadan Diehl C, Dahl G.Formation of hybrid cell-cell channels. Proc Natl Acad Sci U S A 1989;86:5380-5384.

35. Green CR, Harfst E, Gourdie RG, Severs NJ. Analysis ofthe rat liver gap junction protein: clarification of anomaliesin its molecular size. Proc R Soc Lond [Biol] 1988;233:165-174.

36. Beyer EC, Goodenough DA, Paul DL. The connexins, a family of related gap junction proteins. Mod Cell Biol 1988;7:167-175.

37. Beyer EC, Paul DL, Goodenough DA. Connexin family of gap junction proteins. J Membr Biol 1990;116:187-194.

38. Zimmer DB, Green CR, Evans WH, Gilula NB. Topological analysis of the major protein in isolated intact rat liver gap junctions and gap junction-derived single membrane structures. J Biol Chem 1987;262:7751-7763.

39. Hertzberg EL, Disher RM, Tiller AA, Zhou Y, Cook RG. Topology of the Mr 27,000 liver gap junction protein. Cytoplasmic localization of amino- and carboxyl termini and a hydrophilic domain which is protease -hypersensitive. J Biol Chem 1988;263:19105-19111.

40. Goodenough DA, Paul DL, Jesaitis L. Topological distribution of two connexin32 antigenic sites in intact and split rodent hepatocyte gap junctions. J Cell Biol 1988;107:1817-1824.

41. Milks LC, Kumar NM, Houghten R, Unwin N, Gilula NB. Topology of the 32-kd liver gap junction protein determined by site-directed antibody localizations. EMBO J 1988;7:2967-2975.

42. Beyer EC. Molecular cloning and developmental expression of two chick embryo gap junction pro teins. JBiol Chem 1990;265:14439-14443.

43. Beyer EC, Reed KE, Westphale EM, Kanter HL, LarsonDM. Molecular cloning and expression of rat connexin40,a gap junction protein expressed in vascular smooth muscle. J Membr Biol 1992;127:69-76.

44. Haefliger JA, Bruzzone R, Jenkins NA, Gilbert DJ,Copeland NG, Paul DL. Four novel members of the connexin family of gap junction proteins. Molecular cloning, expression, and chromosome mapping. J Biol Chem 1992;267:2057-2064.

45. Hennemann H, Dahl E, White JB, Schwarz HJ, Lalley PA, Chang S, Nicholson BJ, Willecke K. Two gap junction genes, connexin 31.1 and 30.3, are closely linked on mousechromosome 4 and preferentially expressed in skin. J Biol Chem 1992;267:17225-17233.

46. Hennemann H, Schwarz HJ, Willecke K. Characterization of gap junction genes expressed in F9 embryonic carcinoma cells: molecular cloning of mouse connexin31 and -45cDNAs. Eur J Cell Biol 1992;57:51-58.

47. Hennemann H, Suchyna T, Lichtenberg Frate H, Jungbluth S, Dahl E, Schwarz J, Nicholson BJ, Willecke K. Molecular cloning and functional expression of mouse connexin40, a second gap junction gene preferentially expressed in lung. J Cell Biol 1992;117:1299-1310.

48. Gimlich RL, Kumar NM, Gilula NB. Differential regulation of the levels of three gap junction mRNAs in Xenopus embryos. J Cell Biol 1990;110:597-605.

49.   Musil LS, Beyer EC, Goodenough DA. Expression of the gap junction protein connexin43 in embryonic chick lens: molecular cloning, ultrastructural localization, and post-translational phosphorylation. J Membr Biol 1990;116:163-175.

50.   Fishman GI, Spray DC, Leinwand LA. Molecular characterization and functional   expression ofthe human cardiac gap junction channel. J Cell Biol 1990;111:589-598.

51.   Beyer EC, Steinberg TH. Evidence that the gap junction protein connexin-43 is the ATP-induced pore of mouse macrophages. J Biol Chem 1991;266:7971-7974.

52.   Lash JA, Critser ES, Pressler ML. Cloning of a gap junctional protein from vascular smooth muscle and expression in two-cell mouse embryos. J Biol Chem 1990;265:13113-13117.

53.   Kanter HL, Saffitz JE, Beyer EC. Cardiac myocytes express multiple gap junction proteins. Circ Res 1992;70:438-444.

54.   Kanter HL, Saffitz JE, Beyer EC. Molecular cloning of two human cardiac gap junction proteins, connexin40 and   connexin45. J Mol Cell Cardiol 1994;26:861-868.

55.   Essner JJ, Laing JG, Beyer EC, Johnson RG, Hackett PB.Expression of Zebrafish connexin43.4 in the notochord and tail bud of wild-type and mutant no tail embryos. Dev Biol 1996;177:462

56.   Willecke K, Heynkes R, Dahl E, Stutenkemper R, Hennemann H, Jungbluth S, Suchyna T, Nicholson BJ.Mouse connexin37: cloning and functional expression of a gap junction gene highly expressed in lung. J Cell Biol 1991;114:1049-1057.

57.   Reed KE, Westphale EM, Larson DM, Wang HZ,Veenstra RD, Beyer EC. Molecular cloning and functional   expression of human connexin37, an endothelial   cell gap junction protein. J Clin Invest 1993;91:997-1004.

58.   Miller T, Dahl G, Werner R. Structure of a gap junction gene: rat connexin-32. Biosci Rep 1988;8:455-464.

59.   Fishman GI, Eddy RL, Shows TB, Rosenthal L, Leinwand LA. The human connexin gene family of gap junction proteins: distinct chromosomal locations but similar structures. Genomics 1991;10:250-256.

60.   Hennemann H, Kozjek G, Dahl E, Nicholson B, Willecke K. Molecular cloning of mouse connexins26 and -32:similar genomic organization but distinct promoter   sequences of two gap junction genes. Eur J Cell Biol 1992;58:81-89.

61.   Sullivan R, Ruangvoravat C, Joo D, Morgan J, Wang BL, Wang XK, Lo CW. Structure, sequence and expression of the mouse Cx43 gene encoding connexin 43. Gene   1993;130:191-199.

62.   Neuhaus IM, Dahl G, Werner R. Use of alternate promoters for tissue specific expression of the gene coding for connexin32. Gene 1995;158:257-262.

63. Che n Z-Q, Lefebvre D, Bai X_, Reaume A, Rossant J, Lye SJ. Identification of two regulatory elements within the promoter region of the mouse connexin 43 gene. J Biol Chem 1995;270:3863-3868.
64. De Leon JR, Buttrick PM, Fishman GI. Functional analysis of the connexin43 gene promoter in vivo and in vitro. Journal of Molecular & Cellular Cardiology 1994;26:379-389.
65. Yu W, Dahl G, Werner R. The connexin43 gene is responsive to estrogen. Proc R Soc Lond 1994;255:125-132.
66. Geimonen E, Jiang W, Ali M, Fishman GI, Garfield RE,Andersen J. Activation of protein kinase C in human uterine smooth muscle induces connexin-43 gene transcription through an AP-1 site in the promoter sequence. J Biol Chem 1996;271:23667-23674.
67. Dahl G, Miller T, Paul D, Voellmy R, Werner R.Expression of functional cell-cell channels from cloned rat liver gap junction complementary DNA. Science 1987;236:1290-1293.
68. Eghbali B, Kessler JA, Spray DC. Expression of gapjunction channels in communication-incompetent cells afterstable transfection with cDNA encoding connexin 32. Proc Natl Acad Sci U S A 1990;87:1328-1331.
69. Veenstra RD, Wang HZ, Westphale EM, Beyer EC.Multiple connexins confer distinct regulatory and conductance properties of gap junctions in developing heart. Circ Res 1992;71:1277-1283.
70. Barrio LC, Suchyna T, Bargiello T, Xu LX, Roginski RS, Bennett MV, Nicholson BJ. Gap junctions formed byconnexins 26 and 32 alone and in combination are differently affected by applied voltage. Proc Natl Acad Sci U S A 1992;89:4220
71. Spray DC, Moreno AP, Eghbali B, Chanson M, Fishman GI. Gating of gap junction channels as revealed in cells stably transfected with wild type and mutant connexin cDNAs. Biophys J 1992;62:48-50.
72. Liu S, Taffet S, Stoner L, Delmar M, Vallano ML, Jalife J. A structural basis for the unequal sensitivity of the major cardiac and liver gap junctions to intracellular acidification: the carboxyl tail length. Biophys J 1993;64:1422-1433.
73. Elfgang C, Eckert R, Lichtenberg-Frate H, Butterweck A,Traub O, Klein RA, Hulser DF, Willecke K. Specific permeability and selective formation of gap junction channels in connexin-transfected HeLa cells. J Cell Biol 1995;129:805-817.
74. Veenstra RD, Wang HZ, Beblo DA, Chilton MG, Harris AL,Beyer EC,Brink P. Selectivity of connexin-specific gap junctions does not correlate with channel conductance. Circ Res 1995;77:1156-1165.
75. Paul DL, Ebihara L, Takemoto LJ, Swenson KI, Goodenough DA. Connexin46, a novel lens gap junction protein, induces voltage-gated currents in nonjunctional plasma membrane of Xenopus oocytes. J Cell Biol 1991;115:1077-1089.

76.   Harfst E, Severs NJ, Green CR. Cardiac myocyte gap junctions: evidence for
       a major connexon protein with an apparent relative molecular mass of 70,000.
       J Cell Sci   1990;96:591-604.

77.   Davis LM, Kanter HL, Beyer EC, Saffitz JE. Distinct gap junctionphenotypes
       in cardiac tissues with disparate conductino properties. J Am Coll Cardiol
       1994;24:1124-1132.

78.   Bastide B, Neyses L, Ganten D, Paul M, Willecke K, Traub O. Gap junction
       protein connexin40 is preferentially expressed in vascular endothelium and
       conductive bundles   of rat myocardium and is increased under hypertensive
       conditions. Circ Res 1993;73:1138-1149.

79.   Kanter HL, Laing JG, Beau SL, Beyer EC, Saffitz JE. Distinct patterns of
       connexin expression in canine Purkinje fibers and ventricular muscle. Circ Res
       1993;72:1124-1131.

80.   Gros D, Jarry-Guichard T, Ten Velde I, De Maziere A, van Kempen MJA,
       Davoust J, Briand JB, Moorman AFM, Jongsma HJ. Restricted distribution of
       connexin40, a gap   junctional protein, in mammalian heart. Circ Res
       1994;74:839-851.

81.   Davis LM, Rodefeld ME, Green K, Beyer EC, Saffitz JE. Gapjunctionprotein
       phenotypes of the human heart and   conduction   system. J   Cardiovasc
       Electrophysiol 1995;6:813-822.

82.   van Kempen MJA, Ten Velde I, Wessels A, Oosthoek PW, Gros D, Jongsma
       HJ, Moorman AFM, Lamers WH. Differential connexin distribution
       accomodates cardiac function in different species. Microscopy Research and
       Technique 1995;31:420-436.

83.   Kanter HL, Laing JG, Beyer EC, Green KG, Saffitz JE. Multiple connexins
       colocalize in canine ventricular myocyte gap junctions. Circ Res
       1993;73:344-350.

84.   Minkoff R, Rundus VR, Parker SB, Beyer EC, Hertzberg EL. Connexin
       expression in the developing avian cardiovascular system. Circ Res
       1993;73:71-78.

85.   Larson DM, Wrobleski MJ, Sagar GDV, Westphale EM, Beyer   EC.
       Differential regulation of connexin43 and connexin37 in endothelial cells by cell
       density, growth, and TGF-beta1. Am J Physiol (Cell Physiol)
       1997;272:C405-C415.

86.   Dejana E, Corada M, Lampugnani MG. Endothelial cell-to-cell junctions.
       FASEB J 1995;9:910-918.

87.   Christ GJ, Spray DC, El-Sabban M, Moore LK, Brink PR. Gap junctions in
       vascular tissues: evaluating the role of intercellular communication in the
       modulation of vasomotor tone. Circ Res 1996;79:631-646.

88. Spagnoli LG, Villaschi S, Neri L, Palmieri G. Gap junctions in myo-endothelial bridges of rabbit carotid arteries. Experientia 1982;38:124

89. Cuevas P, Gutierrez-Diaz JA, Reimers D, Dujovny M, Diaz FG, Ausman JL. Pericyte endothelial gap junctions in human cerebral capillaries. Anat Embryol 1984;170:155

90. Beny JL, Pacicca C. Bidirectional electrical communication between smooth muscle and endothelial cells in the pig coronary artery. Am J Physiol 1994;266:H1465-H1472.

91. Little TL, Xia J, Duling BR. Dye tracers define differential endothelial and smooth muscle coupling patterns within the arterial wall. Circ Res 1995;76:498-504.

92. Larson DM, Haudenschild CC, Beyer EC. Gap junction messenger RNA expression by vascular wall cells. Circ Res 1990;66:1074-1080.

93. Laing JG, Westphale EM, Engelmann GL, Beyer EC. Characterization of the gap junction protein connexin45. J Membr Biol 1994;139:31-40.

94. Bruzzone R, Haefliger JA, Gimlich RL, Paul DL. Connexin40, a component of gap junctions in vascular endothelium, is restricted in its ability to interact with other connexins. Mol Biol Cell 1993;4:7-20.

95. Little TL, Beyer EC, Duling BR. Connexin43 and connexin40 gap junctio n proteins are present in arteriolar smooth muscle and endothelium in vivo. Am J Physiol 1995;268:H729-H739.

96. van Rijen HVM, van Kempen MJA, Analbers LJS, Rook MB, van Ginneken ACG, Gros D, Jongsma HJ. Gap junctions in human umbilical cord endothelial cells contain multiple connexins. Am J Physiol 1997;272:C117-C130.

97. Christ GJ, Brink PR, Zhao W, Moss J, Gondre CM, Roy C, Spray DC. Gap junctions modulate tissue contractility and alpha 1 adrenergic agonist efficacy in isolated rat aorta. J Pharmacol Exp Ther 1993;266:1054-1065.

98. Carter TD, Chen XY, Carlile G, Kalapothakis E, Ogden D, Evans WH. Porcine aortic endothelial gap junctions: identification and permeation by caged InsP3. J Cell Sci 1996;109:1765-1773.

99. Pepper MS, Montesano R, el Aoumari A, Gros D, Orci L, Meda P. Coupling and connexin 43 expression in microvascular and large vessel endothelial cells. Am J Physiol 1992;262:C1246-C1257.

100. Moore LK, Beyer EC, Burt JM. Characterization of gap junction channels in A7r5 vascular smooth muscle cells. Am J Physiol 1991;260:C975-C981.

101. Campos De Carvalho AC, Roy C, Moreno AP, Melman A, Hertzberg EL, Christ GJ, Spray DC. Gap junctions formed of connexin43 are found between smooth muscle cells of human corpus cavernosum. J Urol 1993;149:1568-1575.

102. M oore LK, Burt JM. Selective block of gap junction channel expression with connexin-specific antisense oligodeoxynucleotides. Am J Physiol 1994;267:C1371-C1380.

103. Polacek D, Lal R, Volin MV, Davies PF. Gap junctional communication between vascular cells. Induction of connexin43 messenger RNA in macrophage foam cells of atherosclerotic lesions. Am J Pathol 1993;142:593-606.

104. Beyer EC, Steinberg TH. Connexins, gap-junction proteins, and ATP-induced pores in macrophages. In: Hall JE, Zampighi G, Davis RM. eds. Gap Junctions (Progress in Cell Reserach, Vol. 3). Amsterdam: Elsevier, 1993:55-58.

105. Jara PI, Boric MP, Saez JC. Leukocytes express connexin43 after activation with lipopolysaccharide and appear to form gap junctions with endothelial cells after ischemia-reperfustion. Proc Natl Acad Sci USA 1995;92:7011-7015.

106. Guinan EC, Smith BR, Davies PF, Pober JS. Cytoplasmic transfer between endothelium and lymphocytes: quantitation by flow cytometry. Am J Pathol 1988;132:406-409.

107. Dorshkind K, Green L, Godwin A, Fletcher WH. Connexin-43-type gap junctions mediate communication between bone marrow stromal cells. Blood 1993;82:38-45.

108. Rosendaal M, Green CR, Rahman A, Morgan D. Up-re regulation of the connexin43+ gap junction network in haemopoietic tissue before the growth of stem cells. Journal of Cell Science 1994;107:29-37.

109. Traub O, Look J, Dermietzel R, Brummer F, Hulser D, Willecke K. Comparative characterization of the 21-kD and 26-kD gap junction proteins in murine liver and cultured hepatocytes. J Cell Biol 1989;108:1039-1051.

110. Moreno AP, Eghbali B, Spray DC. Connexin32 gap junction channels in stably transfected cells: unitary conductance. Biophys J 1991;60:1254-1266.

111. Moreno AP, Fishman GI, Beyer EC, Spray DC. Voltage dependent gating and single channel analysis of heterotypic gap junctin channels formed of Cx45 and Cx43. In: Kanno Y, Katoaka K, Shiba Y, Shibata Y. eds. I n t e r c e l l u l a r Communication through Gap Junctions, Progress in Cell Research, vol. 4. Amsterdam: Elsevier Science Publishers BV, 1995:405press-408.

112. Moreno AP, Laing JG, Beyer EC, Spray DC. Properties of gap junction channels formed of connexin45 endogenously expressed in human hepatoma (SKHep1) cells. Am J Physiol 1995;268:C356-C365.

113. Barrio LC, Suchyna T, Bargiello T, Xu LX, Roginski RS, Bennett MV, Nicholson BJ. Gap junctions formed by connexins 26 and 32 alone and in combination are differently affected by applied voltage. Proc Natl Acad Sci U S A 1991;88:8410-8414.

114. Verselis VK, Ginter CS, Bargiello TA. Opposite voltage gating polarities of two closely related connexins. Nature   1994;368:348-351.
115. White TW, Paul DL, Goodenough DA, Bruzzone R. Functional analysis of selective interactions among rodent connexins. Mol Biol Cell 1995;6:459-470.
116. White TW, Bruzzone R, Wolfram S, Paul DL, Goodenough DA. Selective interactions among the multiple connexin proteins expressed in the vertegrate lens: the second extracellular domain is a determinant of compatibility between connexins. J Cell Biol 1994;125:879-892.
117. Haubrich S, Schwartz H-J, Bukauskas F, Lichtenberg-Frate H, Traub O, Weingart R, Willecke K. Incompatibilty of connexin 40 and 43 hemichannels in gap junctions between mammalian cells is determined by intracellular domains. Mol Biol Cell 1996;7:1995-2006.
118. Verselis VK, Bargiello TA, Rubin JA, Bennett MVL. Comparison of voltage dependent properties of gap   junctions in hepatocytes and in Xenopus oocytes expressing Cx32 and Cx26. In: Hall JE, Zampighi GA, Davis RM. eds. Gap Junctions, Progress in Cell Research, volume 3. Amsterdam: Elsevier, 1993:105-112.
119. Stauffer KA. The gap junction proteins beta(1)-connexin   (connexin-32) and beta(2)-connexin (connexin-26) can form heteromeric hemichannels. J Biol Chem 1995;270:6768-6772.
120. Jiang JX, Goodenough DA. Heteromeric connexons in   lens gap junction channels. Proc Natl Acad Sci USA 1996;93:1287-1291.
121. Brink PR, Cronin K, Banach K, Peterson E, Westphale   EM, Seul KH, Ramanan SV, Beyer EC. Evidence for   heteromeric gap junction channels formed from rat connexin43 and human connexin37. Am J Physiol (Cell Physiol) 1997;(in press):
122. Laird DW. The life cycle of a connexin: gap junction formation, removal, and degradation. J Bioenerg Biomemb 1996;28:311-318.
123. Lau AF, Kurata WE, Kanemitsu MY, Loo LM, Warn-Cramer BJ, Eckhart W, Lampe PD. Regulation of connexin43 function by activated tyrosine protein kinases. J Bioenerg Biomemb 1996;28:357-365.
124. Saez JC, Berthoud VM, Moreno AP, Spray DC. Gap junctions: multiplicity of controls in differentiated and   undifferentiated cells and possible functional implications. In: Shenolikar S, Nairn AC. eds. Advances in Second Messenger and Phosphoprotein Research Vol. 27. New   York: Raven Press, Ltd. 1993:163-198.
125. Crow DS, Beyer EC, Paul DL, Kobe SS, Lau AF. Phosphorylation of connexin43 gap junction protein in uninfected and Rous sarcoma virus-transformed mammalian fibroblasts. Mol Cell Biol 1990;10:1754-1763.

126. Filson AJ, Azarnia R, Beyer EC, Loewenstein WR, Brugge JS. Tyrosine phosphorylation of a gap junction protein correlates with inhibition of cell-to-cell communication. Cell Growth Differ 1990;1:661-668.

127. Jiang JX, Paul DL, Goodenough DA. Posttranslational phosphorylation of lens fiber connexin46: a slow occurrence. Invest Ophthalmol Vis Sci 1993;34:3558-3565.

128. Butterweck A, Gergs U, Elfgang C, Willecke K, Traub O. Immunochemical characterization of the gap junction protein connexin45 in mouse kidney and transfected human HeLa cells. J Membr Biol 1994;141:247-256.

129. Traub O, Eckert R, Lichtenberg-Frate H, Elfgang C, Bastide B, Scheidtmann KH, Hulser DF, Willecke K. Immunochemical and electrophysiological characterization of murine connexin40 and -43 in mouse tissue and transfected human cells. Eur J Cell Biol 1994;64:101-112.

130. Brissette JL, Kumar NM, Gilula NB, Dotto GP. The tumor promoter 12-O-tetradecanoylphorbol-13-acetate and the ras oncogene modulate expression and phosphorylation of gap junction proteins. Mol Cell Biol 1991;11:5364-5371.

131. Reynhout JK, Lampe PD, Johnson RG. An activator of protein kinase C inhibits gap junction communication between cultured bovine lens cells. Exp Cell Res 1992;198:337-342.

132. Berthoud VM, Rook MB, Traub O, Hertzberg EL, Saez JC. On the mechanism of cell uncoupling induced by a tumor promoter phorbol ester in clone 9 cells, a rat liver epithelial cell line. Eur J Cell Biol 1993;62:384-396.

133. Warn-Cramer BJ, Lampe PD, Kurata WE, Kanemitsu MY, Loo LM, Eckhart W, Lau AF. Characterization of the mitogen-activated protein kinase phosphorylation sites on the connexin-43 gap junction protein. J Biol Chem 1996;271:3779-3786.

134. Kanemitsu MY, Lau AF. Epidermal growth factor stimulates the disruption of gap junctional communication and connexin43 phosphorylation independent of 12-0-tetradecanoylphorbol 13-acetate-sensitive protein kinase C: the possible involvement of mitogen-activated protein kinase. Mol Biol Cell 1993;4:837-848.

135. Musil LS, Cunningham BA, Edelman GM, Goodenough DA. Differential phosphorylation of the gap junction protein connexin 43 in junctional communication-competent and -deficient cell lines. J Cell Biol 1990;111:2077-2088.

136. Jongen WM, Fitzgerald DJ, Asamoto M, Piccoli C, Slaga TJ, Gros D, Takeichi M, Yamasaki H. Regulation of connexin 43-mediated gap junctional intercellular communication by Ca2+ in mouse epidermal cells is controlled by E-cadherin. J Cell Biol 1991;114:545-555.

137. Fujimoto K, Nagafuchi A, Tsukita S, Kuraoka A, Ohokuma A, Shibata Y. Dynamics of connexins, E-cadherin and alpha-catenin on cell membranes during gap junction formation. J Cell Sci 1997;110:311-322.

138. Meyer RA, Laird DW, Revel JP, Johnson RG. Inhibition of gap junction and adherens junction assembly by connexin and A-CAM antibodies. J Cell Biol 1992;119:179-189.

139. Wang YJ, Rose B. An inhibition of gap-junctional communication by cadherins. J Cell Sci 1997;110:301-309.

140. Musil LS, Goodenough DA. Biochemical analysis of connexin43 intracellular transport, phosphorylation, and assembly into gap junctional plaques. J Cell Biol 1991;115:1357-1374.

141. Musil LS, Goodenough DA. Multisubunit assembly of an integral plasma membrane channel protein, gap junction connexin43, occurs after exit from the ER. Cell 1993;74:1065-1077.

142. Falk MM, Kumar NM, Gilula NB. Membrane insertion of gap junction connexins: polytopic channel forming membrane proteins. J Cell Biol 1994;127:343-355.

143. Atkinson MM, Menko AS, Johnson RG, Sheppard JR, Sheridan JD. Rapid and reversible reduction of junctional permeability in cells infected with a temperature-sensitive mutant of avian sarcoma virus. J Cell Biol 1981;91:573-578.

144. Azarnia R, Reddy S, Kmiecik TE, Shalloway D, Loewenstein WR. The cellular src gene product regulates junctional cell- to-cell communication. Science 1988;239:398-401.

145. Swenson KI, Piwnica Worms H, McNamee H, Paul DL. Tyrosine phosphorylation of the gap junction protein connexin43 is required for the pp60v-src-induced inhibition of communication. Cell Regul 1990;1:989-1002.

146. Loo LWM, Berestecky JM, Kanemitsu MY, Lau AF. pp60src-mediated phosphorylation of connexin 43, a gap junction protein. J Biol Chem 1995;270:12751-12761.

147. Atkinson MM, Sheridan JD. Altered junctional permeability between cells transformed by v-ras, v-mos, or v-src. Am J Physiol 1988;255:C674-C683.

148. Kurata WE, Lau AF. p130gag-fps disrupts gap junctional communication and induces phosphorylation of connexin43 in a manner similar to that of pp60v-src. Oncogene 1994;9:329-335.

149. Fallon RF, Goodenough DA. Five-hour half-life of mouse liver gap-junction protein. J Cell Biol 1981;90:521-526.

150. Larsen WJ, Tung HN. Origin and fate of cytoplasmic gap junctions in rabbit granulosa cells. Tissue Cell 1978;10:585-598.

151. Ginzberg RD, Gilula NB. Modulation of cell junctions during differentiation of the chicken otocyst sensory epithelium. Dev Biol 1979;68:110-129.

152. Larsen WJ, Tung HN, Murray SA, Swenson CA. Evidence for the participation of actin microfilaments in the internalization of gap junction membrane. J Cell Biol 1979;83:576-587.

153. Murray SA, Larsen WJ, Trout J, Donta ST. Gap junction assembly and endocytosis correlated with patterns of growth in a cultured adrenocortical tumor cell(SW-13). Cancer Res 1981;41:4063-4069.

154. Traub O, Druge PM, Willecke K. Degradation and resynthesis of gap junction protein in plasma membranes of regenerating liver after partial hepatectomy or cholestasis. Proc Natl Acad Sci U S A 1983;80:755-759.

155. Severs NJ, Shovel KS, Slade AM, Powell T, Twist VW, Green CR. Fate of gap junctions in isolated adult mammalian cardiomyocytes. Circ Res 1989;65:22-42.

156. Dermietzel R, Hertberg EL, Kessler JA, Spray DC. Gap junctions between cultured astrocytes: immunocytochemical, molecular, and electrophysiological analysis. J Neurosci 1991;11:1421-1432.

157. Naus CC, Hearn S, Zhu D, Nicholson BJ, Shivers RR. Ultrastructural analysis of gap junctions in C6 glioma cells transfected with connexin43 cDNA. Exp Cell Res 1993;206:72-84.

158. Rahman S, Carlile G, Evans WH. Assembly of hepatic gap junctions. Topography and distribution of connexin 32 in intracellular and plasma membranes determined using sequence-specific antibodies. J Biol Chem 1993;268:1260-1265.

159. Laing JG, Beyer EC. The gap junction protein connexin43 is degraded via the ubiquitin proteasome pathway. J Biol Chem 1995;270:26399-26403.

160. Reaume AG, Desousa PA, Kulkarni S, Langille BL, Zhu DG, Davies TC, Juneja SC, Kidder GM, Rossant J. Cardiac malformation in neonatal mice lacking connexin43. Science 1995;267:1831-1834.

161. Guerrero PG, Schuessler RB, Davis LM, Beyer EC, Johnson CM, Yamada KA, Saffitz JE. Slow ventricular conduction in mice heterozygous for a connexin43 null mutation. J Clin Invest 1997;99:1991-1998.

4 BIOPHYSICS OF GAP JUNCTION CHANNELS

Richard D. Veenstra and Hong-Zhan Wang

*Department of Pharmacology, College of Medicine SUNY at
Syracuse*

1. Introduction

All multicellular organisms require a means for long distance intercellular communication for the purpose of tissue homeostasis, coordinated body movements, and receiving sensory input about its environment. Signals are transmitted long distances primarily by electrical impulses through nerve or muscle tissues, whereas chemical signaling is more localized since it is spatially and temporally limited by the constraints of aqueous diffusion within either the extracellular or intracellular fluid compartments of the organism. Signals arising within the cytoplasm of a cell require a mechanism for transmembrane signal transduction if the message is to be received by neighboring cells. The most direct means of intercellular communication between cells is to form cytoplasmic connections with its neighbors thereby permitting the rapid signaling carried by ions and the more specialized chemical signaling provided by intracellular second messengers. The existence of gap junction channels was first proposed in 1964 by Werner Loewenstein[1] and are now know to occur by the expression of at least 13 cloned connexin proteins.[2,3,4] The ability of many of the connexins to facilitate intercellular communication has been clearly demonstrated by electrical coupling assays in a variety of expression systems.[3,4] To date, some of the elementary channel properties (e.g. unitary conductance, g_j) of at least six of these connexins are known.[5] With so many connexin channels in the mammalian body, we must now begin to discern the unique characteristics of each type of gap junction channel in order to determine the physiological consequences of each connexin and their interactions with other connexins. With this in mind, I want to review the essential theories of channel permeability as it pertains to ion channels and relate this body of knowledge to our developing understanding of connexin channel permeability.

1.1 *General Description of a Gap Junction Channel*

The gap junction channel is commonly portrayed as a weakly selective ion channel capable of passing hydrophilic molecules of nearly 1 kD in molecular mass or 10 to 14 Å in diameter from cell to cell. This general description predates present knowledge about the diversity in the molecular composition of gap junction channels and only superficially acknowledges permeability data known since 1980 that demonstrates differential size permeability limits based on the electronegativity of the permeant molecule.[6,7] Although the size limitation for permeant molecules decreases with increasing electronegativity, the molecular mass of a molecule is a less accurate indicator of the limiting size of a pore than the abaxial width (second largest dimension) of the molecule.[8] Actually the cross sectional area of the largest permeant molecule provides the best estimate of the limiting pore size.[9] In a channel where the molecule remains hydrated for the entire length of the pore, the electrical conductance increases as the square of the pore radius.[9,10] Hence, the larger the channel conductance, the larger the pore radius and the larger the molecular permeability limit should be for a particular channel. While this interpretation has been directly challenged by experimental evidence from at least four different connexins where the permeability to two anionic fluorescein dye derivatives was not correlated with channel conductance,[5] this generic aqueous pore model serves as a convenient starting point for the discussion of gap junction channel selective permeability. This is especially true since most published articles as recent as 1996 still refer to gap junctions as specialized membrane structures that permit the flow of ions and hydrophilic molecules of upto 1 kD in size between mammalian cells. Efforts have already begun to address this issue in a connexin-specific manner.

1.2 *Overview of Ionic Permeability Theory*

No discussion of gap junction channel permeability is complete without considering the initial investigations which provide the existing framework of knowledge of the physical forces that govern ion and nonelectrolyte selective permeability. This subject was extensively reviewed by Diamond and Wright[11] and Eisenman and Horn[12], so only the major elements of ionic selectivity theory will be presented here.

1.2.1. Ionic Selectivity Sequences.

In biological systems, the physiologically most relevant ions to consider are the alkali metal cations (Cs^+, Rb^+, K^+, Na^+, Li^+), the halide anions (I^-, Br^-, Cl^-, F^-), and the alkali earth divalent cations (Ba^{++}, Sr^{++}, Ca^{++}, Mg^{++}). Ironically, the origin of the known selectivity sequences for these ions began in nonliving systems (e.g. soils and aluminum silicate glasses). It is now understood that the same finite set of selectivity sequences exists in nature for living and nonliving systems. This is because the same physical forces act to bind these elements in organic materials (e.g. ion channel proteins) or inorganic materials (e.g. glass). To understand how an ordered ionic selectivity sequence arises from intermolecular attractive and repulsive forces, let us begin with the earliest observations of two oppositely ordered sequences and the physical reasons for the sequence inversion.

1.2.1.1. *Lyotropic sequence.*

In an aqueous solution, the measured mobilities of the alkali cations are the exact opposite of their atomic radii. In order of the smallest to the largest monovalent cation, the sequence is: $Li^+ > Na^+ > K^+ > Rb^+ > Cs^+$. However, the effective radius in water, which can be calculated by the Stokes equation, has the opposite order of $Cs^+ > Rb^+ > K^+ > Na^+ > Li^+$ since the smaller ions are more hydrated.[13] This sequence, called the lyotropic or Hofmeister series, was described around the turn of the century. The corresponding sequences for the halide anions and earth divalent cations are: $I^- > Br^- > Cl^- > F^-$ and $Ba^{++} > Sr^{++} > Ca^{++} > Mg^{++}$. It was initially thought that the most hydrated ion would be the first to be affected by dehydration, i.e. the first ion to become dehydrated.[14] It is now known that this is not the what occurs for reasons that will become more obvious once we consider the second proposed selectivity sequence.

1.2.1.2. *Polarizability sequence.*

An alternative explanation for ionic selectivity was forwarded by Bungenberg de Jong[15] in 1949 that attributed the selectivity to the polarization of water or the binding site by the ion. Since the smallest ion has the highest charge density, ions like Li^+, F^-, and Mg^{++} have the highest relative ability to polarize (orient) the charge on a dipole (e.g. water). Hence, the polarizing sequences are in the exact order of the atomic radii of the monovalent and divalent cations and anions. The result of these two original considerations of how ionic selectivity sequences arise predicts that only Li^+ or Cs^+ would be the most preferred ion under any circumstances. We know this is not the case since K^+ and Ca^{++} channels abound in nature from protozoans to metazoans (Na^+ channels are of metazoan origin). How do these other selectivity sequences arise and what forces are responsible for their occurrence inorganic and inorganic matter? The present understanding for the occurrence of a finite set of transition sequences was provided by George Eisenmans investigations using aluminosilicate glass electrodes.[12]

1.2.1.3. *Transitional sequences.*

Despite the possibility that N! sequences can exist, only a few are commonly observed (seven or eleven respectively). The first sequence always corresponds to the lyotropic sequence and the last sequence in the series for the alkali cations, earth divalent cations, and halide anions always corresponds with the polarizability sequence described above. The intervening sequences, called the transitional sequences, do not have only the smallest or the largest ion of each group as the preferred species. For instance, K^+ channels may correspond to a sequence IV, V or VI while a Na^+ channel may correspond to sequences VII through X. Calcium channels require additional considerations to impart divalent over monovalent selectivity (two closely spaced cation-binding sites) [11], but nonetheless correspond to sequences III through VI for the alkanine-earth cations. So what does this have to do with gap junction channels. The same rules will apply and it will depend on the extent to which the permeant ions are hydrated as they pass through the gap junction channel pore. So it follows that we must consider the mechanisms which determine these series of selectivity sequences.

1.2.2. Mechanisms for Selectivity.

As portrayed in the general definition of a gap junction channel, ions readily pass since they are considerably smaller in diameter than the known permeant molecules of 400 to 900 daltons (or 10 to 14 Å in diameter). Hence, the ionic selectivity should be considerably less than the modest charge selectivity observed for large permeant molecules. This is an oversimplification of the interactions that determine the above mentioned selectivity sequences and implies that only lyotropic sequences would be expected to be observed for gap junction channels given their large diameters. There is even more to consider when a channel is permeable to both cations and anions, as gap junction channels are reported to be, and there are only three published models for anion:cation selectivity presently in existence.[16,17,18,19] Of these three, only one of these models incorporates a central aqueous cylinder within the pore where the ions can electrodiffuse in proportion to their aqueous diffusion coefficients. These models will be considered later in this chapter. The selection of permeant molecules on the basis of physical size alone we will refer to as steric hindrance. A second mechanism for selectivity involves preferences of a related substrates for a specific site or the binding affinity of the ion for the site. Binding sites that result in the observed ionic selectivity of known biological ion channels are more commonly referred to as the selectivity filter of the channel. Selectivity filters for many cation and anion channels have been identified through ionic permeability studies and subsequent structure-function analysis of previously identified pore-forming domains.[20,21,22] Definitive structural models depicting the three-dimensional spatial organization of critical amino acid residues that form the selectivity filter of a particular channel are still forthcoming although the conceptual framework for constructing them already exists. A weak anionic site that selects slightly for cations over anions was suggested by the pioneering molecular permeability studies.[6,7] However, actual ionic binding sites within gap junction (or more precisely connexin) channel pores or the physical dimensions of a gap junction channel ion selectivity filter were not previously investigated until the complete alkali cation selectivity sequences for connexin43 and connexin40 were recently reported by Wang and Veenstra and Beblo and Veenstra.[23,24] These findings will be presented in the context of the three existing models for ion permeation within cation and anion permeable channels later in this chapter. Let us first consider further the mechanisms for steric hindrance and binding affinity.

1.2.2.1. *Steric Hindrance.*

The term steric hindrance implies a physical impediment that separates one molecule from another by its mere presence even though the barrier may not recognize the same locus (pore or site) as the substrate. This is typically less frequent than one might expect, but it forms an essentially insurmountable (absolute) barrier when present. Steric effects involve non-coulomb forces (not involving charge) and are mediated primarily by the relative physical dimensions of, for example, the ion and the pore, and the rigidity of the imposed structure (e.g. the wall of the pore and the crystalline radius of the ion). In the case of two ions where one blocks the other by being impermeant or significantly less permeant, the frequency and order of their occurrence at a common locus is also relevant to the net flux of the ion. For aqueous pores, molecular sieving of the hydrated ion is relevant and results in effectively reducing the mobility of the ion.[25]

1.2.2.2. *Affinity Binding.*

The term binding affinity implies a mutual attraction between two molecules or a molecule for a site. The primary determinant of the binding affinity is the difference in free energy of the ion for water versus the ion for the site. The difference in free energies largely depends on the electrostatic forces involved in the interactions of the ion with water and the binding site. When these interactions are between fixed point charges (not inducible dipoles)[11], the strength of the coulomb forces decreases as the square of the distance between the ion and the site. Hence, local concentration of the ion is also importance in these intermolecular interactions. Ion selectivity implies the preference of a given site for one ion over another. The selectivity of the site is, therefore, relative in regards to the two competing ions. If $\Delta G_{ion} = \Delta G_{site} - \Delta G_{water}$, then it follows that $\Delta G_{ion\,A} - \Delta G_{ionB}$ provides the difference in free energy between the two ions. At low field strengths, the above equation is dominated by the ΔG_{water} terms and at high electrostatic field strengths the equation is dominated by the ΔG_{site} terms for each ion. The electrostatic forces at a distance x from the fixed site are affected by ionic field strength and the water content of the pore. Conventionally, the selectivity of a pore for a series of ions is expressed as the ratio of the ionic permeabilities for two ions calculated from the biionic reversal potential using the Goldman-Hodgkin-Katz (GHK) equation. This form of selectivity measurement is based on the equilibrium established between two ions with oppositely directed electrochemical potentials. Equilibrium selectivity theory has the advantage of not being influenced by kinetic considerations of ion permeation (i.e. channel conductance).[22,26] Selectivity can also be modeled as alternating energy barriers and wells that represent the selectivity barriers and binding sites within the pore with which the ion must interact en route.[12] The kinetic rate constants for an ion are proportional to the energy difference between the barrier height and the site depth, which vary for different ions. Both approaches are model-dependent and are subject to error. Equilibrium selectivity does not account for ion-ion or ion-site interactions that occur in multi-ion single file (long) pores. Barrier models require more specific information and may be subject to error if the barriers (or sites) vary depending on the occupancy state of a site. Hence, all ion permeation models require further verification by direct electrophysiological and/or structure-function analysis. The inherent assumption of ionic independence from equilibrium selectivity theory is not likely to be valid for channels that are permeable to both cations and anions since the likelihood of ion-ion interactions is enhanced unless the ions remain fully hydrated.

2. Review of Gap Junction Channel Permeability

Ionic permeability ratios were performed on many plasmalemmal ion channels as early as 1973 on the sodium current from the frog node of Ranvier.[27] The arrival of the patch clamp recording technique in 1981 permitted investigators to perform selectivity experiments on single channels, rather than whole cell membrane currents, from native cell membranes or cloned ion channels expressed in *Xenopus* oocytes (nAChR and sodium channel clones as first two examples).[28,29,30] Alternatively, intracellular ion channels can be studied using artificial lipid bilayer reconstitution techniques.[31] Similar conductance and permeability experiments performed on native gap junction channels or connexin-specific channels have been less forthcoming owing mostly to the technical difficulties of either recording from the double membrane gap junction channel using the patch clamp technique or attempting to reconstitute the channels into planar lipid bilayers. Hence, knowledge about the ionic permeabilities of gap junction channels is and their subsequent structure-function relationships is comparatively sparse. There exist only two published accounts of ionic permeability ratios from native gap junction channels. How this limited experimental data correlates with previous interpretations of the generic gap junction channel based on molecular permeability investigations will now be considered.

2.1 *Ionic Permeability Ratios*

Biionic reversal potential experiments are more difficult to perform on gap junction channels since they are intercellular channels and are, therefore, not accessible from the extracellular surface of the plasmamembrane. Indeed, the first accounts of gap junction channel recordings required intracellular recordings from two electrically coupled cells.[32,33] Two cell voltage clamp approaches to the recording of net junctional currents existed prior to these dual whole cell patch clamp recordings, but both approaches suffer from the need to modify the intracellular ionic composition of both cells in order to perform the necessary reversal potential experiments. Junctional reversal potential measurements are further hindered by the present knowledge that cells typically express more than one type of gap junction channel and selective blockers necessary to isolate the current of interest are not yet known for gap junction channels. Nonetheless, there are two accounts of ionic permeability ratios from native gap junction channels.

Membrane potential is measured relative to the external ground reference that is taken as 0 mV and assumed to be invariant. Junctional current flows between the interior of two cells and is, by definition, isolated from ground by the input resistance of each cell.[34] Hence, the measurement of ionic reversal potentials imposed across the junction within a cell pair becomes more difficult to ascertain. Typically, one side of the channel-containing membrane is exposed to the bath and the bath ground is maintained essentially constant by the use of a chloride salt bridge that minimizes the junction potentials between the bath and the reference recording electrode. Still, the measurement of net junctional current in coupled cell pairs is determined from the baseline whole cell currents obtained when there is no net transjunctional voltage. The zero junctional current ($I_j = 0$) level is readily ascertained under symmetrical ionic conditions, but is not readily defined under biionic conditions (asymmetric pipette solutions). Neyton and Trautmann reported relative potassium to sodium and potassium to chloride permeability ratios (P_K/P_{Na} and P_K/P_{Cl}) of 1.23 and 1.45 respectively for the rat lacrimal gland gap junction channels by taking the junctional biionic reversal potential as the voltage applied to the prejunctional cell (cell 1) that was required to make the current in the prejunctional cell (cell 1) that was required to make the current in the post-junctional cell (cell 2) equal to zero.[32] This measurement requires knowing the holding current value required to clamp cell 2 to -50 mV in the absence of the biionic- or differential voltage-clamp amplifier-induced transjunctional voltage gradient. Their reported P_K, P_{Na}, and P_{Cl} values of 1.0, 0.81, and 0.69 were consistent with the interpretation of a modest (<2:1) cation:anion selectivity for a mammalian gap junction channel. This investigation remains the only quantitative estimate of the ionic permeabilities of native mammalian gap junction channels to date.

Brink and Fan developed a more novel approach to the patch clamp analysis of gap junction channel currents by directly patching onto the septal membrane of the earthworm axon, a large surface area junctional membrane not typically found between mammalian cells.[35] Using a cocktail of ionic blockers of nonjunctional membrane channels, a 100 pS monovalent permeant ion channel was isolated. This junctional membrane channel had ionic conductance ratios of $K^+ = 1.0$, $Cs^+ = 1.0$, $Na^+ = 0.84$, $TMA^+ = 0.64$, $Cl^- = 0.52$, and $TEA^+ = 0.20$. These conductance ratios can be equated to ionic permeability ratios if the assumption that $P_{ion} = G_{ion}(RT/F^2[K])$ is valid. This expression is derived from the GHK current equation where G is the conductance of the ion and [K] is the ion (K^+) concentration. The similarity of the relative P_K, P_{Na}, and P_{Cl} values to the previous interpretation of gap junction channels was again consistent with the conventional interpretation of the gap junction channel. In either case, the molecular composition of the junctional channels was not known.

2.2 Molecular (Dye) Permeability Limits

The often stated upper size limit of approximately 1 kD is derived from fluorescent tracer studies performed on native gap junction channels performed during the late 1970s until 1980. Of the numerous investigations performed, only a few provide significant information about the selectivity of gap junction channels. To be precise, the largest molecular tracers known to permeate a mammalian gap junction channel are the multiple glycine conjugates of lissamine rhodamine B-200 (LRB).[6] LRB(glycine)$_6$OH (M_r = 901) was permeable in all cultured mammalian cells investigated and LRB(glycine)$_4$OH (M_r = 859) was shown to diffuse through mammalian ventricular myocyte gap junctions.[36] It should be noted that the permeability limit decreased with increasing negative charge on the rhodamine or fluorescein dye conjugates (e.g. FITC(glutamate)$_2$OH, M_r = 665 and 6-carboxyfluorescein, M_r = 376), suggestive of fixed negative charge within the gap junction channel pore.[5,6,7] Precise information about the limiting cross sectional area of the gap junction channel pore and its charge selectivity cannot be determined without knowing the cross-sectional area of the tracer molecule and its permeability coefficient relative to other permeant molecules. Furthermore, most published accounts of fluorescent tracer studies were performed independently of junctional conductance measurements in the observed cell pairs or clusters.[5,10] Suitable tracer molecules should be membrane impermeant and have little or no cytoplasmic binding, which would falsely increase or decrease the dyes observed junctional permeability.[37,38]

What are the physiological consequences of this molecular permeability to cellular function? Activation of membrane-bound receptors by ligand-binding triggers a cytoplasmic cascade of events culminating in modulation of protein kinases or phosphatases and transcription regulatory binding proteins to give only a few general examples. Membrane signal transduction by the generation of physiologically relevant second messengers (e.g. Ca^{++}, cAMP, 1,4,5-inositoltrisphosphate (IP_3)) is vital to cellular function and the integration of neurohumoral signals within a tissue is provided by intercellular chemical signaling via gap junctions. There are reports of cell-to-cell transfer of all of these second messengers in the present gap junction literature,[39,40] although there is increasing evidence that IP_3, and not Ca^{++}, is responsible for the propagation of intercellular calcium waves.[41] Some of these second messengers are also believed to regulate junctional conductance (e.g. cAMP),[42] which is another related area of investigation that has been reviewed elsewhere.[8,43] Without the spatial and temporal signal averaging that occurs via gap junctions, all cells in a tissue would have to receive identical neurohumoral signals in order to coordinate their functional activity. Hence, direct coupling via gap junctions provide for functional homogeneity and tissue homeostasis. The loss of junctional communication is often associated with developmental defects and cellular transformation.[1,44,45,46] The host of potential permeable molecules could also include a variety of metabolites and enzyme products provided that the molecular permeability limit is in excess of 10 Å and $\approx$ 1 kD.[47]

3. Connexin-specific Channel Permeability

All of the above investigations were performed on native gap junction channels from mammalian or invertebrate cells. In 1986, the first gap junction channel protein, connexin32 (Cx32)[48], was cloned and electrophysiological methodologies for recording unitary gap junction channel currents were developed.[32,33,34] With thirteen mammalian connexins identified thus far, the discussion of ionic and molecular permeabilities of gap junctions now must be considered in the context of the specific proteins expressed rather than the conceptualized version of a generic gap junction channel. The use of expression systems for connexins has contributed new evidence that has begun to advance our understanding of gap junction channels from the cellular to the molecular level.[49,50,51] Let us reconsider the previous interpretations about gap junction channels in the context of these most recent findings.

3.1 *Ionic Permeability*

The first approach taken regarding the relative ionic permeabilities of connexin-specific channels was to assess the relative cation:anion selectivity of several connexin channels by substituting glutamate⁻ for Cl⁻ in both patch pipettes and determining the change in unitary channel conductance (g_j) for four different connexin channels.[5] Given the measured aqueous diffusion coefficient for glutamate⁻, a 33% decrease in g_j was predicted.[10] All four cardiovascular connexins examined exhibited decreases in g_j in excess of the predicted value, indicative of a modest cation:anion selectivity of 2:1 or higher. Hence, hCx37, rCx40, rCx43, cCx43, and rCx45 (r = rat, h = human, c = chicken) all fit this one general interpretation of a gap junction channel. However, the predicted inverse correlation of increasing conductance (i.e. pore diameter) and decreasing ionic selectivity expected for an aqueous pore was not observed. In fact, no correlation between channel conductance and cation:anion selectivity was evident at all. This simply implies that conductance and pore diameter need not be directly correlated, as was already known to be true for ion selective channels[9], and/or that the connexin g_j may not be limited by restricted aqueous diffusion alone.

3.2 *Differential Dye Permeability*

These observations were echoed at the molecular level by the differential dye permeability of these five connexin channels to 2,7-dichlorofluorescein (diCl-F) and 6-carboxyfluorescein (6-CF).[5] It was striking to note that the highest g_j channel, hCx37, exhibited only sporadic dye passage while rCx43 (1/3 the g_j of hCx37) was the only connexin channel to 100% permeable to both dyes. It should be noted that only the presence or absence of dye transfer was determined following a 10 min recording period to assess the junctional conductance of the cell pair. Still, this is the only investigation that directly determined the junctional conductance of cells in which dye transfer was assayed. Another key advantage of this investigation was the use of two dyes that were structurally similar except for side-chain substitutions to the fluorescein molecule that minimize the physical constraints (i.e. diameter) and maximize the effect of net surface charge (i.e. valence) on the permeability through a connexin channel.

Evidence in support of the differential permeability of connexin-specific channels also came from Hela-transfected cells expressing Cx26, Cx31, Cx32, Cx37, Cx40, Cx43, and Cx45.[52] Although all connexins were permeable to Lucifer Yellow, a known fluorescent tracer with properties suitable for assaying gap junction permeability (M_r = 443, valence = -2, ≈ 10 Å diameter), differential dye transfer was noted for the less conventional dyes ethidium bromide, propridium iodide, and DAPI. All of these dyes are cationic and are known to bind to DNA, which may limit their junctional permeability. It is also true that the dye transfer assays were performed by dye microinjection into clusters of connexin-transfected Hela cells so the junctional conductances of the dye-coupled or -uncoupled cells was not known. Nonetheless, the data are consistent with a reduced dye permeability of Cx31 and, to a lesser extent, Cx32 to propridium iodide and ethidium bromide relative to the other connexins. There are experimental discrepancies between the above two investigations, particularly regarding the dye permeability of Cx45 to anionic dyes such as Lucifer Yellow that should be investigated further under more closely correlated experimental conditions.

3.3 *Hemichannel Permeability*

Although most connexins appear to form functional channels only when paired with connexins from a partner cell, a few cloned connexins are capable of forming hemichannels where the extracellular domain of the connexin opens to the extracellular space. This allows the investigator to study the voltage gating and permeability of the connexin hemichannel. The lens fiber cell connexins, Cx46, Cx50, and Cx56 are capable of forming functional hemichannels. While their physiological function is not known, hemichannels provide a unique opportunity to investigate the ionic permeability of half a gap junction channel. This information will also be useful when considering heterotypic gap junction channels where each hemichannel is formed from a different connexin. These results will also be considered in the context of the homotypic gap junction channel formed from a single connexin. There is only one such report of connexin hemichannel permeability ratios. Subsequent to the ionic permeability experiments performed on rCx43, rCx40 and others as reported above and to be presented in more detail later in this chapter, biionic reversal potential measurements were performed on Cx46 hemichannels expressed in *Xenopus* oocytes.[53] They found the monovalent cation sequence to follow the aqueous mobility sequence for the alkali cations (minus Rb^+) and the tetraalkylammonium ions tetramethylammonium (TMA) and etraethylammonium (TEA). This corresponds to a selectivity sequence I or II. The P_X/P_K ratios were: Cs^+, 1.19; K^+, 1.00; Na^+, 0.80; Li^+, 0.64; TMA^+, 0.34; and TEA^+, 0.20. The two-fold lower permeability ratios for TMA^+ and TEA^+ relative to Li^+ suggest additional factors (i.e. pore diameter) may be involved in reducing their permeability, although an estimate of pore diameter was not made from these data. These values were based on a P_K/P_{Cl} value of 10.3 and a P_{TEA}/P_{Cl} value of 2.8 as determined from asymmetric KCl and KCl:TEACl salt gradients. Anionic reversal potentials for Cl^-, Br^-, NO_3^-, and acetate⁻ were not reported. The inherent difficulty of measuring relative permeability ratios of a channel that is permeable to monovalent anions and cations will be discussed later in this chapter.

3.4 *Heterotypic Connexin Channel Permeability*

Every connexin cloned to date is capable of forming heterotypic junctions with at least one other connexin.[4] It is not known if heterotypic junctions occur naturally in native cell types, but expression systems permit the investigator to determine if two connexins can couple when brought into contact with one another. This also provides insight into how two connexins interact to form a functional channel, namely, whether each connexin maintains its intrinsic properties or not. Cx26/Cx32 heterotypic pairs were one of the first combinations tested and produced some unique conductance properties not found in the homotypic channels of Cx26 or Cx32. While the voltage gating properties of the heterotypic pair were attributed to the opposite polarity of their transjunctional gating mechanisms, the channel conductance and permeability properties are less well understood. The Cx26/Cx32 channel has a nonlinear conductance with respect to transjunctional voltage similar to the instantaneous junctional current-voltage relationship observed in *Xenopus* oocytes.[54,55] Mutation of a single amino acid residue in the N-terminal cytoplasmic domain (Cx32N2D or Cx26D2N) appears to alter transjunctional voltage-gating polarity (- to + or + to -, respectively) as evidenced by the current-voltage relationships.[56] The voltage sensor was believed to be formed by two residues at the M1-E1 border on the opposite side of the membrane (ES in most connexins, KE in Cx26) since the reciprocal mutations alter the kinetics and sensitivity of the transjunctional voltage-dependent inactivation of current (and conductance). The opposite polarity of the voltage gate for Cx26 and Cx32 (D2 or N2) can explain the rectifying instantaneous junctional current-voltage relationship for the Cx26/Cx32 channel. The similarity of the single channel Cx26/Cx32 I-V relationship lead Bukauskas et al. to propose that the rectifying I-V is due to the asymmetric voltage-sensitivity of the channel open state that are not predicted from the homotypic connexin channels.[55]

In what began as a collaborative effort to investigate the channel properties of the Cx26P87L mutant gap junction[57], we also investigated the properties of the heterotypic Cx26/Cx32 gap junction channels. Our homotypic Cx26 and Cx32 g_j values were nearly identical to those reported by Bukauskas et al.[55] and the heterotypic single channel I-V curve rectified in the same direction as well. In addition to the above experiments, however, we performed the glutamate⁻ for Cl⁻ substitutions described above for Cx43, etc. and estimated their relative cation:anion selectivity.[10] From these results, we concluded that Cx26 and Cx32 also have opposite ionic selectivities. Cx26 favors cations by $\approx$ 2:1 while Cx32 is slightly anionic ($\approx$1.0:1.1). Specific ionic conductances were calculated for Cx26 and Cx32 from the homotypic g_j values and the estimated cation:anion selectivities for each connexin. I-V relations for the heterotypic Cx26/Cx32 channel were calculated using the unidirectional flux equations and by equating ionic conductance and permeability according to the assumption $P_{ion} = G_{ion}(RT/F^2[ion])$. The results are summarized in Figure 1 where the homotypic Cx26, homotypic Cx32, and heterotypic Cx26/Cx32 channel I-V relations are plotted in 115 mM Kglutamate pipette solutions.

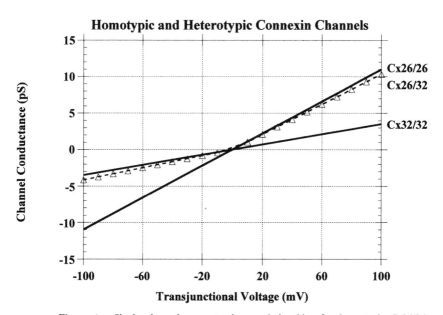

Figure 1. Single channel current-voltage relationships for homotypic Cx26/26, homotypic Cx32/32, and heterotypic Cx26/32 channels in 115 mM Kglutamate. Conductance of the Cx26 channel was 110 pS and 35 pS for Cx32. The heterotypic channel has a nonlinear I-V as illustrated by the data points (Δ). The dashed line is a theoretical fit of the data derived by calculating the unidirectional flux equations for the homotypic Cx26/26 and Cx32/32 channels for each ion where 1 = cell 1, 2 = cell 2, and n = flux coupling coefficient (= 4 for the fitted line). The ionic permeability (P_{ion}) was determined from the channel conductance using the GHK current equation and the relation $P_{ion} = g_{ion} \times RT/F^2$. The cation:anion selectivities of the Cx26/26 and Cx32/32 channel were assumed to be 2.6:1.0 and 0.94:1.0 respectively.[10] For the heterotypic channel the P_{ion} values of Cx26 were assigned to one direct and the P_{ion} values of Cx32 were assigned to the opposite direction flux.

It is apparent upon visual inspection that conductance of the hybrid chanel asymptotes towards the conductance of one connexin hemichannel or another depending on the voltage polarity (negative transjunctional voltage = Cx26 cell negative for Figure 1). The results illustrate one model which describes the asymmetric rectification of a heterotypic gap junction channel based on the intrinsic ionic permeability properties of each connexin to one hemichannel of the junction. While there are further experimental tests of the model that should be performed, this experimental evidence provides an alternative explanation to the asymmetry of the instantaneous I-V of the Cx26/Cx32 channel. It should be noted that gating activity was also observed to be altered in an asymmetric manner across the junction.

4. Mechanisms of Ion Permeation

The details of ion permeation through ion selective channels are being elucidated by site-directed mutagenesis of pore-forming residues and critical sites for ion binding within pore are being identified. Already, key residues involved in determining whether two highly homologous proteins form a Na^+ or Ca^{++} channel are known. Furthermore, the most recent model directly impacts on previous models developed from important Ca^{++} channel conductance and permeability data from the previous decade.[26] The two-site, three-barrier now appears to be a single site model where four glutamate residues only transiently bind the second Ca^{++} ion and form a single high-affinity Ca^{++}-binding site which blocks the monovalent Na^+ current. This model is consistent with all previous permeability and conductance data on the L-type calcium channel and is supported by data from other divalent cation-binding proteins.[58] Permeation models developed from other ion channels may assist us as we continue our investigations into the permeability properties of connexin-mediated gap junction channels.

4.1 *Independent Electrodiffusion*

The GHK current and voltage equations all assume that ions move through the pore independently of other ions. For long single file (narrow multi-ion) pores, this assumption does not hold.[9] Electrodiffusion theory has accounted for ion-ion interactions within the pore by introducing a flux-coupling coefficient to the flux-ratio equation. To experimentally test this theory, one must perform tracer flux experiments measuring both efflux and influx independently, a difficult task.[59] Conventionally, equilibrium selectivity theory is applied to biionic permeability ratios and mole-fraction effects on conductance are employed to determine ion-ion interactions within the pore. If two different ions are competing for a single site within the pore, the reversal potential can accurately reflect the relative affinity of the site for the two ions under biionic conditions. On other occasions, ionic permeability ratios cannot be determined using the GHK voltage equation. This is frequently the case for channel that are permeable to both cations and anions since electrostatic attraction within a restricted space is favored and the binding energies for a fixed electrostatic site will be oppositely-directed. This adds another dimension of complexity to the measurement of ionic permeabilities unless impermeant counterions can be used. There are three examples in the literature that explore the cation:anion selectivity of three different ion channels. In all cases, non-compliance with constant field theory occurred due to ion-dependent permeabilities.

4.2.1 Large channel theory, porin channels.

VDAC is a voltage-dependent anion channel found in the mitochondrial membrane.[19] It is estimated to form an aqueous pore approximately 3 nm in diameter and 5 nm in length. As is expected for a large diameter aqueous pore, any ionic selectivity was not presumed to be due to specific binding sites but rather electrostatic interactions between (partially) hydrated ions and the wall of the channel. It is widely accepted that electrostatic interactions are concentration-dependent and are strongest at low ionic strength. Hence, measuring the concentration-dependence of the cation:anion reversal potential provides a direct test of this facet of the Large Channel Theory (LCT).[19] The two essential features of the VDAC permeability are that (i) the cation:anion reversal potential deviates from linearity as the KCl gradient increases above 5-fold and (ii) the KCl reversal potential decreases with increasing concentration (constant KCl gradient of 2.0). Neither of these observations fit with GHK theory and are indicative of concentration-dependent permeability ratios. A third test is to measure the cation:anion reversal potential using salts with different aqueous mobilities. Whereas GHK theory predicts changes in the reversal potential[5], LCT predicts less change in the biionic reversal potential than expected from the mobility difference between the cations and anions.

The essential feature of the LCT theory is that the pore forms two compartments (Figure 2A). An outer compartment lining the wall of the channel where electrostatic interactions attract permeant ions and reduce their permeability through the channel. This screening of electrostatic charge along the pore wall creates a central aqueous compartment where ions can electrodiffuse through the channel without interacting with the wall of the channel. This screening is more effective at higher ionic strength, thus reducing the cation:anion reversal potential of the channel. The pore diameter and amount of electrostatic charge is critical to this theory since the diameter must be sufficient to allow ions to screen the pore wall and create a central cylinder still sufficient in diameter to allow other ions to electrodiffuse with minimal interaction. Concentration-dependent anion:cation reversal potentials using salts with similar or different aqueous mobilities provide an experimental test of this hypothesis.

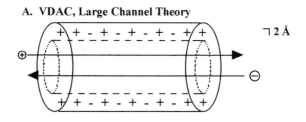

Figure 2. Illustrations of the three different mechanisms for cation and anion permeation through a common pore. **A,** Diagramatic representation of the 30 Å by 50 Å mitochondrial voltage-dependent anion channel (VDAC) channel and the Large Channel Theory for ion permeation.[19] Electrostatic charge associated with the wall of the pore attracts ions of opposite charge creating an outer shell of ions within the pore. This alters the electrostatic profile of the central pore compartment whereby ions (K$^+$ and Cl$^-$ drawn to scale) can diffuse down their electrochemical gradient. **B,** Channels formed by polyene antibiotics are 8 Å in diameter and do not possess fixed charges. Nonetheless, anions are readily permeable while cations can permeate the pore only when a permeant anion is present.[16] **C,** A similar mechanism is proposed for the 7 Å diameter neuronal Cl$^-$ channel except that the cation reversal potentials shift in the opposite direction of their mobilities and are correlated with the anion permeability.[17,18] The anion-dependent cation permeability is consistent with an occassional cation-anion pair transiting through the pore.

4.2.2. Model channels, polyene antibiotic channels (amphotericin B).

A different observation was made on the model channel formed by the polyene antibiotic, amphotericin B.[16] This compound aligns in an end-to-end fashion between the inner and outer membrane leaflets to form a continuous pore of ≈ 8 Å in diameter across the membrane. Again, the cation:anion selectivity are less than an order of magnitude (<1:10). A striking difference between this anion channel and VDAC is that the cation permeability was not observed to be concentration-dependent, but rather dependent on the sum of the monovalent permeant anions on both sides of the membrane. The anion permeability, however, is independent of the monovalent cation concentration. The key experimental test of their hypothesis involved the use of impermeant divalent ions (Mg^{++}, $SO_4 2-$) in combination with permeant monovalent cations and anions. They derived an equation resembling the GHK voltage equation where the cation:anion permeability ratio $r_{ca} = L_{ca}([A_1] + [A_2])$, thus replacing P_c/P_a in the normal GHK equation. In the above modified relative permeability coefficient expression, a = anion, c = cation, [A] is the concentration of anions 1 and 2 respectively, and L_{ca} = the cation:anion selectivity coefficient as determined by the expression $L = a_c/b_a[(b_c/v)+2]$. The terms a, b, and v are model-dependent rate constants for the entry rate (a) of an ion to an electrostatic site, release rate (b) of the same ion from the site, and the rate of cation c and anion a trading places at the same site.

The essential features of the permeation model for the amphotericin B channel is that there is a site that selects highly for anions and does not allow a cation to pass unless a permeant anion is also present (Figure 2B). In other words, the cation permeability of the channel is observed only in the presence of a permeant anion. An anion may occupy this site alone and binds to or dissociates from this site with rate constants a_a and b_a. A cation can bind to and dissociate from the anion-bound site with rate constants a_c and b_c. The cation:anion pair can also exchange places at the site in an electroneutral manner with rate constant v. If the site is anion-selective, a_c is rate limited by a_a and b_a is rate limited by b_c since a cation cannot occupy the site alone. Hence, $L = a_c/b_a[(b_c/v)+2]$. This model can be tested experimentally by examining the counterion-dependent or -independent permeability ratios using the modified GHK equation. These permeability coefficients will also be constant for a given cation-anion pair, in sharp contrast to the LCT theory. It is possible that the permeability ratios could be concentration-dependent if a_a is concentration-dependent, which is only likely if the site is accessible to the bulk solution. The distinguishing characteristic of this model is that the permeability of one ion is dependent on the presence of a permeant counterion whereas the reciprocal relationship is not true.

4.2.3. Background neuronal anion channel.

The data for the third permeation model comes from a background Cl⁻ channel found in nerve and skeletal muscle.[17,18] This channel had been previously found to be permeable to Na⁺ and even large organic cations.[60] Again, the cation permeability was < 1:10 relative to Cl⁻ (0.1-0.35). Originally thought to be a cation-dependent anion channel, this channel exhibited some uniquely interesting characteristics. First, substitution of Na⁺ with a large organic cation had a minimal effect on channel conductance .[17] Biionic cation:Cl⁻ reversal potentials demonstrated that even a large divalent cation, bis-tris-propane (BTP), was permeable through this channel. Second, substitution of Cl⁻ or Br⁻ with the larger and less permeable propionate produced smaller changes in the Na⁺:anion reversal potential than expected from GHK, and the shift was in the opposite direction, indicating a reduced cation permeability in the presence of less permeable anions. Third, the channel was blocked by large hydrophobic cations (benzyltrimethylammonium, BTMA) and anions (9-anthracene carboxylic acid, 9-ACA),but not by the small hydrophobic anion benzoate. Again the anion channel was not permeant to divalent anions ($SO_4{}^{2-}$). So the data suggests a lyotropic sequence for the permeant monovalent anions and a hydrophobic moiety as well. Furthermore, the cation permeability sequence ($Li^+ \approx Cs^+ > K^+ \approx Na^+$) does not correspond to any of the transitional selectivity sequences. Franciolini and Nonner[17,18] interpreted these results as suggestive of a large diameter aqueous pore with only weak electrostatic groups and a strong hydrophobic site. Their molecular model for ion permeation is similar to the Borisova et al.[16] model described above in so far as they propose that a single permeant anion may bind to a site while transiting through the pore while the permeant cation must associate with the bound cation at the site. The difference is that the cation can only dissociate from the site and pass on through the pore by associating with a permeant anion (Figure 2C). This can explain the anion-dependence of the cation permeability and the minimal effect of cation substitution on the channel conductance for a common anion. Hence, the two models involving ion-pairing at a site within the pore are mutually exclusive and can be distinguished by cation:anion reversal potential measurements.[16] In their permeation model, they predicted the pore to be ≈ 7 Å in diameter and 15 Å in length with an anion-binding site that senses 56% of the transmembrane voltage.

4.3 *Connexin Channel Cation/Anion Permeability*

The observation that most connexin channels were slightly cationic (2:1 - 10:1 cation:anion selectivity)[5,10] prompted us to examine the ionic permeabilities of homotypic connexin channels in more detail in order to elucidate the selectivity sequence for the monovalent cations and anions. For this purpose, we chose two related connexins that varied in their relative cation:anion selectivity by a factor of two, rat Cx43 and Cx40. Cx43 was of primary interest since it is expressed in a greater variety of tissues than any other cloned connexin and because it appears to be less selective as demonstrated by its low relative cation:anion permeability ratio and highest permeability to fluorescent dyes.[5] These two connexins are also of interest since they are coexpressed in the mammalian heart and vasculature[61], but are atypical of other connexins as demonstrated by their inability to form heterotypic gap junctions.[4] The results of our most recent investigations are summarized below and speculation as to the favored model for cation and anion permeation based on the above previous three examples of distinct cation and anion permeable channels are presented.

4.3.1. Connexin43.

Previously we had estimated the rCx43 cation:anion selectivity ratio to be 0.77 based on equimolar substitution of Cl⁻ by glutamate⁻.[5,10] To further elucidate the mechanism for this modest selectivity, we performed conductance and permeability ratio experiments on the rCx43 channel using the alkali metal cations and the tetraalkylammonium organic cations.[23] The monovalent cationic g_j and permeability ratios were in close agreement both in magnitude of the ratios and order of the selectivity sequence. For the alkali cations, the equilibrium selectivity sequence was $Rb^+ \geq Cs^+ > K^+ > Na^+ \geq Li^+ > TMA^+ > TEA^+$. This corresponded to a series II sequence and was not indicative of a high affinity cation binding site within the pore. The most significant deviation from the aqueous mobility sequence occurred with Li^+, whose aqueous mobility in bulk solution is lower than that of Na^+ and TMA^+. This discrepancy in the ionic g_j ratios was modeled using the Levitt approximation for the relative reduction (D_x) in the aqueous diffusion coeffient (D_o) based on frictional drag of water molecules associated with the permeant ion within a pore of limited diameter.[25] This effect was expected to be most pronounced for Li^+ since it is the most hydrated ion whereas TMA^+ and TEA^+ are the least hydrated. These results could readily be explained by a limiting diameter of 6.3 ± 0.4 Å (Figure 3) and a weak anionic site within the pore. More importantly, a direct measure of the cation:anion permeability ratio was obtained using an asymmetric LiCl salt gradient using impermeant sugars (e.g. raffinose) to maintain osmotic balance between the two cells.[23] Surprisingly, this yielded a P_{Cl}/P_K value of 0.13, or a cation:anion selectivity of $\approx$ 8:1. Hence, estimation of relative permeabilities based on aqueous diffusion theory appears to underestimate the selectivity of the rCx43 channel. This could be true if stronger ion-site and cation-anion interactions are occurring within the pore (i.e. ionic independence principal is violated).

Even more surprising were the relative anionic permeability measurements. Asymmetric KCl:Kanion equilibrium reversal potential experiments produced anionic reversal potentials of the same magnitude as those observed for the monovalent cations. This is not expected, according to the GHK voltage equation, if the anionic flux is less than 1/8th that of K^+. The anionic reversal potential and permeability ratios are listed in Table 1.

Table 1.   Cx43 Relative Anion Reversal Potentials and Permeability Coefficients

Ion	N	Mean E_{rev} (mV)	Measured E_{rev} (mV)	P_{ion}	Calculated E_{rev} (mV)	g_j Ratio
Br-	4	-0.9±1.2	-1.5	1.08	-1.5	1.08
Cl-	--	------	-----	1.00	-----	1.00
Acetate-	4	+3.8±0.5	+3.6	0.85	+3.6	0.79
glutamate-	3	+13.2±0.5	+13.1	0.52	+13.1	0.63

N = number of cell pairs.

Mean E_{rev} = statistical mean from N experiments ± s.d.

Measured E_{rev} = value obtained from pooled data from N experiments.

Calculated E_{rev} = value from modified GHK voltage equation.

g_j ratio = unitary channel conductance ratios obtained using symmetrical solutions.

Calculation of the relative P_{anion}/P_{Cl} permeability ratios, while taking into account all of the permeant ions and their relative permeability coefficients, required dividing all of the cationic concentration terms by 135 mM, which is equivalent to the total cation concentration of the IPS. The exact equation used was:

where 1 = cell 1, 2 = cell 2, Y = substitute anion, PK = 1.35, P_{Na} = 1.05, P_{Cs} = 1.53, and P_{TEA} = 0.43 (relative to P_{Li} = 1.0).[23] Although emperically derived for the ionic conditions used on the rCx43 channel, this equation is analogous to the one derived by Borisova et al. where L_{ac} = 1 and P_{Cl} and P_Y are multiplied by $([K^+] + [Na^+] + [Cs^+] + [TEA^+] = 135)$.[16] Hence, our solution to the anionic reversal potential measurements requires the same assumption made by Borisova et al. for the amphotericin B channel except that the it is the anion which must pair with one bound cation at the site in order to permeate through the rCx43 pore. This hypothesis for cation:anion selective permeability in the Cx43 channel can be examined experimentally and efforts are underway to distinguish between this model and the other two alternative models for cation:anion permeability.

The rCx43 gj was observed to increase nonlinearly when increasing KCl from 115 mM to 140 mM in subsequent experiments. Based on the above hypothesis of a cation-binding site within the pore, g_j was determined for varying KCl concentrations in the absence of other monovalent cations. The results are summarized graphically in Figure 4 and, although saturating concentrations of KCl were not achieved, extrapolation of the data from the theoretical fit provided by the Hill equation estimates a saturating KCl g_j of 253 pS and a half-maximal g_j concentration (K_d) of 143 mM. This is equivalent to the intracellular [K] in mammalian cells, consistent with the hypothesis that K^+ ions are largely responsible for the electrical coupling between mammalian cells *in situ*.

4.3.2. Connexin40.

Similar experiments were performed on the rCx40 channel and revealed some quantitative differences between these two connexin channels.[24] Although the quantitative differences in the cation g_j and permeability ratios are small relative to rCx43 (series I sequence and P_{Cl}/P_K = 0.14), some notable differences were observed when using impermeant sugars for the asymmetric LiCl reversal potential experiments and the monovalent anion g_j and permeability experiments. Although raffinose produced similar results with both channels, mannitol produced the same result in the rCx40 channel, but not in the rCx43 channel. The reduction in g_j and the 115:30 mM LiCl reversal potential in the presence of mannitol with rCx43, but not rCx40, is consistent with mannitol being permeant through the rCx43 pore and impermeant through the rCx40 channel.[23,24] The concept that the rCx40 pore may be smaller than the rCx43 pore, despite the similarities illustrated in Figure 3, were further substantiated by the observed blocking effect of TBA$^+$ on the rCx40 channel.[24] Even more startling was the observation that the rCx40 g_j did not decrease when Cl$^-$ was replaced with less mobile anions. Furthermore, the asymmetric anion reversal potentials shifted in the opposite direction than expected, which prompted us to examine the effects of even more anions (e.g. aspartate$^-$, nitrate$^-$, F$^-$). Equilibrium reversal potentials for the monvalent cations and anions were determined using the conventional GHK equation provided that glutamate$^-$ was assumed to be more permeable than Cl$^-$. This contrast to the anion results on the rCx43 channel suggests a different mechanism for anion permeation. Again, by analogy to a previously examined model, we hypothesize that the rCx40 channel exhibits the ion-pair permeation scheme forwarded by Franciolini and Nonner.[17,18] The oppositely shifted reversal potentials and the lack of a change in g_j when less mobile anions were used are consistent with this hypothesis. If this is the case, then the anion permeabilities are the reciprocal of the values presented in Table V of Beblo and Veenstra.[24] These model-dependent values for $P_{glutamate}/P_{Cl}$ and $P_{nitrate}/P_{Cl}$ are 0.17 and 0.76 respectively. This hypothesis for cation:anion selective permeability of the rCx40 channel should also be examined experimentally and efforts are underway to distinguish between the three alternative models for cation:anion permeability. The permeability studies of the rCx40 and rCx43 channels are hampered by the lack of a known nonblocking impermeant cation and/or anion for the connexin channels to date.

The rCx40 gj - [KCl] was examined using the same methods employed to examine the rCx43 channel. The results are illustrated in Figure 4 and again indicate that g_j approaches saturation with increasing KCl concentrations in the absence of other monovalent cations. The theoretical fit provided by the Hill equation estimates a saturating KCl g_j of 233 pS and a half-maximal g_j concentration (K_d) of 127 mM. This is slightly lower than the equivalent to the intracellular [K] in mammalian cells, but still consistent with the hypothesis that K^+ ions are largely responsible for the electrical coupling between mammalian cells *in situ*.

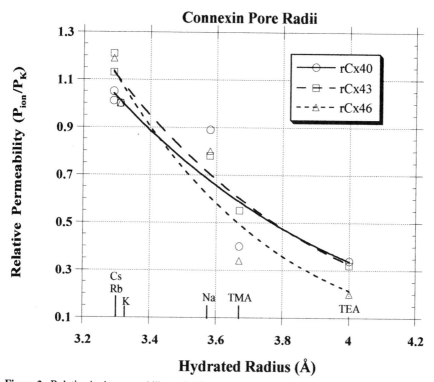

Figure 3. Relative ionic permeability ratios for rCx40, rCx43,and rCx46.[23,24,53] Curved lines are the theoretical fit of the permeability data by the hydrodynamic equation.[23,24,62] Estimates of pore radii in Å are: Cx40, 6.6±0.9; Cx43, 6.3±0.4, and Cx46, 5.5±0.6. Hydrated ionic radii as reported by Nightingale.[63]

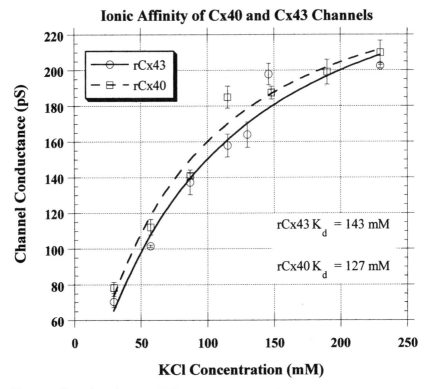

Figure 4. Channel conductance -KCl concentration curves for rCx40 and rCx43. The curved lines are the theoretical fits according to the Hill equation with a Hill coefficient of 1.14 and 1.11, K_d of 127 and 143 mM, and limiting conductance of 233 and 253 pS for rCx40 and rCx40 respectively. Data points are mean ± s.d. of two to six experiments. All conductances were determined from the slope of a single channel current-voltage relationship (Wang and Veenstra, unpublished results).

5. Future Directions

It is apparent from existing permeability theory from channel that are permeable to both cations and anions that simple aqueous diffusion models do not reflect the real situation. Even in large diameter pores, ionic permeabilities are not predicted by constant field (GHK) theory. In channels of diameters approximating a single KCl ion pair ($\approx 7\text{Å}$), complex cation-anion interactions occur within the pore. Connexin pore diameters estimated from ionic permeability ratios are indicative of 11 - 13 Å diameters, or only about 2 to 3 water molecules in addition to the passing ions. Preliminary comparisons to other cation:anion channels are consistent with cation-dependent anion permeabilities, indicative of specific cation-anion interactions occurring within the connexin pores. The cation:anion selectivity of the rat Cx40, Cx43, and Cx46 channels are ≈ 10:1. What remains is to determine the exact mechanisms for cation and anion permeation through connexin pores and identify the pore forming domains and specific residues involved in these interactions.

REFERENCES

1. Loewenstein, WR. Junctional intercellular communication: the cell-to-cell membrane channel. Physiol Rev 1981; 61:829-913.
2. Bruzzone R, White TW, and Goodenough, DA. The cellular internet: on-line with connexins. Bioessays 1996;18:709-718.
3. Willecke K and Haubrich, S. Connexin expression systems: To what extent do they reflect the situation in the animal? J Bioener Biomembr 1996;28:319-326.
4. White TW and Bruzzone R. Multiple connexin proteins in single intercellular channels: Connexin compatibility and functional consequences. J Bioener Biomembr 1996;28:339-350.
5. Veenstra RD, Wang H-Z, Beblo DA, Chilton MG, Harris AL, Beyer EC, and Brink PR. Selectivity of connexin-specific gap junctions does not correlate with channel conductance. Circ Res 1995;77:1156-1165.
6. Flagg-Newton J, Simpson I, and Loewenstein WR. Permeability of the cell-to-cell membrane channels in mammalian cell junction. Science 1979;205:404-407.
7. Brink PR and Dewey MM. Evidence for fixed charge in the nexus. Nature 1980;285:101-102.
8. Brink PR. Gap junction channels and cell-to-cell messengers in myocardium. J Cardiovasc Electrophysiol 1991;2:360-366.
9. Hille B. Ionic Channels of Excitable Membranes, 2nd edition, Sunderland, MA, Sinauer Associates Inc., 1992, 607 pp.
10. Veenstra RD. Size and selectivity of gap junction channels formed from different connexins. J Bioener Biomembr 1996;28:327-337.
11. Diamond JM and Wright EM. Biological membranes: the physical basis of ion and nonelectrolyte selectivity. Annu Rev Physiol 1969;31:581-646.
12. Eisenman G and Horn R. Ionic selectivity revisited: The role of kinetic and equilibrium processes in ion permeation through ion channels. J Membr Biol 1983;76:197-225.

13. Robinson RA and Stokes RH. Electrolyte Solutions, 2nd edition, London, UK, Butterworths, 1965, 571 pp.

14. Jenny H. Studies on the mechanism of ionic exchange in colloidal aluminum silicates. J Physiol Chem 1932;36:2217-2258.

15. Bungenberg de Jong HG, in Kruyt HR (ed.): Colloid Science, II, New York, NY, Elsevier, 1949, pp. 259-334.

16. Borisova MP, Brutyan RA, Ermishkin LN. Mechanism of anion-cation selectivity of amphotericin B channels. J Membr Biol 1986;90:13-20.

17. Franciolini F and Nonner W. Anion-cation interactions in the pore of neuronal background chloride channels. J Gen Physiol 1994a;104:711-723.

18. Franciolini F and Nonner W. A multi-ion mechanism in neuronal background chloride channels. J Gen Physiol 1994b;104:725-746.

19. Zambrowicz EB and Colombini M. Zero-current potentials in a large membrane channel: A simple theory accounts for complex behavior. Biophys J 1993;65:1093-1100.

20. Tomaselli GF, Backx PH, Marban E. Molecular basis of ion permeation in voltage-gated ion channels. Circ Res 1993;72:491-496.

21. Galzi J-L, Devillers-Thiery A, Hussy N, Bertrand S, Changeux J-P, and Bertrand D. Mutations in the channel domain of a neuronal nicotinic receptor convert ion selectivity from cationic to anionic. Nature 1992;359:500-505.

22. Ellinor PT, Yang J, Sather WA, Zhang J-F, and Tsien RW. Ca^{2+} channel selectivity at a single locus for high-affinity Ca^{2+} interactions. Neuron 1995;15:1121-1132.

23. Wang H-Z and Veenstra RD. Monovalent ion selectivity sequences of the rat connexin43 gap junction channel. J Gen Physiol 1997;109:491-507.

24. Beblo DA and Veenstra RD. Monovalent cation permeation through the connexin40 gap junction channel. Cs, Rb, K, Na, Li, TEA, TMA, TBA, and effects of anions Br, Cl, F, acetate, aspartate, glutamate, and NO_3. J Gen Physiol 1997;109:509-522.

25. Levitt DG. General continuum theory for multiion channel. II. Application to acetylcholine channel. Biophys J 1991;59:278-288.

26. Hess P, Lansman JB, and Tsien RW. Calcium channel selectivity sequence for divalent and monovalent cations. Voltage and concentration dependence of single channel current in ventricular heart cells. J Gen Physiol 1986;88:293-319.

27. Hille B. Potassium channels in myelinated nerve. Selective permeability to small cations. J Gen Physiol 1973;61:669-686.

28. Hamill OP, Marty A, Neher E, Sakmann B, and Sigworth FJ. Improved patch-clamp techniques for high-resolution current recording from cells and cell-free membrane patches. Pflügers Arch - Eur J Physiol 1981;391:85-100.

29. Mishina M, Tobimatsu T, Imoto K, Tanaka K-i, Fujita Y, Fukuda K, Kurasaki M, Takahashi H, Morimoto Y, Hirose T, Inayama S, Takahashi T, Kuno M, and Numa S. Location of functional regions of acetylcholine receptor a-subunit by site-directed mutagenesis. Nature 1985;313:364-369.

30. Stühmer W, Methfessel C, Sakmann B, Noda M, and Numa S. Patch clamp characterization of sodium channels expressed from rat brain cDNA. Eur Biophys J 1987;14:131-138.
31. Miller C. Voltage-gated cation conductance channel from fragmented sarcoplasmic reticulum. Steady-state electrical properties. J Membr Biol 1978;40:1-23.
32. Neyton J and Trautmann A. Single channel currents of an intercellular junction. Nature 1985;317:331-335.
33. Veenstra RD and DeHaan RL. Measurement of single channel currents from cardiac gap junctions. Science 1986;233:972-974.
34. Veenstra RD and Brink PR. Patch clamp analysis of gap junctional currents, in Stevenson B, Paul DL, Gallin W (Ed.): Cell-Cell Interactions: A Practical Approach , Oxford, UK, IRL Press, 1992, pp. 167-201.
35. Brink PR and Fan S-F. Patch clamp recordings from membranes which contain gap junction channels. Biophys J 1989;56:579-593.
36. Imanaga I, Kameyama M, and Irisawa H. Cell-to-cell diffusion of fluorescent dyes in paired ventricular cells. Am J Physiol 1987;252:H223-H232.
37. Brink PR and Ramanan SV. A model for the diffusion of fluorescent probes in the septate giant axon of earthworm. Biophys J 1985;48:299-309.
38. Safranyos RGA, Caveney S, Miller JG, and Petersen NO. Relative roles of gap junction channels and cytoplasm in cell-to-cell diffusion of fluorescent tracers. Proc Natl Acad Sci USA 1987;84:2272-2276.
39. Tsien RW and Weingart R. Inotropic effect of cAMP in calf ventricular muscle studied by a cut end method. J Physiol 1976;260:117-141.
40. Saez JC, Conner JA, Spray DC, Bennett MVL. Hepatocyte gap junctions are permeable to the second messenger, inositol 1,4,5-trisphosphate and to calcium ions. Proc Natl Acad Sci USA 1989;86:2708-2712.
41. Sanderson MJ. Intercellular calcium waves mediated by inositol trisphosphate. Ciba Found Symp 1995;188:175-194.
42. DeMello WC. Further studies on the influence of cAMP-dependent protein kinase on junctional conductance in isolated heart cell pairs. J Molec Cell Cardiol 1991;23:371-379.
43. Veenstra RD. Physiological modulation of cardiac gap junction channels. J Cardiovasc Electrophysiol 1991;2:168-189.
44. Guthrie SC and Gilula NB. Gap junctional communication and development. Trends Neurosci 1989;12:12-16.
45. Swenson KI, Piwnica-Worms H, McNamee H, and Paul DL. Tyrosine phosphorylation of the gap junction protein connexin43 is required for the pp60vsrc-induced inhibition of communication. Cell Regulation 1990;1:989-1002.
46. Réaume AG de Sousa PA, Kulkarni S, Langille BL, Zhu D, Davies TC, Juneja SC, Kidder GM, and Rossant J. Cardiac malformation in mice lacking connexin43. Science 1995;267:1831-1834.

47. Hobbie L, Kingsley DM, Kozarsky, KF, Jackman RW, Krieger M. Restoration of LDL receptor activity in mutant cells by intercellular junctional communication. Science 1989;235:69-73.

48. Paul DL. Molecular cloning of cDNA for rat liver gap junction protein. J Cell Biol 1986;103:123-134.

49. Dahl G, Miller T, Paul D, Voellmy R, Werner R. Expression of functional cell-cell channels from cloned rat liver gap junction complementary cDNA. Science 1987;236:1290-1293.

50. Eghbali B, Kessler JA, Spray DC. Expression of gap junction channels in communication-incompetent cells after stable transfection with cDNA encoding connexin32. Proc Natl Acad Sci USA 1990;87:1328-1331.

51. Veenstra RD, Wang H-Z, Westphale EM, and Beyer EC. Multiple connexins confer distinct regulatory and conductance properties of gap junctions in developing heart. Circ Res 1992;75:1277-1283.

52. Elfgang C, Eckert R, Lichtenberg-Frate H, Butterweck A, Traub O, Klein RA, Hülser D, and Willecke K. Specific permeability and selective formation of gap junction channels in connexin-transfected HeLa cells. J Cell Biol 1995;129:805-817

53. Trexler EB, Bennett MVL, Bargiello TA, and Verselis VK. Voltage gating and permeation in a gap junction hemichannel. Proc Natl Acad Sci USA 1996;93:5836-5841.

54. Barrio LC, Suchyna T, Bargiello TA, Xu LX, Roginski R, Bennett MVL, Nicholson B. Gap junctions formed by connexin 26 and 32 alone and in combination are differently affected by applied voltage. Proc Natl Acad Sci USA 1991;88:8410-8414.

55. Bukauskas FF, Elfgang C, Willecke K, Weingart R. Heterotypic gap junction channels (connexin26-connexin32) violate the paradigm of unitary conductance. Pflügers Arch - Eur J Physiol 1995;429:870-872.

56. Verselis VK, Ginter CS, Bargiello TA Opposite voltage gating polarities of two closely related connexins. Nature 1994;368:348-351.

57. Suchyna T, Xu LX, Gao F, Fourtner CR, and Nicholson BJ. Identification of a proline residue as a transduction element involved in voltage gating of gap junction channels. Nature 1993;365:847-849.

58. Matthews BW and Weaver LH. Binding of lanthanide ions to thermolysin. Biochemistry 1974;13:1719-1725.

59. Stampe P and Begenisich T. Unidirectional K^+ fluxes through recombinant Shaker potassium channels expressed in single Xenopus oocytes. J Gen Physiol 1996;107:49-457.

60. Franciolini F and Nonner W. Anion and cation permeability of a chloride channel in rat hippocampal neurons. J Gen Physiol 1987;90:453-478.

61. Gros DB and Jongsma HJ. Connexins in mammalian heart. Bioessays 1996;18:719-730.

62. Dwyer TM, Adams DJ, and Hille B.. The permeability of the endplate channel to orgainc cations in frog muscle. J Gen Physiol 1980;75:469-492.
63. Nightingale ER. Phenomenological theory of ion solvation. Effective radii of hydrated ions. J Phys Chem 1959;63:1381-1387.

5 ON THE CONTROL OF JUNCTIONAL CONDUCTANCE

Walmor C. De Mello

Department of Pharmacology, Medical Sciences Campus, UPR

1. Calcium, junctional conductance and the healing-over process

The idea that the junctional conductance might be modulated was verified in the 1970's (1, 2). It is known since Engelmann (3) that "the death of a cardiac cell does not result in the death of the apposing cells" ("der Tod schreitet nicht von Zelle auf Zelle for"). This important conclusion was based on the observation that the injury potential induced by lesion of cardiac muscle soon vanishes (healing-over) - a phenomenon that was not related to the depolarization of the surface cell membrane because a new lesion applied near the previous one re-established the injury potential (8).

A reasonable explanation for the healing-over process is that an ionic barrier is formed at the site of lesion. Weidmann (4) showed that under normal conditions there is a low resistant pathway between heart cells. The possibility that a new surface cell membrane is quickly established sealing the damaged area received a serious consideration based on the studies of Heilbrunn (5). The fact that healing-over does not occur in skeletal muscle fibers in which the fibers are not communicated through gap junctions ruled out the possibility that the healing-over process is due to a process of reconstitution of the surface cell membrane - a phenomenon seen in damaged skeletal muscle fibers (6). It is interesting to mention that in these muscle fibers exposed to isotonic Ca solution the surface cell membrane becomes liquid and a damage is quickly followed by sealing (6).

A change in ionic concentration at the level of gap junctions located near the lesion might lead to an appreciable increase in junctional resistance and the promotion of healing-over (7, 8). A good candidate was Ca because the ion is required for the healing-over (7, 9) while other ions like Ba had no influence on the process (8). Moreover, the rate of sealing is enhanced in stimulated ventricular muscle (10) - a finding that might be related to the increase in intracellular Ca elicited by the action potential.

In order to test the hypothesis that the healing-over is related to an increase in gap junctional resistance, Ca ions were injected electrophoretically inside a normal heart myocyte and the electrical coupling was measured. The results indicated that an increase in Cai lead to a gradual and reversible decrease of cell coupling (1). The mechanism by which Ca increases the junctional resistance is not known. As discussed previously (11) Ca ions can trigger enzyme reactions closing the channels through a conformational change of the junctional proteins or the ion can bind to negative polar groups of phospholipids and suppress the permeability of the intercellular channels. This idea is supported by the finding that a stronger charged cation like lanthanum when injected intracellularly is more effective than calcium in suppressing the electrical coupling in heart cells (12). These findings had an important implication for heart physiology and pathology because the severe impairment of impulse propagation seen during myocardial ischemia is in great part related to the suppression of cell coupling (13).

The question whether Ca is a physiological modulator of gj has been highly discussed. The finding of Noma and Tsuboi (14) that intracellular dialysis of very small amount of Ca (0.2 uM) causes cell decoupling in mammalian myocardial cells certainly speaks in favor of the idea that the ion can play a role in the modulation of gj under normal conditions (15). Calmodulin seems to play an important role in the Ca-mediated regulation of gj in adult guinea-pig ventricular cells (16) confirming previous findings (17).

2. Protons and the control of gj

Since the work of Turin and Warner (18) it is known that a fall in pHi can elicit a decline in gj. When H ions are injected electrophoretically inside heart cells the electrical coupling is abolished within seconds (19).

The healing-over process can be promoted by protons in absence of Ca ions but only if the pH is reduced to 5.5 (20) (see Figs. 1 and 2). Clearly this is a pH that falls outside the pH range found in a living heart cell. The innefectiveness of pH shifts in the range of 6.5 to 6 on the healing-over process (which requires an appreciable increase in junctional resistance) is in agreement with cable analysis data obtained with Purkinje fibers (21) in which an increase of intracellular resistance of only 30% was found when the pHo was changed from 7.3 to 6.8.

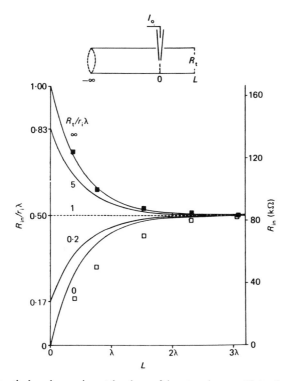

Figure 1. Theoretical and experimental values of input resistance (R_{in}) of a cable in the proximity of a cut end. Distance is normalized in terms of space constants. Theoretical lines are drawn for five ratio of terminal resistance (Rt) to characteristic resistance ($R/ri Å$) of the cable, the ratios being ∞, 5, 1, 0.2 and 0. Experimental values obtained with canine Purkinje fibers are plotted in the same graph. Filled squares indicate healing-over in Ca-containing Tyrode solution; open squares suggest a short circuit at x = 0 in Ca-free solution. From reference 20, with permission.

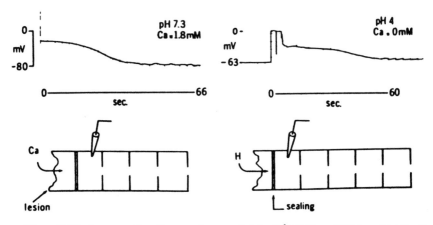

Figure 2. Healing over of cardiac muscle promoted by Ca^{2+} (left) and H^+ ions (right). From reference 59, with permission.

There is information that the sensitivity of gj to acidity is modulated by Ca ions (22). The studies of Noma and Tsuboi (14) indicated that the gap junctions in guinea pig heart have different receptor sites for protons and divalent ions and that intracellular acidity results in a smaller sensitivity of the gap junctions to Ca. These authors interpreted this finding as a competition between H ions and Ca ion for the Ca-receptor site. An interaction between Ca ions and protons on the healing-over process was also found in canine Purkinje fibers. As shown in Table 1 at pHo 7.3 the rate of sealing (mV/s) was proportional to the extracellular calcium concentration. At pHo 6, however, the influence of Ca on the sealing process was smaller for all the concentrations of Ca_o used (23). These findings are in agreement with those of Noma and Tsuboi (14) described above.

TABLE 1
Effect of pH$_o$ on the influence of {Ca^{2+}}$_o$ on the rate of sealing of canine Purkinje fibers

{Ca^{2+}}$_o$	Rate of sealing (mV/s)		
	pH$_o$-7.3		pH$_o$-6
0.4 mM	7.5		1.93
	6.3		-
	6.7		1.80
	9.1		5
	3.2		1.82
	3.6		-
	7		1.5
Mean ± SE of the mean	6.1 ± 0.96	P<0.05	2.4 ± 0.65
0.7 mM	8.4		2.5
	7.7		-
	15.5		8
	6.4		3.2
	9.1		5
Mean ± SE of the mean	9.4 ± 1.56	P<0.05	4.6 ± 1.22
1.3 mM	15		6.8
	18		11.5
	10		6.3
	19		13.1
	25		10
Mean ± SE of the mean	17.4 ± 2.46	P<0.05	9.4 ± 1.32

Recently, studies on the sensitivity of cardiac gap junction proteins connexin43 and connexin45 are more sensitivity to pH than channels built with connexin 43 (24). According to these findings it is possible to conclude that the discrepant results concerning the influence of pH on gj in different preparations might be related to the type of connexin involved (see also 15). The decline in microscopic conductance found at low pHi is related to a decrease in open probability of the channels (24).

3. Na/Ca exchange and metabolic inhibitors alters the electrical coupling

Other observations (58) seems to indicate that lowered pHi uncouples gap junction by a Ca-calmodulin-mediated mechanism.. Furthermore, intramolecular interactions might mediate pH regulation of connexin 43 channels (58).

It is known that the extrusion of Ca from the cytosol of cardiac cells depends on the energy provided by the sodium concentration gradient (25) and that the inward movement of Ca is extremely sensitive to increments in the intracellular sodium concentration. When sodium ions are intophoretically injected into normal heart cells the input resistance is increased and the electrical coupling is abolished (26, 27). Inasmuch, as sodium injection does not produce cell uncoupling in cardiac fibers exposed to Ca-free solution it is assumed that the increment in intracellular sodium concentration activates a Na/Ca exchange with consequent increment of intracellular free-Ca (27). The major implication of this observation is that the inhibition of the sodium pump leads to increase in the intracellular sodium and cell decoupling through the activation of the Na/Ca exchange. Drugs like ouabain that inhibit the sodium pump increases the intracellular resistance (28) and causes cell decoupling (27). Metabolic inhibition or myocardial ischemia can cause cell uncoupling by the elevation of intracellular sodium and calcium or through a drastic decrease of intracellular pH (13). The exposure of normal heart fibers to 2-4-dinitrophenol lead to cell uncoupling-an effect associated with the increment in free Ca because the resting tension is increased (29). The possible role of intracellular acidosis on the decoupling action of dinitrophenol, however, cannot be discarded. It is clear from these observations that the synthesis of ATP is essential for the preservation of low resistance pathways between the cytosol of apposing heart cells.

4. Autonomic regulation of junctional conductance

4.1 Influence of beta-adrenergic receptor activation on gj

Initial studies indicated that epinephrine and theophylline that increment the intracellular cAMP concentration in heart muscle, increases the electrical coupling (30). More direct evidence that cAMP influences gj was found with experiments involving the injection of the nucleotide into the cytosol. In these experiments an increase in electrical coupling of 42% was seen within 30 sec (31). An increase in coupling due to a rise in surface cell membrane resistance is discarded because the input resistance and time constant of the injected cell are slightly reduced. In rat heart cell pairs isoproterenol increase gj within 20 sec. (see Fig. 3). A similar increase in gj was found with isobutyl-methylxanthine-a phosphodiesterase inhibitor (32) as well as with the intracellular dialysis of the catalytic subunit of the cAMP-dependent protein kinase (33). When a cAMP-dependent protein kinase inhibitor was dialyzed into the cell the influence of isoproterenol on gj was totally suppressed (34) (Fig. 4). It is noteworthy that the inhibitor alone reduces gj by 18% what suggests that the junctional proteins are submitted to a phosphorylation tonus - a phenomenon that could be important for the preservation of the physiological characteristics of the gap junctions. The dialysis of the catalytic subunit of protein kinase A into one cell of the pair increased gj and generated rectification of junctional membrane supporting the notion that the absence of rectification depends, in part, on the symmetric phosphorylation of the two hemichannels (33).

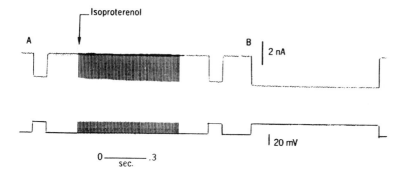

Figure 3. Effect of isoproterenol (10^{-6}M) on gj of ventricular cell pair isolated from normal adult rat heart. Top trace I_2, bottom trace V_1. From reference 32, with permission.

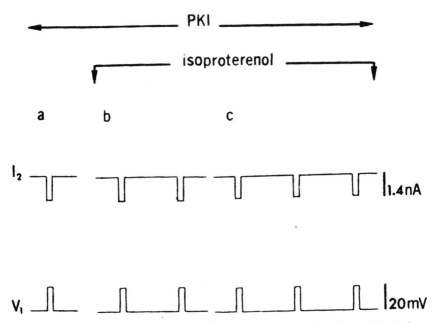

Figure 4. Lack of action of isoproterenol (10^{-6}M) on gj when an inhibitor of PKA (20 ug/ml) was added to internal solution. A - control; B - recorded 1 1/2 min after administration of isoproterenol; C-3 min later. Pulse duration - 100 ms. From reference 34, with permission.

The major conclusion drawn from these findings is that the activation of beta-adrenergic receptors results in the formation of cAMP, activation of PKA and consequent phosphorylation of gap junction proteins which leads to the increment in gj (34, 35).

The phosphorylation hypothesis (31, 36, 37) has been supported by recent studies made on cells transformed by the src oncogene of the Rous sarcoma virus. The results indicated that the decrease in gap junctional communication was elicited by a pp60src-mediated tyrosine phosphorylation of connexin43 (38). The presence of phosphotyrosine on connexin43 is then associated with down regulation of junctional communication. Other studies indicated that connexin 43 serine phosphorylation is also involved in the regulation of gj (see for review 57).

The phosphorylation seems to influence the kinetics but not the steady-state behavior of the gap junction channels (39). According to Burt (40) cell decoupling induced by halothane and acidosis before and after cAMP treatment does not cause any alteration of the single channels conductance what suggests that cAMP does not increase gj by incrementing the single channel conductance.

In intact rat papillary muscle cAMP reduces while high calcium solution (6 mM) increases the intracellular resistance (ri) (41). As it can be seen in Fig. 5 isoproterenol (10^{-5} M) caused an average decline of ri of 25% (SEM ± 2) (n=10) while the conduction velocity was appreciably increased. On the other hand, the exposure of the muscle to high Ca solution (6 mM) caused an increase in ri of 70% (SEM ± 15) (n=9) and the conduction velocity was significantly reduced. The fall in ri seen with forskolin (10^{-5} M) also supports the notion that cAMP is an important modulator of cell communication in intact cardiac muscle (41).

Studies of intercellular diffusion of Lucifer Yellow performed in isolated heart fibers also indicated that dibutyryl-cAMP enhances the diffusion coefficient from 4 x 10^{-7} cm2/s to 2 x 10^{-6} cm2/s (42) what means that the phosphorylation of junctional proteins augments the exchange of chemical signals between heart cells. Acetylcholine that increases the intracellular concentration of cGMP did not cause any change in the diffusion coefficient of Lucifer Yellow in dog trabeculae (42). In isolated heart cell pairs of neonatal rat heart, however, cGMP was seen to reduce gj (43). Recently, similar experiments performed on isolated cell pairs from cardiomyopathic hamsters indicated that dibutyryl-cGMP decreases gj within 30 sec (De Mello, unpublished). The reason for this discrepancy between intact and isolated cells is not known. The effect of cGMP on gj seems related to phosphorylation of junctional proteins with consequent increase in the relative frequency of lowest conductance state and a change in the kinetics of these channels (44).

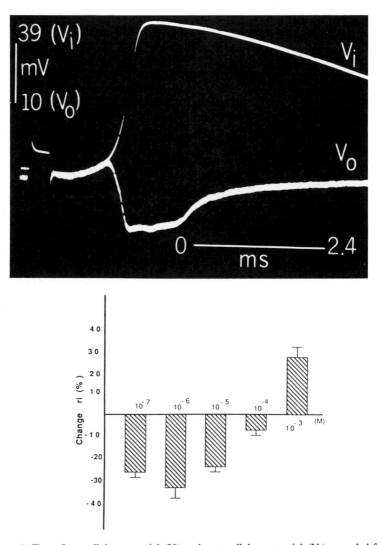

Figure 5. Top - Intracellular potential (V_i) and extracellular potential (V_o) recorded from a single rat trabecula. From reference 41, with permission. Bottom - Effect of different concentrations of isoproterenol on intracellular resistance (ri) keeping the extracellular calcium constant (2.7 mM). From reference 41, with permission.

Previous work of Flagg-Newton et al., (45) has shown that in some cell lines exposed to dibutyryl-cAMP for several hours there is an increased diffusion of fluorescent probes -a result that has been interpreted as an evidence that cAMP induces the synthesis of intercellular channels. In trabeculae isolated form the ventricle of dogs treated chronically with ephedrine (1 mg/Kg/day for a period of 2 weeks) the cAMP levels in heart cells is increased and the longitudinal diffusion of Lucifer Yellow is enhanced -an effect that was seen even after the elimination of the drug (46). These observations indicate that cAMP has long-term effects on cell communication in heart.

4.2 Interaction between Ca and cAMP

The interaction between cAMP and Ca ions is involved in different aspects of hormonal action. Its role on the regulation of junctional communication is demonstrated by the finding that the increase in electrical coupling caused by iontophoretic injection of cAMP in cardiac fibers is followed by a drastic decrease of coupling if the preparation is exposed to a high extracellular (6 mM) Ca concentration (47). The decline in intercellular coupling is due to a rise in Cai because the injection of EGTA into the same cell using a double barreled microelectrode reversed the decrease in electrical coupling. A feedback between Ca and cAMP occurs in part because an increase in Cai decreases the concentration of cAMP through the activation of phosphodiesterase or the inhibition of adenylcyclase. On the other hand, the elevation of intracellular levels of cAMP reduces Cai by enhancing the uptake of Ca ions by the sarcoplasmic reticulum. As mentioned above, measurements of intracellular resistance (ri) made on intact rat papillary muscle indicated that isoproterenol (10^{-5} M) or forskolin (10^{-5} M) reduced ri within 10 sec while high Ca solution (6 mM) incremented ri appreciably (41). Interestingly, in muscles exposed to high Ca solution the administration of isoproterenol to the bath increased ri further what indicates that an increase in Cai can counteract the effect of cAMP or ri.

The major conclusion of all these findings is that the activation of the beta-adrenergic receptor pathway in the heart leads to an increase in electrical synchronization of cardiac myocytes with consequent increment in conduction velocity and quick incorporation of the cells into the mechanical process. By activating simultaneously the processes involved in the control of heart rate, contractility and electrical synchronization the sympathetic nervous system plays a fundamental role on the response of the heart to different stimuli such as stress or exercise. The hormonal system and the intracellular communicating system are, therefore, integrated in the regulation of heart cell function.

4.3 On the influence of alpha-1 adrenergic receptor activation on gj

Recent studies performed on isolated cell pairs from the ventricle of adult rats (48) indicated that the activation of alpha-1 adrenergic receptors with phenylephrine (10^{-6} M) caused a significant reduction (45%; SE $\pm$ 3.4) (p<0.05) of junctional conductance (see Fig. 6). The effect of phenylephrine was abolished by prazosin (10^{-6} M) which is a selective blocking agent of alpha-1 adrenergic receptors (Fig. 7).

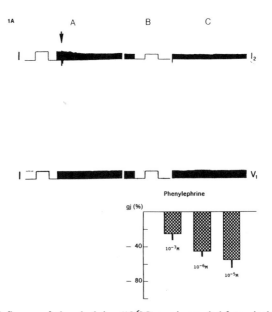

Figure 6. Top - Influence of phenylephrine (10^{-6}M) on gj recorded from single cell pair of rat ventricle. A - control; at arrow phenylephrine was added to the bath. B and C, after 2.5 and 3.5 min. I_2 junctional current (calibration 1.6 nA). V_1 - transjunctional voltage (calibration 40 mV). Bottom - dose - dependent effect of phenylephrine on gj. Each bar - average of 20 cell pairs. Vertical line - SEM; From reference 48, with permission.

Measurements of the time constant of cell membrane (tm) using the electrotonic potentials recorded from single cells under current clamp configuration, showed no significant changes in tm what indicates that a drop in surface cell membrane resistance is unlikely. It was also found that the effect of phenylephrine on gj was dependent on the formation of diacylglycerol and consequent activation of protein kinase C. Indeed, when the pseudo-substrate of the kinase (a potent inhibitor of protein kinase C) was dialyzed into the cell (20 ug/ml) for 4-5 min the effect of phenylephrine on gj was reduced by 95% (p<0.05) (48) (Fig. 7).

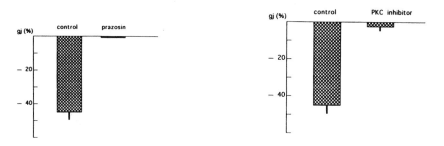

Figure 7. At left - suppression of the effect of phenylephrine (10⁻⁶M) (left bar) on gj caused by prazosin (10⁻⁶M). Bar - average from 15 cell pairs. Vertical line - SEM. At right - influence of the pseudosubstrate of PKC (20 ug/ml) (dialyzed into the cell) on the effect of phenylephrine. Each bar - average of 17 cell pairs. Vertical line - SEM. from reference 48, with permission.

In other experiments it was found that norepinephrine (10^{-6} M) increased gj by 56% (SE ± 5.3) within 15 sec. Since norepinephrine is an alpha-1 and beta-1-adrenergic receptor agonist it is important to know if the activation of both types of receptors are involved in the effect of norepinephrine. This problem was investigated by adding norepinephrine to the bath and as soon as the effect of the drug reached its maximal and steady level prazosin (10^{-6} M) - an alpha-adrenergic blocking agent, was administered to the bath solution containing norepinephrine. The results indicated that prazosin enhanced the effect of norepinephrine on gj by 29.6% (SEM ± 3.7) (p<0.05) within 15-20 sec. (Fig. 8). Similar results were found with epinephrine (10^{-6} M). Prazosin, by itself, had no effect on gj.

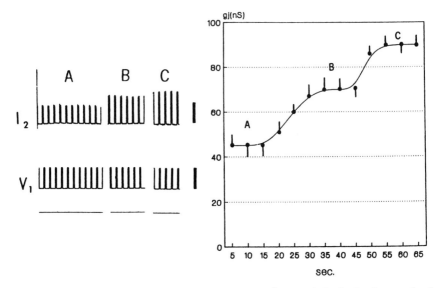

Figure 8. Left - A - control; B - effect of norephrine (10^{-6}M) on gj; C - further increase in gj caused by prazosin (10^{-6}M). I_2 calibration 1.3 nA; V_1 calibration 40 mV. Right - effect of norepinephrine on gj recorded from 12 cell pairs (A - control; B - norepinephrine (10^{-6}M) and C - norepinephrine plus prazosin (10^{-6}M). Vertical line at each point 1/2 SEM.   From reference 48, with permission.

These observations are a clear indication that the activation of alpha-1-adrenergic receptors in the rat ventricle causes a decline in junctional conductance and because the increment in gj elicited by norepinephrine and epinephrine was further enlarged by prazosin it is possible to conclude that the effect of beta-1 receptor activation on gj interacts with the alpha-receptor pathway.

A possible mechanism of interaction between the two receptor pathways is the antagonizing effect of alpha-receptor activation on the increment in cAMP levels caused by beta-adrenergic receptor activation (4, 50, 51). Two possible explanations have been proposed to explain the decline in cAMP levels produced by alpha-receptor agonists: a) inhibition of adenylcyclase or b) activation of phosphodiesterase (49,51). It is conceivable, however, that other mechanisms of interaction can be involved, particularly in the case of junctional communication.

It is known that two major types of receptors are involved in the transduction of information across the cell membrane: one are the receptors related with the cAMP pathway and the other is represented by inositol phospholipids and Ca mobilization. Protein kinase C, Ca mobilization, arachidonate release and cGMP formation are integrated in a single cascade (52). A possible interaction between alpha and beta receptor pathways is the inhibition and desensitization of adenylcyclase caused by protein kinase C as has been described in liver cells (52). No information is available if the same type of interaction occurs in cardiac cells.

There is evidence that phosphorylation of gap junction proteins caused by activation of protein kinase C promotes a decline of gj (53, 54). Since the effect of protein kinase C activation on gj is the opposite of that caused by activation of protein kinase A, it is conceivable that the interaction between the beta-1 and alpha-1 adrenergic receptor pathways occurs at different levels including that gap junction channels themselves.

The remaining question is related to the physiological meaning of these observations. Since both alpha-1 and beta-1 adrenergic receptor pathways are activated by norepinephrine it is conceivable that the activation of the alpha-adrenergic receptor pathway might represent a protective mechanism against excessive activation of the beta-1-adrenergic receptor pathway which is known to cause a remarkable increase in cardiac excitability. Based on these observations it is expected that changes in number of the two types of adrenergic receptors influences the effect of norepinephrine on gj. Certainly, further studies will be required to elucidate this point.

The physiological and pathological implications of these observations are not known. There is evidence that following myocardial ischemia and reperfusion in the cat there is increased ectopy that is prazosin dependent and possibly related to spare alpha-1 receptors (55). The possibility exists that the increased ectopy described under these conditions be related to slow conduction induced by the decline in gj -an appealing subject for future studies.

5. Lipophilic agents and junctional conductance

Lipophilic compounds of several types can decrease the junctional conductance in a reversible fashion. Octanol, heptanol, fatty acids and volatile anesthetics like halothane seems to interact with gap junction proteins at the lipid channel interface and alter the probability of channel opening because single channel conductance is not changed by these agents (40). Some fatty acids like decaoid acid causes cellular uncoupling without altering the cardiac cell excitability suggesting a specificity for the junctional channels (40). During ischemia free fatty acids and short-chain fatty acids accumulate in the cell membrane as a consequence of the effect of cellular lipases and lipid peroxidation -a finding that might be associated with a higher incidence of cardiac arrhythmias (40).

The fluidity of cholesterol-rich domain seems to be important for heart cell coupling (56). Indeed, the decline in gj elicited by heptanol seems related to a reduction of fluidity of the cholesterol-rich domains rather than to an increase in bulk membrane fluidity.

Acknowledgement: I want to thank the American Heart Association and NIH (HL-34148; 2S06GM-08224; RR03651) for support.

References

1. De Mello WC (1975). Effect of intracellular injection of calcium and strontium on cell communication in heart. J Physiol (London) 250:231-245.
2. Rose B and Loewenstein WR (1975). Calcium ion distribution in cytoplasm visualized by aequorin: diffusion in cytosol restricted by energized sequestering. Science, 190:1204-1206.
3. Engelmann TW (1877). Vergleichende Untersuchungen zur Lehre von der Muskel-und Nervenelektricitat. Pflüg Arch ges Physiol 15:116-148.
4. Weidmann S (1952). The electrical constants of Purkinje fibres. J Physiol (London) 118:348-360.
5. Heilbrunn LV. (1956). Dynamics of Living Protoplasm. (Heilbrum, LV, ed). Academic Press, New York.

6. De Mello WC (1973). Membrane sealing in frog skeletal-muscle fibers. Proc Natl Acad Sci, USA, 70:982-984.

7. De Mello WC, Motta G and Chapeau M (1969). A study on the healing-over of myocardial cells of toads. Circ Res 4:475-487.

8. De Mello WC (1972). The healing-over process in cardiac and other muscle fibers. In: Electrical Phenomena in the Heart, (De Mello, W. C. ed) pp 323-351, New York Academic Press.

9. Délèze J (1970). The recovery of resting potential and input resistance in sheep heart injured by knife or laser. J Physiol (London) 208:547-552.

10. De Mello WC and Dexter D (1970). Increased rate of sealing in beating heart muscle of the toad. Circ Res 26:481-489.

11. De Mello WC (1982). Cell-to-cell communication in heart and other tissues. Prog Biophys Molec Biol. 39:147-182.

12. De Mello WC (1979). Effect of intracellular injection of La^{3+} and Mn^{2+} on electrical coupling of heart cells. Cell Biol Int Rep 3:113-119.

13. De Mello WC (1985). Intercellular communication in cardiac muscle; physiological and pathologic implications. In: Cardiac Electrophysiology (Zipes D and Jalife J, eds) pp 65-72, Grume and Straton, Inc New York.

14. Noma A and Tsuboi N (1987). Dependence of junctional conductance on proton, calcium and magnesium ions in cardiac paired cells of guinea pig. J Physiol (London) 382:193-211.

15. Firek L and Weingart R (1995). Modification of junctional conductance by divalent cations and protons on neonatal rat heart cells. J Mol Cell Cardiol 27:1633-1643.

16. Toyama I, Sugiura H, Kmiya K, Kodamma I, Terasawa M, Hidaka H (1994). Ca^{2+} calmodulin mediated modulation of electrical coupling of ventricular myocytes from guinea-pig heart. J Mol Cell Cardiol 26:1006-1015.

17. Peracchia C (1988). The calmodulin hypothesis for gap junction regulation six years later. In: Gap Junctions (Hertzberg EL and Johnson RG, eds) pp 267-282. Alan R Liss, New York.

18. Turin L and Warner AE (1977). Carbon dioxide reversibly abolishes ionic communication between cells of early amphibian embryos. Nature 270:56-57.

19. De Mello WC (1980). Influence of intracellular injection of H^+ on the electrical coupling in cardiac Purkinje fibres. Cell Biol Int Rep 4:51-57.

20. De Mello WC (1983). The influence of pH on the healing-over of mammalian cardiac muscle. J Physiol (London) 339:299-307.

21. Reber W and Weingart R (1982). Ungulate cardiac Purkinje fibres: The influence of intracellular pH on the electrical cell-to-cell coupling. J Physiol (London) 328:87-104.

22. White RL, Verselis VK, Doeller J, Wittenberg BA and Bennett MVL (1987). Acid sensitivity of junctional conductance in pairs of ventricular myocytes is modulated by calcium ions. J Cell Biol 105:307a.

23. De Mello WC (1985). Healing-over of cardiac muscle: Interaction between protons and Ca ions. Biophys J 49:339a.

24. Hermans MM, Kontekaas P, Yongsma HJ and Rook MB (1995). pH sensitivity of the cardiac gap junction protein connexin 45 and 43. Pflugers Arch 431:138-140.

25. Reuter H and Seitz N (1968). The dependence of calcium efflux from cardiac muscle on temperature and external ion composition. J Physiol (London) 195:451-470.

26. De Mello, WC (1974). Electrical uncoupling in heart fibers produced by intracellular injection of Na or Ca. Fed Proc 17:3.

27. De Mello WC (1976). Influence of the sodium pump on intercellular communication in heart fibres: Effect of intracellular injection of sodium ion on electrical coupling. J Physiol (London) 263:171-197.

28. Weingart R (1977). The action of ouabain on intercellular coupling and conduction velocity in mammalian ventricular muscle. J Physiol (London) 264:341-365.

29. De Mello WC (1979). Effect of 2-4 dinitrophenol on intercellular communication in mammalian cardiac fibres. Pfluegers Arch 380:267-276.

30. Estapé E and De Mello WC (1982). Effect of theophylline on the spread of electrotonic activity in heart. Fed Proc 41:1505.

31. De Mello WC (1984). Effect of intracellular injection of cAMP on the electrical coupling of mammalian cardiac cells. Biochem Biophys Res Comm 119:1001-1007.

32. De Mello WC (1989). Effect of isoproterenol and 3-isobutyl-1-methylxanthine on junctional conductance in heart cell pairs. Biochim Biophys Acta, 1012:291-298.

33. De Mello WC (1991). Further studies on the influence of cAMP-dependent protein kinase on junctional conductance in isolated heart cell pairs. J Mol Cell Cardiol 23:371-379.

34. De Mello WC (1988). Increase in junctional conductance caused by isoproterenol in heart cell pair is suppressed by cAMP-dependent protein-kinase inhibitor. Bioch Biophys Res Comm 154, 2:509-514.

35. De Mello WC (1990). Cyclic AMP and junctional communication viewed through -a multi-biophysical approach. In: Biophysics of Gap Junction Channels (C Peracchia, ed) CRC Press, ppp 230-238,, Boca Raton, Fl.

36. De Mello WC (1983). The role of cAMP and Ca on the modulation of junctional conductance: An integrated hypothesis. Cell Biol Int Rep 7:1033-1040.

37. Saez JC, Spray DC, Nairn AC, Herzberg E, Greengard P, Bennett MVL (1986). cAMP increases junctional conductance and stimulates phosphorylation of the 27 KDa principal gap junction peptide. Proc Natl acad Sci, USA, 83:2473-2477.

38. Loo LW, Berestecky JM, Kanemitsu MY and Lau AF (1995). pp60SRC-mediated phosphorylation of connexin 43 -a gap junction protein. J Biol Chem 270:12751-12756.

39. Spray DC, Moreno AP and Campos de Carvalho AP (1993). Biophysical properties of the human cardiac gap junction channels. Braz J Med Biol Res 26:541-552.

40. Burt J (1990). Modulation of cardiac gap junction channel activity by the membrane lipid environment. In: Biophysics of Gap Junction Channels (C Peracchia, ed) pp 76-90, CRC, Boca Raton, Fl.

41. Xiao RP and De Mello WC (1991). Intracellular resistance in rat papillary muscle; interaction between cyclic AMP and calcium J Cardiovasc Pharmacol 17:754-760.

42. De Mello WC and van Loon P (1987b). Further studies on the influence of cyclic nucleotides on junctional permeability in heart. J Mol Cell Cardiol 19:763-771.

43. Burt JM and Spray DC (1988). Inotropic agents modulate gap junction conductance between cardiac myocytes. Am J Physiol 254:H1206-H1210.

44. Kwak BR, Saez JC, Wilders R, Chanson M, Fishman GI, Hertzberg E, Spray DC and Yongsma HJ (1995). Cyclic GMP modulates phosphorylation of rat Cx43 but not human. Pflugers Arch 430:770-778.

45. Flagg-Newton JL, Dahl G and Loewenstein WR (1981). Cell junctions and cyclic AMP: Upregulation of junctional membrane permeability and junctional membrane particles by administration of cyclic nucleotide or phosphodiesterase inhibitor. J Membr Biol 63:105-121.

46. De Mello WC (1988). Cyclic nucleotides and gap junctional permeability. Brazilian J Med Biol 21:1225.

47. De Mello WC (1986). Interaction of cAMP and Ca in the control of electrical coupling in heart fibers. Biochim Biophys Acta 888:91-99.

48. De Mello WC (1997). Influence of alpha-adrenergic-receptor activation on junctional conductance in heart cells; interaction with beta-adrenergic agonists. J Cardiovasc Pharmacol 29:273-277.

49. Watanabe A, Hathaway DR and Besch HR, Jr. (1974). Alpha-adrenergic reduction of cyclic adenosine monophosphate concentrations in rat myocardium. Circ Res 40:596-602.

50. Berridge MJ (1988). Inositol triphosphate and diacylglycerol; two interacting second messengers. Ann Rev Biochem 56:159-193.

51. Buxton ILO and Brunton LL (1985). Action of alpha-1-adrenergic receptor: activation of cyclic AMP degradation. J Biol Chem 260:6733-6737.

52. Nishizuka Y (1984). Turnover of inositol phospholipids and signal transduction. Science, 225:1365-1370.

53. Takeda A, Hashimoto E, Yamamura H, and Shimazu I (1987). Phosphorylation of liver gap junction protein by protein kinase C. FEBS Lett 210:169-172.

54. Münster PN and Weingart R (1993). Effect of phorbol ester on gap junctions of neonatal rat heart cells. Pflugers Arch 423:181-188.

55. Corr PB Shayman JA, Kramer JB et al (1981). Increased alpha-adrenergic receptors in ischemic cat myocardium. A potential mediator of electrophysiological derangements. J Clin Invest 67:1232-1236.

56. Bastiaanse EM, Jongsma HJ, van-der-Laarse A, Takens A and Kwak BRC (1993). Heptanol- induced decrease in cardiac gap junction conductance is mediated by a decrease in the fluidity of membraneous-cholesterol rich domains. J Membr Biol 136:135-145.

57. Beyer EC (1993). Gap junctions. Intern Rev Cytology, 137C:1-34.

58. Peracchia C, Wang X and Peracchia LL (1966). Inhibition of calmodulin expression prevents low pH - induced gap junction uncoupling in Xenopus oocytes. Pflüegers Arch 431: 379-387.

59. De Mello WC (1984). Modulation of junctional permeability. Fed. Proc 43:2692-2696.

6 GAP JUNCTIONS AND THE SPREAD OF ELECTRICAL EXCITATION

Robin Shaw and Yoram Rudy

Cardiac Bioelectricity Research and Training Center,
Department of Biomedical Engineering
Case Western Reserve University, Cleveland, Ohio

1. Introduction

Historically, cardiac electrical activity has been separated into "passive" and "active" components; the passive component has included the membrane capacitance and tissue resistivity, and the active component has been defined in terms of the non-linear membrane ionic currents. We are now learning that there is little functional separation between passive and active components. Ionic currents (the "active component) are important in every phase of the cardiac action potential, from peak excitation to rest [1, 2]. Cardiac structural properties (a contributor to the "passive component) can be highly variable during action potential propagation, changing with fiber orientation[3, 4], non-myocyte inhomogeneities[5], and disease state[6-9]. Cardiac structure may also indirectly modulate the membrane ionic currents[10, 11], altering their function during action potential generation and propagation.

As an alternative to an active/passive distinction, cardiac electrical function may be separated into membrane and structural factors. Membrane factors encompass all aspects of membrane electrical function including membrane capacitance, membrane resistance, and ionic currents. Most basic research in cardiac electrophysiology is presently focused on determining the structure, kinetics, regulation and subtypes of membrane ionic channels. This focus is warranted because membrane factors are responsible for action potential generation and its beat-to-beat variation. Also, present pharmacological interventions are based on altering the functional properties of membrane ion-channels[12]. It is important, however, to recognize that structural factors can have a profound influence on the cellular action potential and its propagation. At a microscopic level, the determinant of structural effects is cell-to-cell communication through gap junctions[13-16].

In this chapter we explore the role of gap-junctions in cardiac excitability and action potential propagation. The focus is on theoretical studies that we have performed, with comparison to experimental findings. We discuss the mechanisms by which electrical excitation travels down a cardiac fiber. The theoretical fiber contains the appropriate anatomical distinction between cells and gap junctions. This permits analysis of the relative roles of membrane factors and structural (gap-junction) factors in cardiac propagation.

The chapter begins with a brief discussion of how cardiac cells and multicellular fibers are modeled mathematically. Theoretical studies are becoming increasingly important to elucidate mechanisms in cardiac electrophysiology, especially when studying the interplay between membrane and structure, and this section is provided as a background to the theoretical approach. We then explore the function of membranes and gap-junctions in conduction with typical coupling; conditions that occur in normal myocardium. This section leads into a section that provides analysis of mechanisms underlying slow conduction and conduction block. We also explore changes in propagation safety (as manifest in the maximum upstroke velocity of the action potential) under normal and pathological conditions which alter gap-junction function. Finally, the insights obtained into the mechanisms of conduction are applied to arrhythmogenesis in a discussion of the influence of membrane factors and gap-junction factors on the vulnerable window for unidirectional block and reentry. The chapter compiles results from previously published articles that can be consulted for further detail[11, 17-25].

2. The Theoretical Approach to Action Potential Propagation in a Multicellular Cardiac Fiber

2.1 Modeling Individual Cardiac Cells- the Elements of the Fiber

The membrane of an intact isolated cell can be assumed to be space-clamped because there is minimal spatial spread of current. It follows that a model of the cell's electrical activity consists of transmembrane current densities and intracellular processes that affect these membrane currents. In electrical terms the membrane functions as a parallel RC (resistance-capacitance) circuit in which the resistance is determined by non-linear gating kinetics of ion channels and the lipid bilayer maintains charge separation, providing capacitance. Total membrane current is the sum of its ionic and capacitive components:

$$I_m = I_c + I_{ion} \qquad (1)$$

where I_m is membrane current density ($\mu A/cm^2$), I_c is capacitive current ($\mu A/cm^2$) and I_{ion} is ionic current ($\mu A/cm^2$). As with any capacitor, the transmembrane voltage (by convention inside minus outside) is proportional to the charge separation across the membrane; and I_c, the time derivative of charge, is proportional to the time derivative of voltage:

$$I_c = C_m * dV_m/dt \qquad (2)$$

where the constant C_m is membrane capacitance per unit area ($\mu F/cm^2$) and dV_m/dt is the rate of membrane voltage change over time (V/s). Due to conservation of current, total (net) transmembrane current, I_m, is zero. Combining this conservation principle with equations (1) and (2):

$$dV_m/dt = -I_{ion} / C_m \qquad (3)$$

Equation (3) is the principal relation for mathematical simulation of excitable membranes. The difficult task is to accurately determine I_{ion} which is the sum of all individual ionic currents. For each time increment, once I_{ion} is determined the change in voltage can be determined, leading to a new membrane voltage. By repeating this process, the entire action potential can be constructed. Most present membrane and cellular models[26-32] use

Hodgkin-Huxley type equations[33-36] to quantitatively represent the ionic currents.

2.2 Modeling a Multicellular Fiber- Combining the Cellular Elements

The theoretical fiber (Figure 1) is composed of a series of individual cell models spatially interconnected through an axial resistivity. The fiber introduces a spatial dimension to the flow of current such that the cells are no longer space-clamped. The spatial spread of current along the fiber is mathematically related to the transmembrane current by equations known alternatively as either the cable equations or reaction-diffusion equations[37, 38]. These equations state the conservation law in the multicellular fiber. That is, the transmembrane current I_m (zero in the case of an isolated cell) is equal to the change (gain or loss) of axial current that flows down the fiber. The equation of this relationship is:

$$I_m = f(2, aR_i) \; f(\partial^2 V_m, \partial x^2) = C_m \; f(\partial V_m, \partial t) + I_{ion} \quad (4)$$

where a is fiber radius (cm), R_i is axial resistivity (Ωcm), and ∂x is (when discretized) the spatial discretization element of the fiber. The right side of equation (4) is obtained from equations (1) and (2) above which describe the membrane current components. The middle part of equation (4) is a computation of axial current flowing into the cell (or into a discretization element of the cell) less axial current leaving the cell, i.e. the net loss or gain of axial current. From the conservation principle, this net change in axial current must be equal to the current that crosses the membrane, I_m.

When modeling cardiac fibers, it is critical to recognize that the fiber is not continuous but is composed of discrete cells interconnected by gap junctions[13, 14, 39]. Gap junctions are represented as ohmic (resistive) pathways based on the evidence that the interaction between cells is passive[40, 41] and that junctional resistance is constant over a wide range of voltages[42]. In addition, the purely resistive model of the gap-junctions neglects capacitive shunting. This approximation reflects the short time constant associated with nexus membranes[43, 44]. This chapter focuses on the role of gap junctions in the spread of electrical excitation. For numerical implementation of the cable equations in a fiber that contains gap-junctions, the readers are referred to References[18, 38, 45, 46].

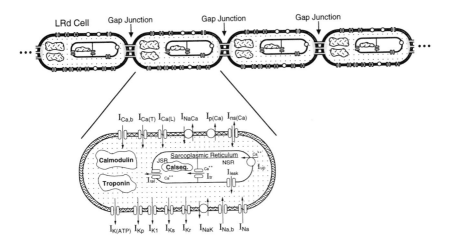

Figure 1. Schematic diagram of the multicellular fiber model. Multicellular cardiac fiber composed of a series dynamic Luo-Rudy (LRd) ventricular cell models interconnected by resistive gap junctions. Fiber is typically 7 mm (70 cells) long. Conduction is initiated by an external stimulus applied to the proximal end of the fiber, and conduction proceeds to the distal end autonomously. Enlarged section is a schematic of the LRd cell model, one of the several cell models that can be used in the fiber. The LRd model contains: I_{Na}, fast sodium current; $I_{Ca(L)}$, calcium current through L-type calcium channels; $I_{Ca(T)}$, calcium current through T-type calcium channels; I_{Kr}, fast component of the delayed rectifier potassium current; I_{Ks}, slow component of the delayed rectifier potassium current; I_{K1}, inward rectifier potassium current; I_{Kp}, plateau potassium current; $I_{K(ATP)}$, ATP sensitive potassium current; I_{NaK}, sodium-potassium pump current; I_{NaCa}, sodium-calcium exchange current; $I_{p(Ca)}$, calcium pump in the sarcolemma; $I_{Na,b}$, sodium background current; $I_{Ca,b}$, calcium background current; $I_{ns(Ca)}$, nonspecific calcium-activated current; I_{up}, calcium uptake from the myoplasm to network sarcoplasmic reticulum (NSR); I_{rel}, calcium release from junctional sarcoplasmic reticulum (JSR); I_{leak}, calcium leakage from NSR to myoplasm; I_{tr}, calcium translocation from NSR to JSR. For details on the LRd cell model see references[29, 30, 56].

2.3 Influence of Loading

Even with an identical ionic composition, there are differences between the action potential upstroke of a single isolated (space-clamped) cell and the same cell coupled to other cells in a multicellular fiber. A cell undergoing depolarization experiences electrical load from its neighboring cells. This phenomenon is illustrated in Figure 2 in which the action potential upstroke (V_m, dashed line) and its rate of rise (dV_m/dt, solid line) are shown for a single isolated cell (Panel A) and the middle cell of a multicellular fiber (Panel B). The maximum upstroke velocity, $(dV_m/dt)_{max}$, in the coupled cell is significantly smaller than that of the isolated cell (212 V/s versus 380 V/s) and occurs earlier, at less depolarized potential (at -12 mV versus -2 mV). The differences in upstrokes are not due to different membrane currents. Peak membrane ionic current, I_{ion}, of the isolated cell is 380 $\mu A/\mu F$ which is actually slightly smaller than peak I_{ion} of 398 $\mu A/\mu F$ for the coupled cell. Peak I_{ion} of the coupled cell also occurs at $V_m = -1$ mV, close to $V_m = -2$ mV for the single cell.

Reduction in upstroke velocity of the coupled cell is due to load from unexcited downstream fiber. The cartoon on the bottom right of each panel of Figure 2 compares the flow of current during the upstroke of an isolated cell and of a coupled cell. In the isolated cell the entire I_{ion} is used to discharge local membrane capacitance. Thus the single cell I_{ion} is equal to the capacitive current and, therefore, the rate of depolarization is directly related to I_{ion} (equation 3). In contrast, the charge generated by I_{ion} during depolarization of the coupled cell is divided between discharging local membrane capacitance (as in the isolated cell) and depolarizing downstream membrane (equation 4). As a result of charge loss to downstream fiber, the rate of depolarization of the coupled cell is reduced. The earlier occurrence of $(dV_m/dt)_{max}$ in the coupled cell indicates that as soon as the cell achieves significant depolarization, much of its generated charge is delivered downstream.

Figure 2 illustrates that fiber load can have a major effect on the characteristics of the cardiac action potential upstroke. Because intercellular conductance is regulated by gap-junction function, gap-junctions are important determinants of propagation and excitation in the heart. The remaining sections in this chapter explore the role of gap-junction function in cardiac propagation and excitation.

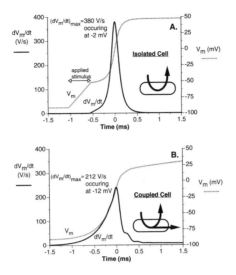

Figure 2. The effect of loading on the action potential upstroke. Action potential upstroke (V_m, dashed line, in mV) and its rate of rise (dV_m/dt, solid line, V/s) for a single isolated cell (Panel A) and the middle cell of a multicellular fiber (Panel B) with gap-junction conductance at $g_j = 2.5$ μS. The isolated cell requires an applied stimulus for excitation. In the fiber, a depolarizing cell receives excitatory current from upstream cells. Load by downstream cells significantly reduces maximum upstroke velocity, $(dV_m/dt)_{max}$.

3. Mechanisms of Conduction, Slow Conduction, and Conduction Failure

3.1 Cellular Conduction Time and Gap-Junction Delays

It is intuitively clear that a decrease in intercellular (gap-junctional) conductance will decrease propagation velocity. However the role of gap-junctions in determining conduction, even under normal conditions, is often under appreciated. Figure 3 shows action potential profiles in two neighboring cells under conditions of normal gap-junction coupling (Panel A) and a marginal (tenfold) decrease in coupling (Panel B). For normal intercellular coupling, the gap-junction conductance between cells ($g_j = 2.0$ μS) is roughly equal to the myoplasmic conductance of the entire cell. The result is a similar conduction time (~ 0.1 ms) between cells and in crossing the entire cell length (note, however, that the ratio of cell length to gap-junction dimension is 100 μm : 80 Å). On a macroscopic (many cells) scale, the result is an apparent uniform spread of excitation as seen in Figure 3A. With only tenfold reduction in coupling (Panel 3B) a large (~ 0.5 ms) conduction delay is introduced at each intercellular junction, while the entire cell depolarizes almost simultaneously.   The almost simultaneous depolarization of the cell is due to increased confinement of depolarizing current to the cell when intercellular coupling is reduced.   In this case cells in a fiber regain some of their isolated space-clamped characteristics and the entire cell membrane becomes essentially isopotential. Note (Figure 3B) that propagation under these conditions is nonuniform ("discontinuous) with long delays at gap-junctions.   In fact, the macroscopic conduction velocity over many cells is determined by the gap-junction delays rather than by the (negligible) time spent in traveling across individual cells.   With further reduction in gap-junction coupling, the intercellular delay can be on the order of milliseconds.

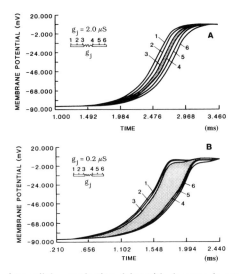

Figure 3. Increase in intercellular conduction delay with decrease in gap-junction coupling. Action potential upstrokes from the edge elements (see inset) of two adjoining cells for intercellular conductance of 2.0 μS (Panel A) and intercellular conductance of 0.2 μS (Panel B). The Beeler and Reuter[26] model was used for membrane kinetics and discretization was 20 patches per cell. For control coupling (Panel A), intercellular conduction delay is approximately equal to intracellular (myoplasmic) conduction time.   A tenfold decrease in intercellular conductance (Panel B) increases intercellular conduction time and decreases intracellular conduction time dramatically, resulting in gap junction dominance of overall conduction velocity. (From Reference[23] by permission).

The relationship of intracellular and intercellular conduction velocity to gap-junction conductance can be seen in Figure 4. Two different velocities are defined: microscopic velocity (q_{mic}), representing the velocity of propagation inside a single cell, and macroscopic velocity (q_{mac}) (or average velocity, q), representing the average velocity of propagation over many cells. Both velocities are defined in terms of time of arrival of $(dV_m/dt)_{max}$. As the gap-junction conductance is varied from 0.5 μS to 0.005 μS, q_{mic} and q_{mac} exhibit opposite changes. The microscopic velocity increases with decreasing gap-junction conductance, reflecting the fact that the current is more confined to the single cell and, therefore, more current is available to depolarize the cellular membrane. The macroscopic (average) velocity, on the other hand, decreases with decreasing gap-junction conductance as a result of increased time delays at the gap-junctions.

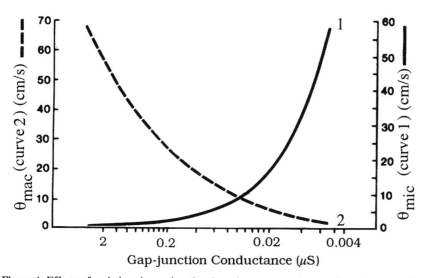

Figure 4. Effects of variations in gap-junctional conductance on microscopic and macroscopic velocities. Macroscopic average velocity over many cells (q_{mac}, dashed line) decreases whereas microscopic intracellular velocity (q_{mic}, solid line) increases with decreasing gap-junction conductance. Membrane elements are formulated with the Beeler and Reuter equations[26]. (From Reference[18] by permission of the American Heart Association, Inc.).

3. 2 Ionic Mechanisms of Conduction Failure

Conduction block due to gap-junction decoupling occurs when coupling is restricted to the point that upstream cells cannot excite downstream cells. Yet, failure of conduction is not instantaneous, rather conduction can be decremental prior to block. Figure 5 contains action potentials of cells 13-17 of a multicellular fiber computed with a stimulus at cell 1 and two degrees of gap-junction conductance; $g_j = 0.006$ μS (Panel A) and $g_j = 0.005$ μS (Panel B). Each cell in the fiber is of LRd formalism. Conduction down the fiber fails at $g_j = 0.0057$ μS. The action potentials of Panel A correspond to non-decremental conduction at very low degree of intercellular coupling. The subthreshold phase for each cell (e.g. time 390-420 ms for cell 14) is very long. However, once activation threshold is reached, membrane depolarization occurs rapidly. As a cell fires, the voltage gradient between it and the adjoining upstream cell is rapidly reduced. The decreased gradient removes the load on the upstream cell, an event reflected by a slight depolarization during its plateau that coincides with excitation of the downstream cell (time 420 ms for cell 13). Beyond this brief depolarization, both the newly excited cell and its upstream neighbor repolarize in concert (time 440-455 for cells 13 and 14), until the next cell downstream (e.g. cell 15) reaches threshold. The non-decremental conduction in panel A is also evidenced by the constant $(dV_m/dt)_{max}$ of all cells in the fiber beyond the proximal end (empty circles of panel C, elevated $(dV_m/dt)_{max}$ in the first 5 cells is due to stimulus and end effects).

An important aspect of non-decremental conduction is that once a cell excites, it becomes isopotential with its upstream neighbor. Thus the only loading it experiences is from downstream fiber- in the direction of propagation. In the case of decremental conduction leading to block, intercellular conduction time is prolonged so much that the upstream source cell is significantly repolarized when the adjacent cell fires. Under such conditions, a cell during early plateau is loaded by both downstream and upstream cells. For instance, cell 14 in Panel 5B not only delivers current to cell 15 after reaching threshold (time=500 ms), but also delivers current *upstream* to cell 13. As a result, the plateau of cell 14 repolarizes faster which decreases the voltage gradient from this cell to its downstream neighbor. Decreased gradient lowers the axial source current which further increases intercellular conduction time. Ultimately, as occurs with cell 15, the source cell repolarizes before the downstream cell can reach threshold, and conduction block occurs. Failure to reach threshold is associated with dynamic inactivation of sodium channels during the very long sub-threshold depolarization process when axial source current is limited by the very small gap-junction conductance. The progressive decrease of $(dV_m/dt)_{max}$ with propagation (filled circles, panel C) indicates that sodium channel availability is successively reduced, resulting in decremental conduction and, ultimately, conduction failure.

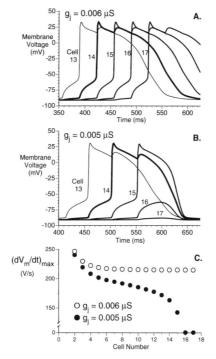

Figure 5. Borderline conduction and conduction failure in a multicellular fiber. In the multicellular fiber model composed of LRd cells, conduction fails at gap-junction conductance $g_j = 0.0057$ μS. Panel A contains action potentials of cells 13-17 for a fiber with barely successful conduction, $g_j = 0.006$ μS. Panel B contains action potentials from the same cell, but with $g_j = 0.005$ μS. In both panels, the action potential of cell 14 is highlighted in bold. Long intercellular delays in Panel B result in significant upstream repolarization of cells prior to excitation of their downstream neighbor. By the time the neighbor cell fires, the upstream cell is so repolarized that it constitutes a load for the downstream neighbor. Bidirectional (upstream and downstream) loading ultimately results in conduction failure. Maximum upstroke velocity, $(dV_m/dt)_{max}$, for the cells of interest are shown in Panel C (empty and filled circles correspond to fibers with $g_j = 0.006$ μS and $g_j = 0.005$ μS, respectively). Note attainment of constant, non-decremental, conduction for $g_j = 0.006$ μS and decremental conduction for $g_j = 0.005$ μS.

3.3 Propagation Safety and Gap-Junction Coupling

The functional effects of the structural discontinuities introduced by the gap-junctions increase with decreases in intercellular gap-junctional conductance. It follows that a greater degree of gap-junction decoupling will produce greater deviation from the conduction properties of a continuous fiber. A comparison of the behavior of a discontinuous fiber where gap junctions are distinctly located between cells and that of a continuous fiber helps illustrate gap-junction function in the context of action potential propagation. Figure 6, panel A contains the maximum rate of rise of the action potential (($dV_m/dt)_{max}$, curve 1) and the average macroscopic velocity of its propagation (q_{macro}, curve 2) as a function of gap-j unction conductance. The continuous case is shown for comparison in panel 6B. In the discontinuous fiber (panel A), ($dV_m/dt)_{max}$ displays a biphasic behavior. In the range of gap-junction conductance from 2 to 0.06 μS, ($dV_m/dt)_{max}$ increases and conduction velocity decreases. This paradoxical behavior is opposite to the direct relation between ($dV_m/dt)_{max}$ and conduction velocity that is observed when velocity is slowed due to decreased membrane excitability[21, 38, 47].

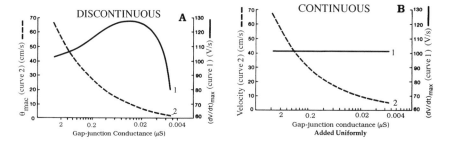

Figure 6. Propagation down discontinuous and continuous fibers. Panel A. Effects of variations in gap-junction conductance on the macroscopic velocity of propagation (curve 2) and on the maximum rate of rise of the action potential, ($dV_m/dt)_{max}$ (curve 1). Panel B. ($dV_m/dt)_{max}$ (curve 1), and conduction velocity (curve 2) as a function of gap-junction conductance that is uniformly spread across the cell and combined with myoplasm conductance to form a continuous fiber (i.e., gap-junction discontinuities are not present). Membrane elements are formulated with the Beeler and Reuter equations[26]. (From Reference[18] by permission of the American Heart Association, Inc.).

For high degrees of coupling (high values of gap-junction conductance), velocity is high and $(dV_m/dt)_{max}$ levels off, approaching the value associated with propagation in a continuous fiber (see panel B). For low coupling (low values of gap-junction conductance) a second phase is exhibited, and $(dV_m/dt)_{max}$ decreases with decreasing gap-junction conductance. This part of the curve reflects the transition to decremental conduction and eventually to complete conduction block. For a certain value of gap-junction coupling (0.02 μS), $(dV_m/dt)_{max}$ attains a maximum. For this low coupling value, the cell is separated to a large degree from its neighbors, and $(dV_m/dt)_{max}$ approaches the value that could be attained in an isolated cell or under space-clamp conditions. In the continuous case (panel 6B) the velocity also decreases with decreasing axial conductance, but $(dV_m/dt)_{max}$ remains constant, independent of variations in conductance.

$(dV_m/dt)_{max}$ is a parameter that reflects both the magnitude of the depolarizing membrane current and the effect of electrical load on the membrane. Due to the fact that it is influenced by the major factors that determine propagation of the action potential, $(dV_m/dt)_{max}$ is often used as an indication of conduction safety. From the results in Figure 6A, we learn that moderate reduction of gap-junction coupling increases propagation safety. This seems paradoxical, however the mechanism is intuitively clear: less coupling limits current flow to neighboring cells, conserving it for local depolarization. Only when coupling is highly reduced does restricted axial flow limit subthreshold depolarization, decreasing $(dV_m/dt)_{max}$ and safety.

The results of Figure 6A also indicate that by lowering gap-junction coupling, conduction velocity can be reduced to velocities on the order of 1 cm/s before conduction failure occurs. A likely consequence of decoupling is the presence of conduction that is slow but safe. Ursell et al.[8] and Dillon et al.[7] recorded conduction velocities of less than 1 cm/s in zones of a healed (2 month old) myocardial infarction. This is in contrast to conduction in the presence of reduced membrane excitability, which can lower velocity to only one third of control values before causing failure[11, 21, 48].

Some of the experimental literature reports conflicting conclusions on whether conduction slowing due to reduced coupling occurs with higher or lower safety. In a classic study, Spach et al.[13] found that cardiac conduction in the longitudinal (well-coupled) direction had higher conduction velocity but was less safe than conduction in the transverse (less-coupled) direction. Safety was evaluated by susceptibility to block with premature stimulation. Delgado et al.[49] observed the opposite, that conduction failed preferentially in the transverse direction. In Delgado's study, block was obtained by elevation of extracellular potassium concentration. A possible reason for the disparity between the two studies is the technique used to obtain block. Elevation of extracellular potassium concentration, unlike premature stimulation, alters the potassium reversal potential and depolarizes the resting membrane potential[50, 51]. As a result, not only do sodium channels inactivate, but distance between resting potential and threshold potential is reduced[51, 52]. In addition, conduction near block due to elevated extracellular potassium depends on the L-type calcium current to aid in excitation[21]. Therefore an evaluation of safety factor based on elevating $[K]_o$ may include important contribution from the L-type calcium current and might differ from the safety factor evaluated by premature stimulation. In further support of the positive effect of uncoupling on propagation safety, Rohr et al.[53] recently found that partial uncoupling restored successful conduction in discontinuous cardiac tissue structures exhibiting unidirectional conduction block. Unidirectional block is discussed further below.

4. Role of Gap-Junction Coupling in Unidirectional Block and Reentry

4.1 Unidirectional Block and the Vulnerable Window

Unidirectional block is a prerequisite to reentrant arrhythmias. The phenomenon of unidirectional block involves successful propagation in one direction and failure of propagation in the other direction. Unidirectional block can occur on the tail of a prior action potential in an otherwise uniform and homogeneous tissue. A directional asymmetry is created by the dispersion of excitability that exists in the wake of the prior action potential. We define the "vulnerable window" (TW) as the time interval in the refractory period (between plateau and diastole) of a propagating action potential during which unidirectional block can be induced (Figure 7). The vulnerable window can also be represented as a distance in the space domain (SW) or as a range of membrane potentials in the voltage domain (VW). Outside this window, it is impossible to induce unidirectional block; an action potential induced by a premature stimulus either propagates or blocks in both directions. When a premature stimulus is applied inside the window, the membrane generates a critical sodium current, giving rise to an action potential that propagates incrementally in the retrograde direction and decrementally in the antegrade direction. This is because in the retrograde direction the tissue is progressively more recovered as the distance from the window increases in this direction, while in the antegrade direction the membrane is progressively less excitable as the distance from the window increases. Figure 8 provides examples of responses to differently timed stimuli. For stimuli outside the window, bidirectional block (Panel A) or bidirectional conduction (Panel C) occur. When the stimulus falls inside the vulnerable window, unidirectional block develops.

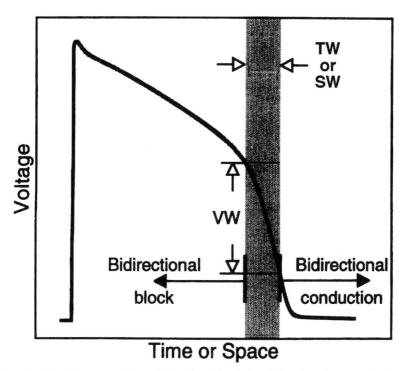

Figure 7. Schematic representation of the vulnerable window during the refractory period of a propagating action potential. TW, SW and VW represent the vulnerable window in the time domain, space domain and voltage domain, respectively. (From Reference[20], by permission).

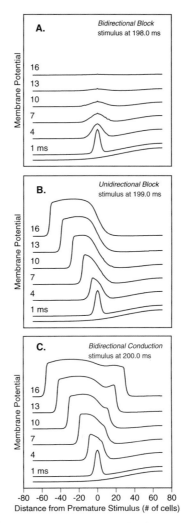

Figure 8. Three types of responses to a premature stimulus. (A) Bidirectional block occurred when the premature stimulus was applied 198 ms after initiation of the conditioning action potential and resulted from an inability of the premature stimulus to excite the fiber in either direction. (B) Unidirectional block at 199 ms resulted from successful retrograde, but not antegrade, excitation. (C) Bidirectional conduction at 200 ms when both retrograde and antegrade fiber were excited. The bottom trace in each panel represents membrane potential immediately prior to stimulus. Gap junction conductance $g_j = 0.9$ μS. (From Reference[19], by permission).

4.2 Gap Junction and Membrane Factors as Modulators of the Vulnerable Window

The size of the vulnerable window in the time domain (TW) provides a measure of the vulnerability of the tissue to the induction of unidirectional block and reentry. TW is a convenient working definition of the vulnerable window. For a large TW the time interval during which unidirectional block can be induced is long. Therefore, the probability that a premature stimulus (e.g. during clinical electrophysiology study in the catheterization laboratory, or a naturally occurring triggering event in the diseased heart) will fall inside the window and induce reentry is high. In Figure 9 we examine the effects of cellular uncoupling at gap junctions and of membrane excitability on the tissue vulnerability to unidirectional block. Vulnerability (TW) is shown as a function of gap junction resistance (solid curve). As the gap junction resistance increases, vulnerability increases as well, with accompanying decrease in propagation velocity (dashed curve). For normal cellular coupling ($g_j = 2.5$ μS), the vulnerability is about 0.4 msec. Very precise timing (TW<0.5 msec) of a premature stimulus is required for induction of unidirectional block and reentry. The vulnerability is increased to 3.7 ms at $g_j = 0.09$ μS, and can get as high as 30 msec for a high degree of cellular uncoupling ($g_j = 0.025$ μS). For such a wide window, unidirectional block can be easily induced.

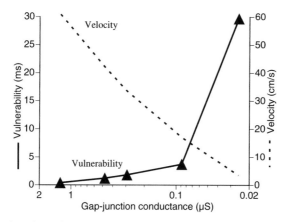

Figure 9. Changes in vulnerability due to changes in gap junction conductance g_j. Solid curve shows an increase in vulnerability when gap-junction conductance decreases. Dashed curve shows decreasing velocity of propagation as gap-junction conductance decreases. (compiled from Reference[19], with permission).

The simulations demonstrate, therefore, that as the degree of cellular uncoupling is increased, velocity of propagation decreases (due to long delays at gap junctions) and vulnerability to reentry increases. In other studies[17, 19] we show that the vulnerability is determined by the degree of spatial functional inhomogeneity of excitability at the vulnerable window. As regional propagation delay increases, due to long delays at gap junctions, the degree of spatial functional inhomogeneity in the state of the membrane increases as well. This increased asymmetry at the vulnerable window reflets an increase in the spatial gradient of sodium channel inactivation.

In contrast to the effect of cellular uncoupling described above, uniform reduction throughout the entire fiber in sodium channel conductance (intrinsic membrane excitability) resulted in slow propagation with decreased vulnerability to the induction of reentry (not shown). This is because a uniform reduction in membrane excitability produces a shift of the vulnerable window to a more recovered portion of the action potential where repolarization is slower and variation of membrane potential and dynamic properties is reduced (for a less excitable membrane, similar conditions to those under a non-compromised membrane are produced at a more recovered region). This shift to a less steep portion of the action potential reduces spatial inhomogeneities in the state of membrane excitability at the vicinity of the window. The result is lower vulnerability to the induction of unidirectional block and reentry. Quantitatively, the effect is small and operatively negligible[17]; 50% reduction of sodium channel conductance brings about a decrease of the vulnerable window from 0.5 msec to 0.1 msec. In comparison, a reduction of cellular coupling that causes similar decrease in conduction velocity is accompanied by a large increase of vulnerability from 0.5 msec to 30 msec.

5. Conclusions

Both membrane factors and gap-junction factors are involved in the spread of cardiac excitation. Their interaction is intimate and bi-directional, making it difficult to define cause-and-effect relationships that govern properties of propagation. However, it is possible to determine the relative influence of the membrane and of gap-junctions on cardiac conduction. In this chapter, we demonstrated that the load associated with normal coupling reduces maximum upstroke velocity of the action potential by almost 50%. At an extreme degree of uncoupling, cellular action potentials appear normal, yet axial current is limited by the gap-junctions to the point that subthreshold sodium channel inactivation occurs, leading to decremental conduction and ultimately conduction failure. Moderate (or even high) degree of uncoupling increases the safety factor of conduction, independent of the state of the membrane, and has a much greater influence on the vulnerable window of unidirectional block than uniform decrease of membrane excitability.

As a consequence of reduced membrane excitability (e.g., due to acute ischemia)[21], velocity can only be reduced by a factor of about 3 (to $\sim$ 17 cm/s) before block occurs. In comparison, reduced intercellular coupling at gap junctions can support very slow conduction velocities ($\sim$ 1 cm/s). This suggests that cellular decoupling plays an important role in very slow conduction that can be observed during reentry[7] while reduced membrane excitability plays a more important role in the development of conduction block. Note, however, that conduction block can result from elevated gap-junction resistance, without compromised membrane excitability (Figure 5), but this requires an extreme degree of uncoupling. We emphasize that to support very slow conduction velocities, gap-junction uncoupling must be present. This implies that uncoupling plays an important role in anisotropic reentry where extremely slow conduction is observed across a line of apparent block[54]. Uncoupling must also be important to the development of reentry in short pathways ("microreentry"). This is because slow conduction shortens the wavelength of the reentrant action potential (defined as velocity x refractory period) to adapt to the short pathway without excessive degree of head-tail interaction that leads to instabilities and termination of reentry[20, 55].

Based on the simulations presented in this chapter, one may conclude that membrane processes generate cardiac action potentials and play a major role in determining their morphology, while structural factors of which gap-junction coupling is a very important component, play an important role in controlling the spread of excitation. These principles suggest that pharmaceutical intervention aimed at altering intercellular coupling may be a promising target for future antiarrhythmic therapy, especially when propagation-type arrhythmias (e.g., reentry) are involved.

References

1. PM Spooner, AM Brown, WA Catterall, GJ Kaczorowski, and HC Strauss, Ion channels in the cardiovascular system: function and dysfunction. Armonk: Futura Publishing Company, Inc., 1994, pp. 580.
2. GT Wetzel and TS Klitzner, Development cardiac electrophysiology: recent advances in cellular physiology, *Cardiovasc Res*, vol. 31, pp. E52-E60, 1996.
3. MS Spach, WT Miller, PC. Dolber, J. M. Kootsey, J. R. Sommer, and C. E. Mosher, Jr., The functional role of structural complexities in the propagation of depolarization in the atrium of the dog. Cardiac conduction disturbances due to discontinuities of effective axial resistivity, *Circ Res*, vol. 50, pp. 175-91, 1982.
4. VG Fast and AG Kleber, Microscopic conduction in cultured strands of neonatal rat heart cells measured with voltage-sensitive dyes, *Circ Res*, vol. 73, pp. 914-25, 1993.
5. VG Fast, BJ Darrow, JE Saffitz, and AG Kléber, Anisotropic activation spread in heart cell monolayers assessed by high resolution optical mapping. Role of tissue discontinuities, *Circ Res*, vol. 79, pp. 115-27, 1996.
6. JM de Bakker, FJ van Capelle, MJ Janse, AA Wilde, R Coronel, AE Becker, KP Dingemans, NM van Hemel and RN Hauer, Reentry as a cause of ventricular tachycardia in patients with chronic ischemic heart disease: electrophysiologic and anatomic correlation, *Circulation*, vol. 77, pp. 589-606, 1988.
7. SM Dillon, MA Allessie, PC Ursell, and AL Wit, Influences of anisotropic tissue structure on reentrant circuits in the epicardial border zone of subacute canine infarcts, *Circ Res*, vol. 63, pp. 182-206, 1988.
8. PC Ursell, PI Gardner, A Albala, JJ Fenoglio Jr. and AL Wit, Structural and electrophysiological changes in the epicardial border zone of canine myocardial infarcts during infarct healing, *Circ Res*, vol. 56, pp. 436-51, 1985.
9. MJ Janse and AG Kleber, Propagation of electrical activity in ischemic and infarcted myocardium as a basis of ventricular arrhythmias, *J Cardiovasc Electrophys*, vol. 3, pp. 77-87, 1992.
10. RW Joyner, R Kumar, R Wilders, HJ Jongsma, EE Verheijck, DA Golod, ACG van Ginneken, MB Wagner and WN Goolsby, Modulating L-type calcium current affects discontinuous cardiac action potential conduction, *Biophys J*, vol. 71, pp. 237-45, 1996.
11. RM Shaw and Y Rudy, Ionic mechanisms of propagation in cardiac tissue. Roles of the sodium and L-type calcium currelts during reduced excitability and decreased gap-junction coupling, *Circ Res*, vol. submitted, 1997.
12. Task Force of the Working Group on Arrhythmias of the European Society of Cardiology, The sicilian gambit: a new approach to the classification of antiarrhythmic drugs based on their action on arrhythmogenic mechanisms, *Circulation*, vol. 84, pp. 1831-51, 1991.

13. MS Spach, WT Miller III, DB Geselowitz, RC Barr, JM Kootsey and EA Johnson, The discontinuous nature of propagation in normal canine cardiac muscle. Evidence for recurrent discontinuities of intracellular resistance that affect membrane currents, *Circ Res*, vol. 48, pp. 39-54, 1981.

14. FS Sjöstrand and E Anderston, Electron microscopy of the intercalated discs of cardiac muscle tissue, *Experientia*, vol. 10, pp. 369-72, 1954.

15. WR Lowenstein, Junctional and intercellular communication: the cell-to-cell membrane channel, *Physiol Rev*, vol. 61, pp. 829-913, 1981.

16. DC Spray, Structure-activity relations of the cardiac gap-junction channel, *Am J Physiol*, vol. 258, pp. C195-205, 1990.

17. W Quan and Y Rudy, Unidirectional block and reentry of cardiac excitation: a model study, *Circ Res*, vol. 66, pp. 367-82, 1990.

18. Y Rudy and WL Quan, A model study of the effects of the discrete cellular structure on electrical propagation in cardiac tissue, *Circ Res*, vol. 61, pp. 815-23, 1987.

19. RM Shaw and Y Rudy, The vulnerable window for unidirectional block in cardiac tissue: Characterization and dependence on membrane excitability and intercellular coupling, *J Cardiovasc Electrophys*, vol. 6, pp. 115-31, 1995.

20. Y Rudy, Reentry: insights from theoretical simulations in a fixed pathway, *J Cardiovasc Electrophysiol*, vol. 6, pp. 294-312, 1995.

21. RM Shaw and Y Rudy, Electrophysiologic effects of acute myocardial ischemia: A mechanistic investigation of action potential conduction and conduction failure, *Circ Res*, vol. 80, pp. 124-38, 1997.

22. WL Quan and Y Rudy, Termination of reentrant propagation by a single stimulus: a model study, *PACE Pacing Clin Electrophysiol*, vol. 14, pp. 1700-6, 1991.

23. Y Rudy and WL Quan, Propagation delays across cardiac gap junctions and their reflection in extracellular potentials: A simulation study, *J Cardiovasc Electrophys*, vol. 286, pp. 177-210, 1991.

24. Y Rudy and W Quan, Effects of discrete cellular structure on propagation of excitation in cardiac tissue: A model study, in *Cell interactions and gap junctions*, vol. 2, N. Sperelakis and W. C. Cole, Eds. Boca Raton: CRC Press, Inc., 1989, pp. 123-142.

25. Y Rudy, Models of continuous and discontinuous propagation in cardiac tissue, in *Cardiac electrophysiology: From cell to bedside*, D. P. Zipes and J. Jalife, Eds. Philadelphia: WB Saunders Co, 1994, pp. 326-334.

26. GW Beeler and H Reuter, Reconstruction of the action potential of ventricular myocardial fibres, *J Physiol (Lond)*, vol. 268, pp. 177-210, 1977.

27. D DiFrancesco and D Noble, "A model of the cardiac electrical activity incorporating ionic pumps and concentration changes, *Phil Trans R Soc Lon (Biol)*, vol. 307, pp. 353-98, 1985.

28. CH Luo and Y Rudy, A model of the ventricular cardiac action potential. Depolarization, repolarization, and their interaction, *Circ Res*, vol. 68, pp. 1501-26, 1991.

29. CH Luo and Y Rudy, A dynamic model of the cardiac ventricular action potential. I. Simulations of ionic currents and concentration changes, *Circ Res*, vol. 74, pp. 1071-96, 1994.

30. CH Luo and Y Rudy, A dynamic model of the cardiac ventricular action potential. II. Afterdepolarizations, triggered activity, and potentiation, *Circ Res*, vol. 74, pp. 1097-113, 1994.

31. D Noble, Ionic mechanisms determining the timing of ventricular repolarization: significance for cardiac arrhyhtmias, *Ann NY Acad Sci*, vol. 644, pp. 1-22, 1992.

32. C Nordin, Computer model of membrane current and intracellular Ca2+ flux in the isolated guinea pig ventricular myocyte, *Am J Physiol*, vol. 265, pp. H211-36, 1993.

33. AL Hodgkin and AF Huxley, Current carried by sodium and potassium ions through the membrane of the giant axon of Logligo, *J Physiol*, vol. 116, pp. 449-72, 1952.

34. AL Hodgkin and AF Huxley, The components of membrane conductance in the giant axon of Loglio, *J Physiol*, vol. 116, pp. 473-96, 1952.

35. AL Hodgkin and AF Huxley, The dual effect of membrane potential on sodium conductance in the giant axon of Loglio, *J Physiol*, vol. 116, pp. 497-506, 1952.

36. AL Hodgkin and AF Huxely, A quantitative description of membrane and its application to conduction and excitation in the nerve, *J Physiol*, vol. 117, pp. 500-44, 1952.

37. AL Hodgkin and WAH Rushton, The electrical constants of a crustacean nerve fibre, *Proc Roy Soc B*, vol. 133, pp. 444-79, 1946.

38. JJB Jack, D Noble, and RW Tsien, *Electric current flow in excitable cells*. Oxford: Clarendon Press, 1975.

39. JE Saffitz, LM David, BJ Darrow, HL Kanter, JG Laing and EC Beyer, The molecular basis of anisotropy: Role of gap junctions, *J Cardiovasc Electrophys*, vol. 6, pp. 498-510, 1995.

40. JW Woodbury and WE Crill, On the problem of impulse conduction in the atrium, in *Nervous inhibition*, L. Florey, Ed. New York: Plenum Press, 1961, pp. 24.

41. RD Veenstra and R. L. DeHaan, Measurement of single channel currents from cardiac gap junctions, *Science*, vol. 233, pp. 972-4, 1986.

42. E Page and Y Shibata, Permeable junctions between cardiac cells, *Ann Rev Physiol*, vol. 43, 1981.

43. WH Freygang and W Trautwein, The structural implications of the linear electrical properties of cardiac Purkinje strands, *J Gen Physiol*, vol. 55, pp. 524-47, 1970.

44. JB Chapman and CH Fry, An analysis of the cable properties of frog ventricular myocardium, *J Physiol (Lond)*, vol. 283, pp. 263-82, 1978.
45. CS Henriquez and R Plonsey, Effect of resistive discontinuities on waveshape and velocity in a single cardiac fibre, *Med Biol Eng Comput*, vol. 25, pp. 428-38, 1987.
46. R. W. Joyner, Effects of the discrete pattern of electrical coupling on propagation through and electrical syncytium, *Circ Res*, vol. 50, pp. 192-200, 1982.
47. PJ Hunter, PA McNaughton and D Noble, Analytical models of propagation in excitable cells, *Prog Biophys Mol Biol*, vol. 30, pp. 99-144, 1975.
48. Y Kagiyama, JL Hill, and LS Gettes, Interaction of acidosis and increased extracellular potassium on action potential characteristics and conduction in guinea pig ventricular muscle, *Circ Res*, vol. 51, pp. 614-23, 1982.
49. C Delgado, B Steinhaus, M Delmar, DR Chialvo and J Jalife, Directional differences in excitability and margin of safety for propagation in sheep ventricular epicardial muscle, *Circ Res*, vol. 67, pp. 97-110, 1990.
50. AS Harris, A Bisteni, RA Russel, JC Brigham and JE Firestone, Excitatory factors in ventricular tachycardia resulting from myocardial ischemia: Potassium a major excitant, *Science*, vol. 119, pp. 200-3, 1954.
51. G Dominguez and HA Fozzard, Influence of extracellular K+ concentration on cable properties and excitability of sheep cardiac Purkinje fibers, *Circ Res*, vol. 26, pp. 565-74, 1970.
52. LS Gettes, JW Buchanan Jr, T Saito, Y Kagiyama, S Oshita and T Fujino, Studies concerned with slow conduction, in *Cardiac electrophysiology and arrhythmias*, D. P. Zipes and J. Jalife, Eds. Orlando: Grune and Stratton, 1985, pp. 81-7.
53. S Rohr, JP Kucera, VG Fast, and AG Kleber, Paradoxical improvement of impulse conduction in cardiac tissue by partial cellular uncoupling, *Science*, vol. 275, pp. 841-4, 1997.
54. AL Wit, SM Dillon and J Coromilas, Anisotropic reentry as a cause of ventricular tachycardias in myocardial infarction, in *Cardiac electrophysiology, from cell to bedside*, DP Zipes and J Jalife, Eds. Philadelphia: W.B. Saunders Co., 1995, pp. 511-526.
55. LH Frame and MB Simson, Oscillation of conduction, action potential duration and refractoriness: A mechanism for spontaneous termination of reentrant tachycardias, *Circulation*, vol. 78, pp. 1277-87, 1988.
56. J Zeng, KR Laurita, DS Rosenbaum and Y Rudy, Two components of the delayed rectifier K^+ current in ventricular myocytes of the guinea-pig type: theoretical formulation and their role in repolarization, *Circ Res*, vol. 77, pp. 140-52, 1995.

7 CELL TO CELL COMMUNICATION IN THE FAILING HEART

Walmor C. De Mello

Department of Pharmacology, Medical Sciences Campus, UPR

It is known that myocytes from the failing heart present several abnormalities of ion pumps, calcium re-uptake by the sarcoplasmic reticulum, hormone receptors, etc (1).

In cardiomyopathic hamsters a calcium overload of the heart cells has been considered a possible etiologic factor. The mechanism of this overload is not completely clear but there is evidence that the calcium uptake by the cell is enhanced (2, 3) leading to a calcium-determined necrotic process with myocytolysis and typical fibrillar disarray (4). As emphasized by Weismand and Weinfeldt (5) the cardiomyopathic hamster represents an important model for cardiomyopathy and hypertrophy in humans. Indeed, ventricular hypertrophy followed by progressive cardiac dilation and death by congestive heart failure is usually seen in cardiomyopathic hamsters at late stage of the disease (6, 7).

Our present knowledge of the electrophysiological properties of the failing heart is meager, particularly of the alterations in cell coupling. In the present chapter I will discuss some relevant aspects of this problem and recent findings.

Measurements of gj performed in cell pairs isolated from normal hamsters (11 months old) indicated predominant values in the rage from 40 to 100 nS (Fig. 1). These values are not smaller than those found in younger animal (6-7 months old) but are higher ($p < 0.05$) than those found in the ventricle of cardiomyopathic (CM) hamsters at late stage of the disease (11 months old) in which the cell pairs can be classified in two major groups according to the value of gj: one in which the value of gj is very low (0.8-2.5 nS) and the other in which the values are higher (7-35 nS) but still smaller than the controls (see Fig. 1) (8).

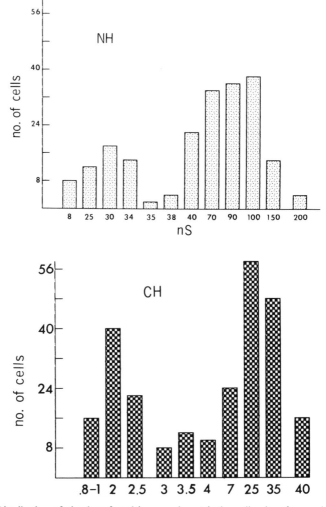

Figure 1. Distribution of gj values found in several ventricular cell pairs of normal hamsters (NH, top) and CM hamsters (CH, bottom). From reference (8) with permission.

These two major populations of CM myocytes were classified not only by their different values of gj but also by some morphological characteristics. The group of cells presenting very low values of gj showed clear alterations in cross striations as previously described by Sen et al (15) while the other group with higher values of gj showed an internal normal structure but the cell length was increased. In normal hamsters of same age (11 months old) no such morphological abnormalities were found among the ventricular myocytes. Histological studies performed in normal and CM hamsters indicated extensive areas of interstitial fibrosis and calcification in the myopathic ventricle but not in the normal animal (see Figs. 2 and 3) (9) and severe destruction of intercellular contacts can be seen in the right and left ventricle of cardiomyopathic hamsters (11 months old) using confocal microscopy (10). This alteration of ventricular morphology, which is more pronounced near calcified zones or in areas in which intense interstitial fibrosis can be detected, represents an important detrimental factor for electrical synchronization and ventricular contractility. Electronmicroscopic studies performed on the myocardium of another strain of cardiomyopathic hamsters (UM-X7.1) indicated smaller intercalated discs with an abnormal orientation and distribution (11).

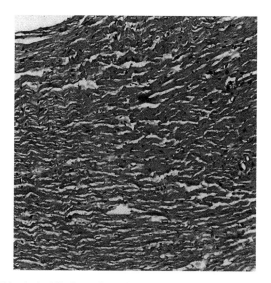

Figure 2. Normal histological findings of the right ventricle of control hamster (11 months old) Haematoxylon-eosin; magnification 50x. From reference 9, with permission.

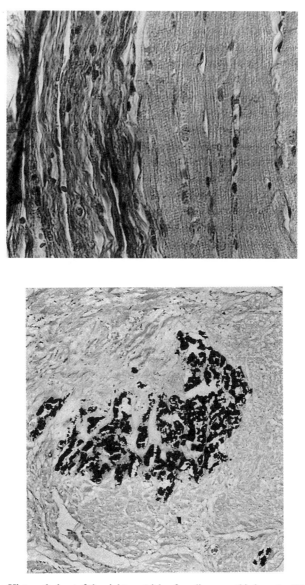

Figure 3. Top-Histopathology of the right ventricle of cardiomyopathic hamster (11 months old) showing extensive interstitial fibrosis with Masson trichrome. Magnification 50x. Bottom-Von Kossa's stain of the left ventricle of cardiomyopathic hamster (11 months old) showing central lesion with Ca depots. From reference 9, with permission.

The mechanism of the impairment of cell coupling in the failing myocardium is not known.

Electrophysiological observations performed on transfected cell pairs showed that different connexins form gap junctions with different channel gating properties (12) (see also Chapters 3 and 4). In the hypertensive rat heart, for instance, the expression of connexin 43 is reduced but by the expression of connexin 40 is enhanced (13). The possibility exists that the impairment of cell coupling seen in the failing heart (8) be in part related to an alteration in the expression of different connexins. A decline in the expression of connexin43 has been considered by Severs (14) as responsible for some electrophysiological abnormalities of the diseased heart (see Chapter 8). An alternative explanation of the decline in gj is the is the calcium overload which is one of the characteristics of this cardiomyopathy. The intracellular calcium concentration measured in isolated myocytes from the BIO-TO2 cardiomyopathic hamsters at late stage of the disease (11 months), for instance, indicated an average value of 480 (SEM ± 28) nM compared with 143 (SEM ± 24) nM in the control hamster (F1B) of the same age (Fig. 4). This result is in accord that those found in other strain of myopathic hamster (BIO 14.6) (8 months old) (15). The mechanism of the calcium overload is not known. An increase in the permeability of the surface cell membrane to calcium has been described (15) but the possibility that excess catecholamine damage of surface cell membrane with consequent increase in intracellular calcium has been proposed by Fleckenstein (16). A deficiency of ATP caused by excessive activation of calcium-dependent ATPases an mitochondrial damage by excessive calcium accumulation in cardiomyhopathic heart might not be related to a primary defect of the sarcolemma but due to a exhausted hypokinetic state that favor Ca accumulation with progressive deterioration of structural proteins (4). Measurements of the time constant of surface cell membrane made in isolated myocytes from CM hamsters indicated no significant change when compared with controls what suggests that the surface cell membrane resistance is not greatly altered. Recently, it has been found that during depolarization a large slowly inactivating inward current is activated in ventricular myocytes of cardiomyopathic hamsters and that this current seems to be generated by the Na-Ca exchanger (17) suggesting that the Na-Ca exchanger plays a major role in the regulation of heart contractility and calcium sequestration in the cardiomyopathic hamsters (17).

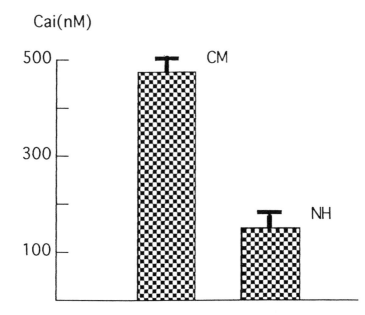

Figure 4. Values of intracellular free Ca concentration (Cai) found in isolated cell of CM hamsters (11 months old) and normal (NH) hamsters of same age at rest. Each bar is the average from 35 cells. Vertical line at the bars-SEM.

Since it is known that an increment in Cai lead to a decline in gj (18, 19) it is justified to think that the fall in gj seen in the myopathic ventricle be related to calcium overload. Although there is an increment in the intracellular calcium concentration in myopathic myocytes it has been found that these cells present a remarkable capacity to buffer changes in Ca_i induced by changes in Ca_o (15). This enhanced buffer capacity for Ca might be in part related to an increased sarcoplasmic reticulum described in these cells (20).

Experiments performed in our laboratory indicated that when cell pairs from cardiomyopathic animals are dialyzed with high Ca solution the junctional conductance is less affected when compared with normal hamsters of same age. As shown in Fig. 5 (De Mello, unpublished) the dialysis of Ca (0.5 uM) into the cells of normal hamster caused a suppression of cell coupling within 12 min while in cardiomyopathic hamster the administration of the same concentration of Ca to the cytosol and using pipettes with the same tip diameter, caused a decline of gj of only 65% in about 18 min. (p<0.05). It is not known if that the gap junction proteins in myopathic hamsters are less sensitive to calcium or whether the buffer capacity of the cytosol for Ca, particularly near the junctions is enhanced in this model of heart failure. Considering that there is a fall in pHi in the myopathic cells it is reasonable to think that the smaller effect of high Cai on gj might be related to the intracellular acidity (19).

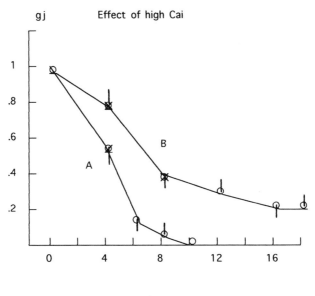

Figure 5. Effect of intracellular dialysis of 0.5 uM Ca on gj of normal hamsters (A) and cardiomyopathic hamster (B) 11 months old. Values of gj were normalized. Vertical line at each point - SEM.

1. The control of junctional conductance by beta-adrenergic receptor activation is impaired in the failing heart.

It is well known that the adrenergic receptors-G protein-adenyl cyclase complex is involved in an important signaling system entailed in the control of heart contractility (21, 22, 23).

Evidence is available that cardiac failure is accompanied by changes in autonomic regulation including a decreased parasympathetic tonus and an enhanced sympathetic control (24, 25).   It is also known that with the progress of the disease the cardiac muscle becomes quite insensitive to sympathetic stimulation (26, 27, 28) -a finding that has been attributed to the down regulation of beta-adrenoreceptor activation in the failing heart and also to a defective coupling of G-proteins to adenyl cyclase (29). An increase in the alpha - subunit of the inhibitory G protein was confirmed by pertussis toxin-catalyzed ADP ribosylation (30, 31). Moreover, myocardial Gi mRNA levels are elevated in terminal cardiac failure (30).

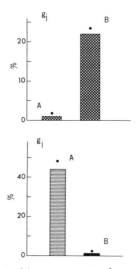

Figure 6. Bottom-Negligible effect of isoproterenol (10^{-6} M) on gj of CM cell pairs from hamsters 11 months old (B). At A-effect of the drug on gj of control of same age. Each bar is the average of 15 experiments. Black dot indicate SEM. Top - Small effect of forskolin (10^{-7} M) on gj of myopathic cell pairs (A) and controls (B) (n=14). From reference 32, with permission.

Recent studies made on the influence of beta-adrenergic receptor activation in cell pairs isolated from the ventricle of cardiomyopathic hamsters at late stage of the disease (11 months) indicated that isoproterenol (10^{-6} M) or forskolin (10^{-7} M) had no influence on gj as shown in Fig. 6 (32). These findings contrast with those obtained in cell pairs of normal hamsters of same age in which isoproterenol and forskolin at the same drug concentration increased gj by 45 ± 3% (n=13) and 23 ± 2.8% (n=16), respectively. The inhibition of phosphodiesterase with isobutyl-methylxanthine (10^{-6} M) which increased gj in the controls by 38 ± 1.5% (n=12) was unable to increment gj in the myopathic cell pairs (32). However, dibutyryl-cAMP (10^{-6} M)incremented gj by 58 ± 2.1% (n=14) in the cardiomyopathic hamster - an effect similar to that found in the normal hamster (Fig. 7; 32). This finding indicates that the activation of cAMP-dependent protein kinase by cAMP is able to increment gj as found in the normal heart (32, 34) supporting the notion that the lack of control of gj by the cAMP cascade is related to down regulation of beta adrenergic receptors and to a defect in the adenyl cyclase. Measurements of the time constant of cell membrane performed in isolated myocytes before (21 ± 3 ms) and after (20.7 ± 2.1 ms) dibutyryl cAMP (10^{-7} M) indicated that the drug is not altering the surface cell membrane resistance (p>0.05). The effect of the compound on gj, however, is inhibited by intracellular administration of an inhibitor of cAMP-dependent protein kinase (32) (Fig. 7).

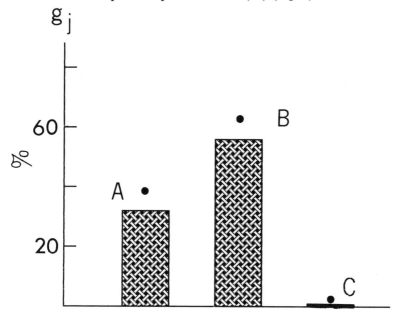

Figure 7. Effect of dibutyryl-cAMP (10^{-7} M) on gj of CM cell pairs from 11 months old hamsters (A) and controls of same age (B). At C suppression of the effect of dB-CAMP caused by intracellular dialysis of an inhibitor of PKA (20 ug/ml). Each bar is the average from 14 experiments. Black dot - SEM. From reference 32, with permission.

These observations indicate that sympathetic stimuli are unable to increase gj in cardiomyopathic myocytes at a late stage of the disease and that the enhanced conduction velocity and electrical synchronization usually seen under beta-adrenergic activation in the normal heart (35) is not present in the failing myocardium what creates a serious impairment of autonomic regulation preventing cardiovascular adjustments that are essential for cardiovascular homeostasis.

2. The role of the renin-angiotensin system on the regulation of gj and impulse propagation

Evidence is available that a local renin-angiotensin system exists in the heart (36, 37). Moreover, angiotensin II and renin activity have been demonstrated in aphrenic patients (38).

There are several lines of evidence supporting the notion that there is a local renin-angiotensin system in the heart: 1) angiotensin II receptors have been localized in cultured heart cells (39); 2) angiotensin I is converted to angiotensin II in the isolated and perfused rat heart (40); 3) genes of renin and angiotensinogen are coexpressed in cardiac muscle (41). An additional and important finding is that the beneficial effect of angiotensin converting enzyme inhibitors in patients with essential hypertension and congestive heart failure is not only dependent on the blockade of the plasma RAS but is also due to an effect on he cardiac RAS (40).

Although there is information concerning the effect of angiotensin II on heart contractility (42) the influence of the peptide and of the renin-angiotensin system as a whole on intercellular communication was not known at the moment we started these studies.

2.1 Influence of extracellular angiotensin II on heart cell coupling

In cell pairs isolated from normal adult rats angiotensin II (Ang II) (1 ug/ml) added to the bath caused a decline in gj of 60% within 45 sec (Fig. 8). The effect of the peptide was blocked by losartan what indicates that the activation of AT1 receptors is essential for the effect of Ang II (43). Moreover, the effect of the peptide on gj requires the activation of protein kinase C because staurosporine abolished the effect of angiotensin II. The activation of the kinase was probably related to the hydrolysis of phosphatidyl-inositol-4-5-biphosphate with consequent formation of diacylglycerol. Since the synthesis of inositol triphosphate leads to the release of calcium from intracellular stores the possibility that the increment in Cai be involved in the effect of the peptide cannot be discarded. However, in our experiments the use of high concentration of EGTA (10 mM) and HEPES (10mM) in the internal solution seems to indicate that the participation of changes in (Ca)i or pHi on the decline of gj is unlikely.

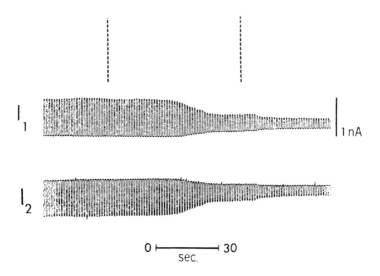

Figure 8. Effect of angiotensin II (1 ug/ml) on gj of normal and adult rat heart cell pair. Dotted lines indicate moment of drug administration. The holding potential for both cells was -40 mV. V$_1$ not shown. From reference 43, with permission.

The conclusion from these experiments was inescapably that the activation of the plasma renin-angiotensin system influences the degree of cell-to-cell communication in the normal myocardium. Conceivably, the decline in cell-to-cell coupling caused by Ang II can increase the intracellular resistance in muscle trabeculae with consequent impairment of impulse propagation. We have carried on studies on the influence of the peptide on the electrical properties of intact normal rat heart muscle and the results showed that the peptide causes a decrease in conduction velocity from 59.5 ± 2.5 cm/s to 35 ± 3.5 cms (44) while enalapril -an angiotensin converting enzyme inhibitor, reduced the intracellular resistance and increased the conduction velocity (45).

In cardiomyopathic hamsters (11 months old) Ang II (1 ug/ml) added to the extracellular fluid also reduced gj as shown in Fig. 9. An average decline of 53 ± 6.6% was seen with the peptide in cell pairs isolated from the CM ventricle and showing a gj of 7-35 nS. However, in the other population of cell pairs with very low values of gj (0.8-2.5 nS) cell uncoupling was seen with the same dose of Ang II within 2 min (Fig. 8). The effect of Ang II on cell communication is not related to a fall in surface cell membrane resistance because the peptide did not change the time constant of cell membrane determined in single cells under current-clamp configuration (8).

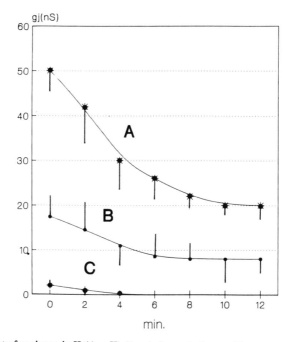

Figure 9. Effect of angiotensin II (Ang II) (1 ug/ml) on gj of normal hamsters (A) (n=14) and CM cell pairs with very low gj (C) and higher gj (7 to 35 nS) (B) (n=18). Vertical line at each point SEM. From reference 8, with permission.

2.2 Angiotensin converting enzyme inhibitors, cardiac failure and cell communication

Several clinical studies indicate that angiotensin converting enzyme (ACE) inhibitors reduce the mortality of patients with congestive heart failure (46). The mechanism of action of these compounds is not limited to the decline in afterload and preload, because there is evidence that these drugs prevent or reduce the ventricular hypertrophy elicited by aortic banding using low doses of the compounds which do not cause a decline of the arterial blood pressure (40). These findings might indicate that a decrease in the synthesis of Ang II in the heart is involved in the effect of the ACE inhibitors.

In rats with left ventricular infarction, for instance, the content of angiotensin converting enzyme as well as the mRNA levels of angiotensinogen and ACE are enhanced in the hypertrophied myocardium (47, 48). In cardiomyopathic hamsters (TO-2) similar increment of ACE activity was found during the late stages of the disease (Crespo and De Mello, unpublished). Furthermore, it is known that Ang II is a growth factor even in cultured heart cells. The peptide enhances the expression of proto-oncogenes such as c-myc and c-fos-an effect mediated by the activation of protein kinase C (49).

Recently, it has been shown that enalapril-an angiotensin converting enzyme inhibitor, increases the junctional conductance in rat isolated heart cell pairs (43). The effect of enalapril was seen within 4 in after its addition to the bath solution -a period of time probably needed to its conversion in enalaprilat. The effect of the ACE inhibitor is not related to cAMP formation or to an effect on bradykinin metabolism. It is then conceivable that in presence of elevated levels of Ang II in plasma enalapril can change gj by suppressing the synthesis of Ang II.

The increment in gj with enalapril (1 ug/ml) was also seen in normal and cardiomyopathic hamsters. In cardiomyopathic ventricle, the effect of enalapril was appreciable ($219 \pm 20.3\%$) in cell pairs with very low values of gj (0.8-2.5 nS) compared with controls ($33 \pm 5.4\%$) (see Fig. 10) while in cell pairs of the myopathic ventricle showing larger values of gj (7-35 nS) the increment in gj elicited by enalapril was of $80 \pm 10.8\%$ (8). Although the mechanism of action of enalapril is not clearly defined the possibility exists that the compound is increasing gj by inhibiting the synthesis of Ang II in the myocardium.

gj(%)

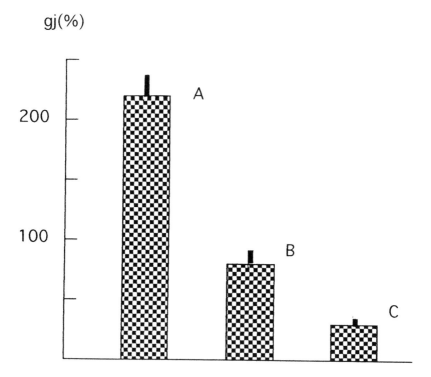

Figure 10. Effect of enalapril -an angiotensin converting enzyme inhibitor, (1 ug/ml) on gj of CM cell pairs with very low gj (0.8 - 2.5 nS) (A), in CM pairs with higher gj (7-35 nS) (B) and in control hamsters (C). Each bar is the average of 18 experiments. From reference 8, with permission.

The effect of the ACE inhibitor on gj is probably responsible, at least in part, for the increase in conduction velocity seen with the drug in muscle trabeculae isolated from the ventricle of CM hamsters (9) (see Table 1) and represents an important mechanism of prevention of slow conduction and reentry-two major components of cardiac arrhythmias. This finding and the increment in cardiac refractoriness elicited by enalapril in the ventricle of cardiomyopathic hamsters (9) indicate that the drug has antiarrhythmic properties.

TABLE 1

Conduction velocity (cm/s) of normal and cardiomyopathic isolated right ventricular muscle

Control		CM
42.7		36.9
(±1)		(±3)
(n=5)		(n=5)
	p<0.05	

Difference between the influence of enalapril on conduction velocity in control and cardiomyopathic ventricular muscle

Control*		CM*
22.5		77.1
(±0.75)		(±2.1)
(n=5)		(n=5)
	p<0.05	

*Numbers indicate increase in conduction velocity elicited by enalapril. An average of 4 measurements were made in each animal. From reference 9, with permission.

Furthermore, enalapril caused a hyperpolarization (6.8 mV) (p<0.05) of myopathic ventricular fibers with consequent increase of the action potential amplitude and facilitation of impulse propagation.

These observations seem to indicate that the activation of the cardiac RAS plays an important role on the impairment of cell coupling found in the ventricle of cardiomyopathic hamsters.

2.3 Is an intracellular renin-angiotensin system involved in the control of gap junction conductance?

The major difficulty of characterizing local renin-angiotensin systems was the possibility of contamination with the plasma RAS and the lack of appropriate biochemical methods.

The use of recombinant DNA technology has provided definitive information on the cardiac RAS. Renin and angiotensinogen transcripts have been localized in atria and ventricles of neonatal rat heart (50) and angiotensin I (Ang I), angiotensin II (Ang II) as well as the angiotensin converting enzyme (ACE) have been found inside cultured cardiac myocytes using immunofluorescent technique (51). The fact that these peptides have been found using in situ hybridization indicates that the elements needed for the synthesis of the compounds are inside the heart cell.

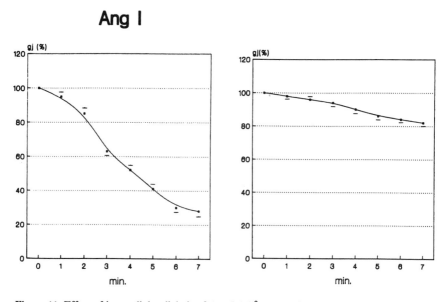

Figure 11. Effect of intracellular dialysis of Ang I (10^{-8} M) on gj of normal adult rat heart cell pairs (Left). At right the peptide was administered after enalapril (10^{-8} M). Each point average from 10 experiments. Vertical line - SME. From reference 52, with permission.

To study the role of an intracrine RAS on the control of junctional conductance studies were initially performed on ventricular myocytes isolated from normal adult rats. The results indicated that the administration of Ang

I (10^{-8} M) into the cytosol reduced gj by 76% within seven minutes (52). The possibility that this effect of Ang I on gj was related to its conversion to Ang II was investigated by adding enalaprilat to the pipettes solution prior to the addition of Ang I to the internal solution. In these experiments an electrode similar to that described by Irisawa and Kokubun (56) was used. Since the effect of Ang I was greatly reduced (but not abolished) by enalaprilat (Fig. 11) it is reasonable to think that the effect of Ang I on gj was mainly related to its conversion to Ang II. The finding that the effect of Ang I was not completely suppressed by enalaprilat probably means that other enzyme (probably a chymase) is also involved in the conversion of Ang I to Ang II (53).

The remaining question is whether Ang II, by itself, is able to reduced gj. The dialysis of Ang II into the cell also reduced gj by 60% within 45 sec (52) - an effect abolished by losartan given intracellularly. This result was quite appealing because not only indicates that the synthesis of Ang II inside the cardiac myocyte can control intercellular communication but also suggests that the activation of an intracellular receptor similar to AT1 is required for the effect of Ang II on gj. Moreover, the activation of protein kinase C is also involved in the effect of Ang II because the dialysis of the pseudo-substrate of protein kinase C (20 ug/ml) - an inhibitor of the kinase, into the cell abolished the effect of the peptide on gj (52). The fall in gj elicited by the activation of this kinase is probably related to the phosphorylation of gap junction proteins (33, 34). Indeed, in isolated cell pairs of the rat heart inhibitors of the protein kinase C increases gj (54).

Further support to the hypothesis that there is an intracrine RAS in the heart was provided by studies of the intracellular dialysis of renin (55). When renin (0.2 pmol/L) was added to the pipette solution and the compound was dialyzed in to the cell a fall in gj of 29 ± 3.8% (p<0.05) was found in seven minutes (see Fig. 55) (Fig. 12). Enalaprilat dialyzed previously into the cell reduced appreciably the effect of renin on gj what indicates that the effect of renin on gj was related to the synthesis of Ang II.

The simultaneous dialysis of angiotensinogen (0.4 pmol/L) and renin (0.2 pmol/L) caused an much greater decline of gj (see Fig. 12). These observations which are not related to a fall in surface cell membrane resistance or series resistance, might indicate that when the genes of renin and angiotensinogen are concomitantly expressed in heart cells an appreciable decline in gj is produced, particularly when the ACE activity is enhanced like in the case of heart failure.

The question whether the activation of the cardiac RAS is in part responsible for the abnormalities of cell communication and impulse propagation seen in the failing heart is of capital importance.

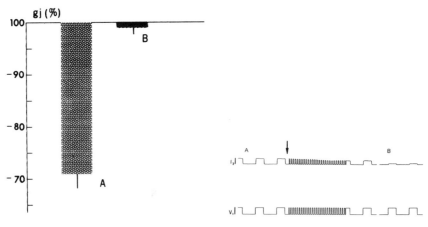

Figure 12. Left - (A) Effect of intracellular dialysis of renin (0.2 pmol/L) on gj of normal adult rat heart cell pairs. B - reduction of the effect of intracellular renin on gj elicited by enalaprilat. Each bar is the average from 11 experiments. Vertical line at each bar SEM. From reference 55, with permission.   Right - effect of intracellular dialysis of renin (0.2 pmol/L) plus angiotensinogen (0.4 pmol/L) on gj of single ventricular cell pair of the rat. I_2 - junctional current; V_1 - transjunctional voltage.   The polarity of I_2 was changed at the recorder. Calibration at I_2 - and V_1 - 2 nA and 20 mV, respectively.   From reference 55, with permission.

In studies made on isolated cell pairs from CM hamsters the intracellular dialysis of Ang I (10^{-8} M) caused cell uncoupling within 2 min in cell pairs with very low values of gj (see Fig. 13) while in the other group of cell pairs isolated from the same ventricle but presenting higher values of gj (7-35 nS) the decline in gj was of 66 ± 1.7% (n=12) within 9 -an effect greater than that seen in the controls hamsters of same age in which a decrease in gj of 50 ± 3.2% (n=5) was seen. In these experiments the influence of variations in dialysis rate was minimized by using pipettes with the same tip diameter.

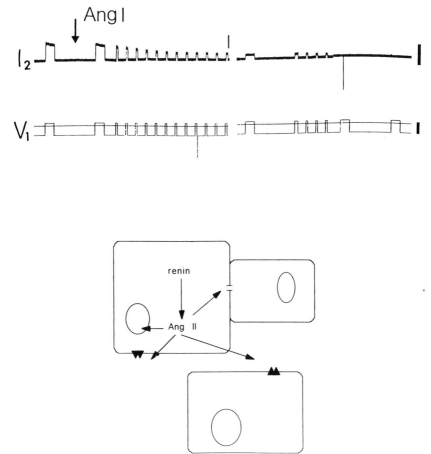

Figure 13. Top - Cell uncoupling elicited by intracellular dialysis of Ang I (10^{-8} M) in single cell pair of CM ventricle (11 months old). Calibration at I_2 - 0.05 nA; at V_1 - 40 mV. Polarity of I_2 changed at the recorder. From reference 8 with permission. Bottom - diagram illustrating the intracrine and paracrine action of Ang II. Small triangles at cell membrane represent Ang II receptors. From reference 55 with permission.

As in the case of normal cell pairs the effect of intracellular administration of Ang I was reduced by previous administration of enalaprilat (10^{-9} M) (see Fig. 14) and the intracellular dialysis of Ang II (10^{-8} M), by itself, reduced gj by 48 ± 4.2% (n=8) within 2.5 min. This effect of Ang II was similar to that seen in the control animals (40 ± 5.6%; n=9).

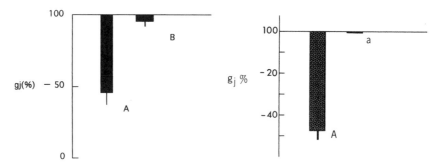

Figure 14. Left - A - effect of intracellular dialysis of Ang II (10^{-8} M) on gj of CM cell pairs. B - decrease of the effect of Ang I caused by enalaprilat (10^{-9} M). Each bar - average from 7 experiments. Vertical line - SEM. Right - suppression of the effect of intracellular administration of Ang II (10^{-8} M) on gj caused by losartan (10^{-8} M). From reference 8, with permission.

Here as in the case of normal controls, the effect of Ang I or Ang II seems to be unrelated to changes in Cai or pHi because high concentrations of EGTA and HEPES were used in the internal solution.

The interesting aspect of these experiments is that the effect of intracellular administration of Ang II was suppressed by the addition of losartan (10^{-8} M) to the cytosol (see Fig. 13). Since losartan is an specific AT1 Ang II receptor antagonist it is possible to conclude that in the failing heart as well as in the controls there is an intracellular Ang II receptor similar to AT1 whose activation is essential for the effect of the peptide on cell communication. Further studies will be necessary to clarify the physiological and pathological role of this receptor on the alteration of cell coupling seen in the failing heart.

3. Conclusion

The development of heart failure is a complex process involving different aspects. The present review provides evidence that the process of cell communication is greatly impaired, especially at late stages of the disease, when a decrease in gap junction conductance associated with severe destruction of the ventricular parenquima represent important factors in the generation of slow conduction, cardiac arrhythmias and the decline in heart contractility. The sequestration of large masses of ventricular myocytes from the normal process of excitation induced by the decrease in gj reduces the number of active cells involved in the process of ventricular contraction and contributes to the impairment of ventricular function. Moreover, the down regulation of beta-adrenergic receptors and the impairment in function of adenyl cyclase prevent the extrinsic regulatory mechanism of cardiac adjustment so necessary for the cardiovascular homeostasis.

Acknowledgements

The author wish to thank Ms. María González for technical help and Ms. Lagnny Jacobo Brito for the preparation of this manuscript. Moreover, I want to thank the American Heart Association and the National Institute of Health (HL 34148, 2S06GM-08224 and RR-03651) for their support.

REFERENCES

1. Morgan ME and Baker MM (1991). Cardiac hypertrophy: mechanical, neural and endocrine dependence. Circulation 1991; 83:23-25
2. Lossnitzer K, Janke J, Hein B, Stauch M and Fleckenstein A (1975). Disturbed myocardial calcium metabolism: a possible pathogenic factor in the hereditary cardiomyopathy of the Syrian hamster. In Fleckenstein A, Rona G, eds., Recent Advances in Studies on Cardiac Metabolism. Baltimore; Vol. VI, 207-215, University Park Press.
3. Wrogemann K and Nylen EG (1978). Mitochondrial calcium overloading in cardiomyopathic hamsters. J Mol Cell Cardiol; 10:185-195.
4. Jasmin G and Proschek L (1984). Calcium and myocardial cell injury. An appraisal in the cardiomyopathic hamster. Can J Physiol Pharmacol; 62:891-900.
5. Wesmand HF and Weinfeldt ML (1987). Toward an understanding of the molecular basis of cardiomyopathies. J Am Cell Cardiol; 10:1135-1138.
6. Bajusz E (1969). Dystrophic calcification of myocardium as conditioning factor in genesis of congestive heart failure: an experimental study. Am Heart J; 78:202-209.
7. Gertz EW (1992). Cardiomyopathic Syrian hamster; a possible model of human disease. Prog Exp Tumor Res 16; 242-247.
8. De Mello WC (1996). Renin-angiotensin system and cell communication in the failing heart. Hypertension, 27:1267-1272.
9. De Mello WC, Cherry R and Manivannan S (1997). Electrophysiologic and morphologic abnormalities in the failing heart; effect of enalapril on the electrical properties. Cardiac Failure 3:53-62.
10. Cherry JR and De Mello WC (1996). Confocal microscopy and intercellular communication in failing cardiomyopathic heart. FASEB J, April 14th, Abstract 2275.
11. Luque EA, Veenstra R, Beyer E and Lemanski LF (1994). Localization and distribution of gap junctions in normal and cardiomyopathic hamster heart. J Morphol 222:203-213.
12. Kanter HL, Laing JG, Beyer EC, Greeen KG and Saffitz JE (1993). Multiple connexins colocalize in canine ventricular myocyte gap junctions. Circ Res 73:344-350.
13. Bastide B, Neyses L, Ganten D and Traub O (1993). Gap junction protein connexin 40 is preferentelly expressed in vascular endothelium and conductive bandles of rat myocardium and is increased under hypertensive condictions. Circ Res, 73:1138-1149.
14. Severs NJ (1994). Pathophysiology of gap junctions in heart disease. J Cardiac Electrophysiol, 5:462-475.

15. Sen L, O'Neill M, Marsh JD and Smith TW (1990). Myocyte structure, function and calcium kinetics in the cardiomyopathic hamster heart. Am J Physiol; 259:H1533-H1543.

16. Fleckenstein A (1971). Specific inhibitors and promoters of calcium action in the excitation-contraction coupling of heart muscle and their role in the prevention or production of myocardial lesions. In: calcium and the Heart, P Harris and LH Opie, Eds pp 135-188, Londong Academic Press.

17. Hatem SN, Sham JSK and Morad M (1994). Enhanced Na^+-Ca^{2+} exchange exchange activity in cardiomyopathic Syrian hamster. Circ Res, 74:253-261.

18. De Mello WC (1975). Effect of intracellular injection of calcium and strontium on cell communication in heart. J Physiol (London) 250:231-245.

19. Noma A and Tsuboi N (1987). Dependence of junctional conductance on proton, calcium and magnesium ions in cardiac paired cells of guinea pig. J Physiol (London), 382:193-201.

20. Lazarus ML, Colgen JA and Sachs HG (1976). Quantitative light and electron microscopic comparison of the normal and cardiomyopathic Syrian hamster heart. J Mol Cell Cardiol, 31:431-441.

21. Epstein SE, Skelton CL, Levey GS and Entman M (1970). Adenyl cyclase and myocardial contractility. Ann Intern Med; 70:561-578.

22. Drummond GE and Severson DL (1979). Cyclic nucleotides and cardiac function. Circ Res; 44:145-152.

23. Brown AM and Birnbaumer L (1980). Ionic channels and their regulation by G protein subunits. Ann Rev Physiol; 52:197-213.

24. Eckberg DL (1980). Parasympathetic cardiovascular control in human disease; a critical review of methods and results. Am J Physiol; 239:H581-H593.

25. Francis GS and Cohn JN (1986). The autonomic nervous system in congestive heart failure. Ann Rev Med; 37:235-247.

26. Covell JW, Chidsey CA and Braunwald E. Reduction in the cardiac response to postganglionic sympathetic nerve stimulation in experimental heart failure. Circ Res 1966; 19:51-66.

27. Bristow MR, Ginsburg R, Minobe WA, Cubicciotti RS, Sageman WS, Luric K, Billingham ME, Harrison DC and Stinson EB (1982). Decreased catecholamine sensitivity and beta-adrenergic receptor density in failing human hearts. N Engl J Med; 307:205-211.

28. Fowler MB, Laser JA, Hopkins GL, Minobe W and Bristow MR (1986). Assessment of the beta-adrenergic receptor pathway in the intact failing human heart: Progressive receptor down-regulation and subsensitivity to agonist response. Circulation, 74:1290-1302.

29. Feldman AM, Rowena GT, Kessler PD, Weisman HF, Schulman SP, Blumenthal RS, Jackson KDG and Van Dop C (1990). Diminished beta-adrenergic receptor responsiveness and cardiac dilation in heart of myopathic Syryan hamsters are associated with functonal abnormality of the G stimulatory protein. Circulation, 81:1341-1352.

30. Bohm M, Gierschik P, Jakobs KH, Pieske B, Schnabel P, Ungerer M, Erdmann E (1990). Increase in Giσ in human heart with dilated but not ichemic cardiomyopathy. Circulation, 82:1249-1265.

31. Feldman AM, Cates AE, Veazey WB, Hershberger RE, Bristow M, Baughman KL, Baungartner WA and van Dop C (1988). Increase in the 40.000-mol-wt pertussis toxing substrate (G-protein) in the failing human heart. J Clin Invest, 82:189-197.

32. De Mello WC (1996). Impaired regulation of cell communication by beta-adrenergic receptor activation in the failing heart. Hypertension, 27:265-268.

33. De Mello WC (1984). Effect of intracellular injection of cAMP on the electrical coupling of mammalian cardiac cells. Biochem Biophys Res Commun, 119:1001-1007.

34. De Mello WC (1988). Increase in junctional conductance caused by isoproterenol in heart cell pairs is suppressed by cAMP-dependent protein kinase inhibitor. Biochem Biophys Res Comm, 154:509-514.

35. De Mello WC (1984). Modulation of junctional permeability. Fed Proc, 43:2692-2696.

36. Dzau VJ (1988). Cardiac renin-angiotensin system. Am J Med, 84:22-27.

37. Lindpaintner K, Jin M, Niedermaier N, Wilhelm MJ, Ganten D (1990). Cardiac angiotensinogen and its local activation in the isolated perfused beating heart. Circ Res, 67:564-573.

38. Campbell DJ (1985). The site of angiotensin production. J Hypertens, 3:199-207.

39. Rogers TB, Gaa AH and Allen IS (1986). Identification and characterization of functional angiotensin II receptors on cultured heart myocytes. J Pharmacol Exp Ther, 36:438-444.

40. Linz W, Scholkens BA, Han JF (1986). Beneficial effects of the converting enzyme inhibitor ramipril in ischemic rat hearts. J Cardiovasc Pharmacol 8: (Suppl 10) S91-S99.

41. Dzau VJ, Ingelfinger J, Pratt RE and Ellison KE (1986). Identification of renin and angiotensinogen RNA sequences in mouse and rat brains. Hypertension, 8:544.

42. Koch-Weser J (1965). Nature of the inotropic action of angiotensin on ventricular myocardium. Circ Res, 16:230-237.

43. De Mello WC and Altieri P (1992). The role of the renin-angiotensin system in the control of cell communication in the heart; effects of angiotensin II and enalapril. J Cardiovasc Pharmacol 20:643-651.

44. De Mello WC and Crespo M (1993). Effect of angiotensin II and enalapril on cardiac refractorinesss and conduction velocity. American Heart Association, 66th Scientific Session, November.

45. De Mello WC, Crespo MJ and Altieri P (1993). Effect of enalapril on intracellular resistance and conduction velocity in rat ventricular muscle. J Cardiovasc Pharmacol 22:259-263.

46. CONSENSUS Trial Study Group (1987) Effects of enalapril on mortality in severe congestive heart failure: Results of the Cooperative North Scandinavian Enalapril Survival Study. N Engl J Med 1987, 316:1429-1435.

47. Fabris B, Jackson B, Kohzuki M, Perich R and Johnston CI (1990). Increased cardiac angiotensin-converting enzyme activity in rats with chronic heart failure. Clin Ex Pharmacol Physiol 1990, 17:309-314.

48. Hirsh AT, Talsness CE, Schunkert H, Paul H and Dzau V (1991). Tissue-specific activation of cardiac angiotensin converting enzyme in experimental heart failure. Circ Res, 69:475-482.

49. Izumo S, Nadal-Ginard B and Mahdavi V (1988). Proto-oncogene induction and reprogramming of cardiac gene expression produced by pressure overload. Proc Nat Acad Sci, USA, 85:339-343.

50. Dostal DC, Rothblum KN, Conrad KM, Cooper GR and Baker KM (1992). Detection of angiotensin I and II in cultured rat cardiac myocytes and fibroblasts. Am J Physiol, 263:C851-C863.

51. Dostal DE, Rothblum KN, Chernin MI, Cooper GR and Baker K (1992). Intracardiac detection of angiotensinogen and renin: a localized renin-angiotensin system in the neonatal rat heart. Am J Physiol, 263:C838-C850.

52. De Mello WC, 1994. Is an intracellular renin-angiotensin system involved in the control of cell communication in heart? J Cardiovasc Pharmacol 23:640-646.

53. Urata H, Kinoshita A, Hisono KS, Bumpus FM and Husain A (1990). Identification of a highly specific chymase as the major angiotensin II - forming enzyme in the human heart. J Biol Chem, 265:22348-22357.

54. De Mello WC (1991). Effect of vasopresin and protein kinase C inhibitors on junctional conductance in isolated heart cell pairs. Cell Biol Int Rep, 15:467-78.

55. De Mello WC (1996). Influence of intracellular renin on heart cell communication. Hypertension, 25:1172-1177.

56. Irisawa H and Kokubun S (1983). Modulation by intracellular ATP and cyclic AMP of the slow inward current in isolated single ventricular cells of the guinea-pig. J Physiol (London) 338:321-337.

8 GAP JUNCTIONS AND CORONARY HEART DISEASE

Nicholas J. Severs

Imperial College School of Medicine at the National Heart and Lung Institute, Royal Brompton Hospital, Sydney Street, London SW3 6NP, England

Coronary heart disease, the generic term for ischemic heart disease, myocardial infarction and other manifestations of atherosclerosis of the coronary arteries, is the leading cause of death and disability in most industrialized countries of the developed world. Atherosclerosis is the process by which portions of the inner layer (intima) of an artery become thickened with fibromuscular material, lipid and calcium, forming plaques which lead to narrowing or occlusion of the vessel lumen.[1] The earlier stages of this disease process are silent, clinical symptoms usually only becoming apparent after decades of plaque progression. As the vessel lumen becomes obstructed with plaque, the blood supply to the portion of heart muscle served by the diseased artery becomes progressively restricted, eventually causing transient ischemia, which is commonly experienced as angina. Although this condition may persist in chronic stable form for many years, lipid-rich atherosclerotic plaques are prone to rupture, even when of a relatively small size and before angina becomes apparent. Plaque rupture precipitates coronary thrombosis, the acute, direct cause of life threatening unstable angina and myocardial infarction. Sudden death from myocardial infarction may occur without warning in individuals who have no prior overt symptoms. Alternatively, under the burden of repeated episodes of non-fatal infarction or less prolonged ischemia, progressive structural changes to the myocardium lead to gradually deteriorating cardiac function and end-stage heart failure. Whether the course of the disease is acute or chronic, arrhythmias are a common complication and the major immediate cause of sudden death. As gap junctions are the subcellular structures responsible for mediating the orderly cell-to-cell spread of action potentials which governs synchronous contractile activity in the healthy heart, a knowledge of these junctions forms an integral part of the framework for understanding the mechanisms of arrhythmogenesis in the diseased heart.[2-4]

The role of gap junctions in coronary heart disease may not be confined to cardiac dysfunction, however, but may start with the primary initiating events of disease in the arterial wall itself.[5,6] Atherosclerosis is a multifactorial disease process involving complex sets of interacting events at the cellular level, in particular, endothelial dysfunction, lipid accumulation in the intima, infiltration of monocyte/macrophages and conversion of macrophages into foam cells.[7] The net effect of these events is release of growth factors, cytokines and mitogens which act on smooth muscle cells, transforming them from their normal contractile form to a synthetic phenotype capable of migration, proliferation and active synthesis of the large quantities of fibrotic material that leads to bulk growth of the plaque. Recent indirect evidence raises the possibility that gap-junction mediated intercellular communication, in addition to extracellular signalling mechanisms, participates in the early cellular interactions of the atherogenic process.

The theme of this chapter, then, is that gap junctions in both their guises — as pathways for intercellular signalling in arterial cells and for electrical coupling in the myocardium — potentially have important roles respectively in the genesis of the primary disease process afflicting the artery and in the resultant arrhythmic dysfunction of the heart. Selected aspects of these dual aspects of gap junction function in coronary heart disease will be outlined, with emphasis on recent studies from the author's laboratory.

1. GAP JUNCTIONS AND CONNEXIN EXPRESSION IN THE ARTERIAL WALL

1.1 The Healthy Artery

In the healthy artery, gap-junctional communication between vascular wall cells is implicated in the local modulation of vasomotor tone and maintenance of circulatory homeostasis.[8-11] In arteries and arterioles, the endothelium is typically more extensively linked by gap junctions than is the underlying medial smooth muscle. The endothelium on the venous side of the vascular tree has fewer, smaller gap junctions than that on the arterial side, and gap junctions are rare in small coronary veins and absent in collecting venules and capillaries.[9] Contacts between endothelial cells and superficial smooth muscle cells are formed through breaks in the internal elastic lamina, especially in smaller coronary arteries and arterioles, and heterocellular gap junctions, implicated in communication between endothelium and smooth muscle, may be found at these sites.[8,9,12] Dye tracer studies in isolated arterioles indicate that gap-junctional coupling between endothelial cells is more extensive than that between the underlying smooth muscle cells, and that heterocellular communication is predominantly one directional, from endothelium to smooth muscle, rather than the reverse.[13]

The connexin composition of vascular cell gap junctions varies according to cell type and location. Smooth muscle cells of larger arteries *in situ* normally express only connexin43, though in some arterioles (e.g., rat brain) and in the A7r5 aortic smooth muscle cell line, connexin40 has also been reported.[6,14-16] Arterial and arteriolar endothelial cells express connexin40, connexin37 and, in some instances, connexin43.[15-17] Recent studies applying specific cell markers to permit unequivocal localization of connexins to the endothelium by confocal microscopy of sections of the intact arterial wall have demonstrated that the precise combinations and amounts of these three connexins vary in different arteries. For example, connexin43 is present in pulmonary artery and aortic endothelium, together with abundant connexin40 and heterogeneous, scattered connexin37; coronary artery endothelium, on the other hand, lacks connexin43.[16] By multiple immunogold label electron microscopy applied to pulmonary artery endothelium, individual gap-junctional plaques have been shown to contain all three connexin types.[18] Within a given vascular site, substantial regional variation in connexin expression may occur; for example, in the rat endocardium, a zone just below the mitral valve region is marked by conspicuous expression of connexin43 compared with surrounding areas.[16] As gap junction channels composed of different connexin types expressed *in vitro* are documented to show distinctive molecular permeability, ionic selectivity and conductance properties,[19-23] differential expression of connexins has been hypothesized to contribute to the modulation of endothelial gap junction function in different segments and sub-zones of the arterial system.[16]

1.2 The Diseased and Injured Arterial Wall

Endothelial gap junction coupling has been implicated in the coordination of endothelial cell migration and replication during repair of the injured artery,[8,24] but little information is available on the extent to which endothelial connexin expression patterns of the intact artery are modulated during disease or injury processes. Recent studies on arterial smooth muscle, by contrast, demonstrate that a conspicuous upregulation of connexin43 gap junctions goes hand-in-hand with the phenotypic transformation of smooth muscle cells responsible for intimal growth in arterial injury and atherosclerosis. In cultured smooth muscle cells, immunodetectable connexin43 expression is high in synthetic-type cells but low in contractile-type cells,[25] and this relationship is paralleled in human coronary atherosclerosis, where a marked increase in expression of connexin43-gap junctions between intimal smooth muscle cells occurs in the early stages of disease (Fig. 1). With further lesion growth and accumulation of extracellular matrix material, gap junction quantity subsequently declines[6] in line with reduced intercellular communication reported in cultured smooth muscle cells isolated from atherosclerotic lesions.[26] A prominent upregulation of connexin43 gap junctions, similar to that observed in the early stages of atherosclerosis, is also found in smooth muscle cells of the neointima formed after injuring the rat carotid artery using a balloon catheter (Fig. 2). In this procedure, inflation of a balloon within the artery removes the endothelium and stimulates rapid proliferation of smooth muscle cells.[27,28] Similar intraluminal balloons are used in balloon angioplasty, an intervention designed to restore coronary artery patency in patients with arteries blocked with plaque, and a common complication of this procedure is restenosis due to injury-provoked smooth muscle cell proliferation.[29,30]

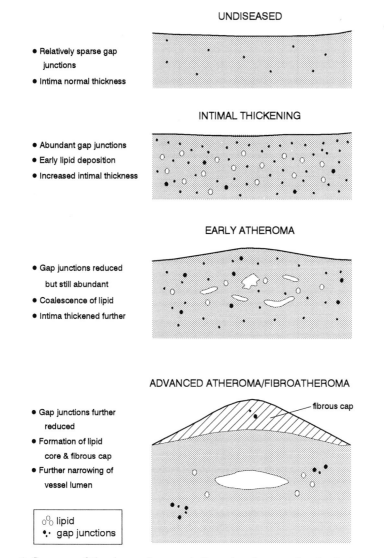

UNDISEASED

- Relatively sparse gap junctions
- Intima normal thickness

INTIMAL THICKENING

- Abundant gap junctions
- Early lipid deposition
- Increased intimal thickness

EARLY ATHEROMA

- Gap junctions reduced but still abundant
- Coalescence of lipid
- Intima thickened further

ADVANCED ATHEROMA/FIBROATHEROMA

- Gap junctions further reduced
- Formation of lipid core & fibrous cap
- Further narrowing of vessel lumen

fibrous cap

lipid
gap junctions

Figure 1. Summary of the changes in connexin43-gap junction quantity, distribution and size during the pathogenesis of human coronary atherosclerosis. (Adapted from Blackburn, J. et al., Arterioscler Thromb Vasc Biol 1995; 15:1219-1228).

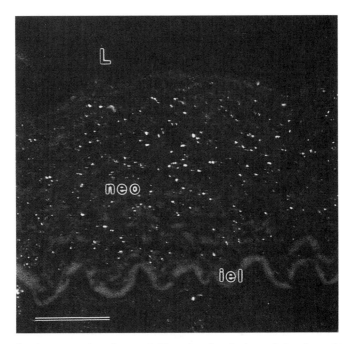

Figure 2. Abundant expression of connexin43 gap junctions in the neointima formed two weeks after balloon catheter injury in the rat carotid artery, as seen by immunoconfocal microscopy. L, lumen; neo, neointima; iel, internal elastic lamina. (From Severs, N.J. et al., Annual of Cardiac Surgery, 9th Edition, Eds. Yacoub, M.H. and Carpentier, A.F., pp.31-44, Rapid Science Publishers, London, 1996). Scale bar: 50 m.

In the rat carotid model, a transient increase in smooth muscle cell gap junction expression occurs prior to neointimal formation, in the innermost (subluminal) medial zone, the major site from which the cells subsequently found in the neointima are recruited.[31] Enhanced connexin43 gap junction expression by arterial smooth muscle cells *in vivo* thus features as an early event both in the slowly evolving intimal growth of atherosclerotic disease, and in the much more rapid intimal growth induced by balloon injury. This increased potential for gap-junctional communication between smooth muscle cells appears to be closely linked both to the phenotypic transition process itself and subsequent maintenance of the synthetic state. The precise relationship between connexin43 upregulation and the migratory and proliferative properties associated with the synthetic phenotype in smooth muscle cells appears complex, however. To migrate, smooth muscle cells would be expected to shed their links with their neighbors, and cell division is associated with gap junction down-regulation. Thus, while connexin43 gap junction upregulation in smooth muscle cells is clearly a correlate of the synthetic phenotype and intimal growth, not all synthetic state smooth muscle cells necessarily have an abundance of connexin43 gap junctions at all times. Increased gap junction formation may occur as a transient event in the cell cycle of the asynchronously dividing populations of smooth muscle cells and/or may be a more permanent feature of specific sub-populations of synthetic cells that are neither actively migrating nor undergoing division. Why smooth muscle cells might need to communicate under these circumstances, the nature of the putative signalling molecules involved, and the possible significance of gap junctions as a growth control mechanism in this setting, are key questions for further investigation. Recent evidence that connexin expression is influenced by growth factors in cultured smooth muscle cells[32,33] raises the possibility of interactions between extracellular signalling and direct cell-to-cell communication in the modulation of smooth muscle cell behavior in arterial injury and disease. Thrombin, in particular, has been found to be a potent simulator of connexin43 expression in cultured arterial smooth muscle cells,[33,34] and could plausibly mediate similar effects in prothrombogenic sites denuded of endothelium after balloon injury *in vivo*.

2. GAP JUNCTION ORGANIZATION AND CONNEXIN EXPRESSION IN THE MYOCARDIUM

2.1 The Normal Heart

As is emphasized throughout this volume, cardiac myocytes are extensively interconnected by gap junctions. In working myocytes of the ventricular myocardium, the gap junctions are characteristically organized, together with two types of anchoring junction, the fascia adherens and desmosome, in intercalated disks (Fig. 3). The fasciae adherentes and desmosomes are responsible respectively for attachment of the contractile filaments and the cytoskeleton to sites of adherence between the adjoining plasma membranes. Between them, the three types of junction of the disk act in concert to integrate cardiac electromechanical function. The size and abundance of gap junctions, their organization within the intercalated disks, and the overall distribution pattern of gap junctions and their component connexins in the tissue as a whole, are key contributors to the normal uniform anisotropic pattern of impulse spread of the healthy adult heart.[3,4,35-37] In the atrioventricular node, where conduction is slowed to ensure sequential contraction of atria and ventricles, gap junctions are sparse and small, whereas in Purkinje fibres and working myocardium, where rapid spread of depolarization throughout the ventricles is required, gap junctions are abundant and large. Such gap junction features are in part a product of the overall tissue architecture, in which variation in shape and size of myocytes results in variations in morphology (or lack) of intercalated disks. A specific feature of myocytes with well defined intercalated disks (as in left ventricular working myocardium) is the presence of a population of large gap junctions at the periphery of the disk circumscribing an inner zone containing smaller gap junctions (Fig. 4), an arrangement thought to contribute to efficiency of propagation of the impulse in the longitudinal axis.[36,38,39]

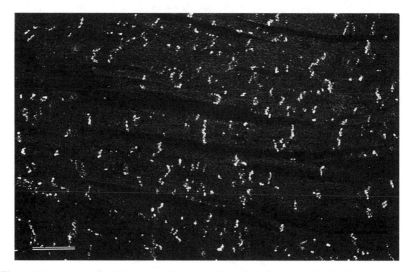

Figure 3. Immunoconfocal detection of connexin43 gap junctions in longitudinally sectioned left ventricular myocardium (rat), illustrating the characteristic organization of gap junctions in the intercalated disks at the end-on abutments between the cells. (From Severs, N.J. et al., J. Microsc. 1993; *169*:299-328). Scale bar: 100 m.

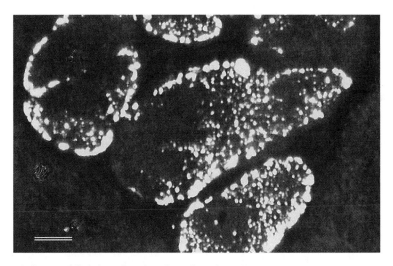

Figure 4. Immunolabeled gap junctions in *en face*-viewed intercalated disks. Note ring of large gap junctions at the disk periphery (image reconstructed from stack of serial optical sections from transversely sectioned human left ventricular myocardium; from Severs, N.J. et al., Annual of Cardiac Surgery, 9th Edition, Eds. Yacoub, M.H. & Carpentier, A.F., pp. 31-44, Rapid Science Publishers, London, 1996). Scale bar: 10 m.

2.2 Spatial Distribution of Connexins in Heart

Three principal connexins are expressed by cardiac muscle cells, connexin43, connexin40 and connexin45.[40-50] Connexin43, the predominant isoform, is expressed in abundance in the ventricles, while connexin40 is preferentially expressed by specialized myocytes of the atrioventricular conduction system. Large quantities of both connexin40 and connexin43 are present in the Purkinje fibres and bundle branches, and small amounts of connexin40 are sometimes detectable (with the usual large quantities of connexin43) in a limited zone of ventricular myocardium just beneath the endocardium.[41,42,51,52] In atrial myocardium, connexin40 is commonly co-expressed with connexin43.[45,52-54] Connexin45 is reported to occur more or less ubiquitously throughout the heart[43,44,46,54] though information on this connexin is less complete than that for connexins 43 and 40, and the possibility of distinct, spatially defined patterns of expression should not be excluded. While this generalized outline applies to most species, some interspecies variation does occur[45] (e.g., connexin40 is not abundant in the atrium of all species, and the guinea pig lacks connexin40 in the bundle branches and Purkinje fibres[52]). Variations in the pattern of expression of these three cardiac connexins are hypothesized to contribute to electrophysiological specialization in defined tissue regions of the heart. As noted earlier, gap junction channels constructed from different connexin types *in vitro* have distinctive properties; studies on cells stably transfected with cDNAs encoding different connexins show that while connexin45 channels have low unitary conductances (26 pS) compared with connexin43 channels ($\sim$60pS), connexin40 channels have high conductance values (typically, $\sim$160 pS).[20,22,23,55] The high levels of connexin40 in the Purkinje fibre system have, accordingly, been implicated in rapid distribution of the impulse throughout the working ventricular myocardium.

2.3 Coronary Heart Disease, Gap junctions and Arrhythmia

Reentrant electrical circuits form the underlying mechanisms of most cardiac arrhythmias. Macro-reentry due to an accessory atrioventricular conduction pathway (Wolff-Parkinson White syndrome) would be predicted to involve aberrant gap junction distribution such that a coupled link is established between the atrium and ventricle where one would not normally occur. Some surgically-resected pathways have indeed been shown to comprise strands of myocytes connected by intercalated disks containing connexin43 gap junctions similar to those of working ventricular myocytes.[56] Micro-reentry arrhythmias are a major cause of sudden death in patients with coronary heart disease, and although alterations in the active ionic membrane properties of the myocyte may contribute to the genesis of these arrhythmias, abnormal intercellular conduction appears, in many instances, to be the key underlying factor.[4,57-61] The initiating causes of re-entrant arrhythmia are heterogeneous wavefront propagation, reduced conduction velocity and localized uni-directional block, and a number of studies have identified gap junction defects that could plausibly give rise to these conditions.[3,4,58]

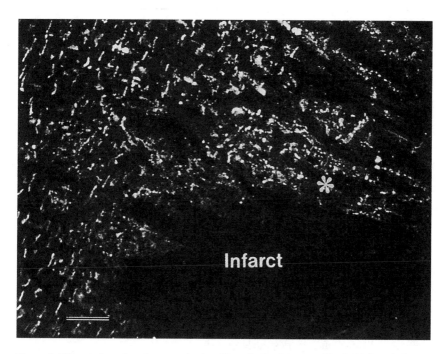

Figure 5. Disrupted gap junction organization (*) at the border zone of healed infarct in human left ventricular myocardium. Elsewhere (e.g., top and bottom left of field), gap junction organization is similar to that observed in normal myocardium (Figure 3). From Severs, N.J. et al., J. Microsc. 1993; *169*:299-328). Scale bar: 50 m.

In the zones adjacent to healed canine infarcts, which are prone to develop re-entry arrhythmia, reduced size and frequency of gap junctions combined with fewer intercalated disk contacts per myocyte have been reported from quantitative electron and light microscopical studies.[4,59,62] A conspicuous abnormality at the border of infarct scar tissue in human ischemic heart disease is loss of the normal ordered distribution of connexin43 gap junctions; instead of being confined to intercalated disks at the end-on abutments between the myocytes (Fig. 3), immunoconfocal microscopy reveals the junctions to be spread chaotically over the lateral surfaces of the cells (Fig. 5).[63] Such abnormalities in gap junction distribution are not solely due to late stages in myocardial degeneration and remodelling associated with fibrosis, but are detectable within a few days after myocardial infarction in dog and rat models.[64,65] By correlating gap junction distribution visualized by confocal microscopy with activation maps obtained using a high resolution electrode array in the surviving epicardial border zone overlying 4-day old anterior canine infarcts, such disordered patterns of gap junction distribution have been shown to correspond to the location of the common central pathway of re-entrant ventricular tachycardia circuits.[64] Abnormal patterns of gap junction localization have also been reported in other pathological settings associated with an increased arrhythmic tendency, in particular hypertrophic cardiomyopathy in humans[66] and in the cardiomyopathic hamster.[67]

In addition to disrupted patterns of gap junction organization in the immediate vicinity of the infarct, quantitative immunoconfocal microscopy reveals a generalized decrease in the quantity of connexin43 gap junctions per myocyte throughout the left ventricular myocardium of ischemic heart disease patients undergoing coronary by-pass operations,[68] and quantitative northern blotting of left ventricular samples from transplant patients with end-stage ischemic heart disease shows a corresponding reduction in connexin43 mRNA levels.[69] Reduced immunodetectable connexin43 is found both in angina patients with exercise-induced reversible ischemia[68] and in patients with documented hibernating myocardium,[70] a state in which myocardial function is persistently impaired at rest due to severely reduced coronary blood flow but which is reversible after by-pass surgery.[71] However, the reduction in immunolabeled gap junctions is greater in hibernating myocardium than in reversibly ischemic myocardium, with loss of the large gap junctions at the disk periphery featuring prominently in the hibernating group.[70] Apart from coronary heart disease, reduced expression of connexin43 in the left ventricular myocardium may contribute to arrhythmogenesis in other cardiac disease settings such as end-stage dilated cardiomyopathy[69] and human hypertrophy in the absence of ischemia,[68] as well as in animal models (e.g., transgenic hypertensive rats[51]) and in a cell culture-model of Chagas' disease[72] (the most common cause of heart disease in South America).

Apart from changes in the distribution of immunolocalized gap junctions and down-regulation of connexin43, the hypothesis that altered expression of other connexin types may contribute to electrophysiological

dysfunction in cardiac disease has been raised.[36,51] In the left ventricle of hypertensive rats and in the infarcted rat heart, increased connexin40 has been discussed as a possible compensatory response to down-regulation of connexin43.[51,73] Some evidence that connexin40 mRNA may be upregulated in the left ventricle of transplant patients with end-stage ischemic heart disease is apparent from northern and dot blot analysis, but if any increase in the corresponding protein does occur, this remains at levels too low to be detectable by western blotting or immunocytochemistry.[74] Connexin45 mRNA is found only at very low levels in the ventricles of these patients and, like connexin43, appears to be reduced in end-stage human heart disease; however, as connexin45 protein is found only in trace quantities by immunoconfocal microscopy, the significance of this connexin in the diseased heart is difficult to assess. The possibility that distinctive alterations in the pattern of expression of multiple connexins may contribute to arrhythmic tendency in ischemic and other human heart disease remains to be more fully investigated.

3. GRAFTING, SURGERY, AND RESTORATION OF GAP-JUNCTIONAL COMMUNICATION IN THE DISEASED HEART

Compared with the adult heart, the developing heart has a greater capacity to remodel and self-repair. Post-natal development is marked by a progressive, coordinated patterning of connexin43 gap junctions and fasciae adherentes from an initially dispersed distribution to the polar organization within intercalated disks found in the fully differentiated working myocyte. This process of gap junction organization is not completed until approximately 3 months of age in the rat and 6 years of age in the human,[75,76] and at the functional level, correlates with increasing anisotropy and altered mechanics.[75,77] Cardiac plasticity, allowing further growth and development, is thus associated with the dispersed gap junction distribution, while the adult ventricle, though functionally more efficient, appears less able to adapt to altered hemodynamics. These observations may have relevance to the timing of corrective cardiac surgery for congenital malformations since early reconstructive operations are associated with fewer late postoperative arrhythmias and with improved cardiac function compared with late surgery. Such advantages may stem from greater ability of the still-developing ventricle to remodel.

In the adult, however, cardiac muscle cells are unable to regenerate, or at best have only a restricted capacity to do so, and hence the capacity for self-repair of myocardium damaged by acquired disease is limited. A series of studies has therefore explored the feasibility of grafting healthy myocytes or myocardial tissue into host hearts to repair damage caused by disease or other injury.[78,79] Success with this strategy depends on the full and complete integration of the graft with host myocardium by formation of intercalated disks and establishment of gap junctions. Grafted fetal myocytes in the mouse heart have been shown to form intercalated disks and gap junctions with host myocytes, and connexin43 expression has been demonstrated at the donor-host myocyte border in a dystrophic dog model.[78,79] Furthermore, cardiac transplant patients eventually show restoration of synchronized electromechanical activity between host and donor regions of the left atrium, further demonstrating that integration at the level of the gap junction is feasible in practice.[3]

4. CONCLUDING COMMENT

Research in the gap junction field continues to develop at great pace. Some of the aspects highlighted in this chapter reflect a gathering interest in research aimed at bridging the gap between fundamental gap junction science and the role of gap junctions in the pathogenesis of human cardiovascular disease. We may be permitted to hope that this synthesis may bring eventual benefits in the form of practical clinical applications.

ACKNOWLEDGMENTS:

Work reported and illustrated here from the authors' laboratory was supported by The Wellcome Trust (Grant No. 046218/Z/95) and the British Heart Foundation (Grant No. PG 93136). I thank all those who have contributed to the development of this work, in particular Dr C.R. Green, Dr. R.G. Gourdie, Dr E. Harfst, Dr N.S. Peters, Mr J. Smith, Mr J. Blackburn, Dr H-I Yeh, Dr. E. Dupont, Dr R.R. Kaprielian, Dr Y-S Ko and Mr S. Rothery.

REFERENCES

1. Fuster V, Ross R and Topol EJ: Atherosclerosis and Coronary Artery Disease. Volume 1 & 2. Lippincott-Raven, Philadelphia, 1996; 1-1661.
2. Gros DB, Jongsma HJ: Connexins in mammalian heart function. BioEssays 1996; 18:719-730.
3. Severs NJ, Dupont E, Kaprielian RR, et al. Gap junctions and connexins in the cardiovascular system. In Yacoub MH, Carpentier A, Pepper J, et al, eds: Annual of Cardiac Surgery 1996: 9th edition. Current Science, London, 1996; 31-44.
4. Saffitz JE, Davis LM, Darrow BJ, et al: The molecular basis of anisotropy; role of gap junctions. J Cardiovasc Electrophysiol 1995; 6:498-510.
5. Navab M, Ross LA, Hama S, et al: Interactions of human aortic wall cells in co-culture. Atherosclerosis Reviews 1991; 23:153-160.
6. Blackburn JP, Peters NS, Yeh H-I, et al: Upregulation of connexin43 gap junctions during early stages of human coronary atherosclerosis. Arterioscler Thromb Vasc Biol 1995; 15:1219-1228.
7. Ross R: The pathogenesis of atherosclerosis: A perspective for the 1990s. Nature 1993; 362:801-809.
8. Larson DM. Intercellular junctions and junctional transfer in the blood vessel wall. In Ryan U, ed: Endothelial Cells III. CRC Press, Boca Raton, 1988; 75-88.
9. Severs NJ. Constituent cells of the heart and isolated cell models in cardiovascular research. In Piper HM, Isenberg G, eds: Isolated Adult Cardiomyocytes. volume 10. CRC Press Inc., Boca Raton, 1989; 3-41.
10. Severs NJ, Robenek H. Constituents of the arterial wall and atherosclerotic plaque: an introduction to atherosclerosis. In Robenek H, Severs NJ, eds: Cell Interactions in Atherosclerosis. CRC Press, Boca Raton, 1992; 1-49.
11. Christ GJ, Spray DC, El-Sabban M, et al: Gap junctions in vascular tissues - Evaluating the role of intercellular communication in the modulation of vasomotor tone. Circ Res 1996; 79:631-646.
12. Rhodin JAG. Architecture of the vessel wall. In Bohr DF, Somlyo AP, Sparks HV, eds: Handbook of Physiology. The Cardiovascular System. American Physiological Society, Bethesda, 1980; 1-31.
13. Little TL, Xia J, Duling BR: Dye tracers define differential endothelial and smooth muscle coupling patterns within the arteriolar wall. Circ Res 1995; 76:498-504.
14. Beyer EC, Reed KE, Westphale EM, et al: Molecular cloning and expression of rat connexin40, a gap junction protein expressed in vascular smooth muscle. J Membr Biol 1992; 127:69-76.
15. Little TL, Beyer EC, Duling BR: Connexin 43 and connexin 40 gap junctional proteins are present in arteriolar smooth muscle and endothelium in vivo. Am J Physiol Heart Circ Physiol 1995; 268:H729-H739.

16. Yeh H-I, Dupont E, Coppen S, et al: Gap junction localization and connexin expression in cytochemically identified endothelial cells from arterial tissue. J Histochem Cytochem 1997; in press.

17. Reed KE, Westphale EM, Larson DM, et al: Molecular cloning and functional expression of human connexin37, an endothelial cell gap junction protein. J Clin Invest 1993; 91:997-1004.

18. Ko Y-S, Yeh H-I, Rothery S, et al: Conexin make-up of the endothelial gap junction probed by triple label immunoelectron microscopy. J Mol Cell Cardiol 1997; in press: (Abstract).

19. Beblo DA, Wang HZ, Beyer EC, et al: Unique conductance, gating, and selective permeability properties of gap junction channels formed by connexin40. Circ Res 1995; 77:813-822.

20. Bukauskas FF, Elfgang C, Willecke K, et al: Biophysical properties of gap junction channels formed by mouse connexin40 in induced pairs of transfected human HeLa cells. Biophys J 1995; 68:2289-2298.

21. Veenstra RD, Wang HZ, Beblo DA, et al: Selectivity of connexin-specific gap junctions does not correlate with channel conductance. Circ Res 1995; 77:1156-1165.

22. White TW, Paul DL, Goodenough DA, et al: Functional analysis of selective interactions among rodent connexins. Mol Biol Cell 1995; 6:459-470.

23. White TW, Bruzzone R: Multiple connexin proteins in single intercellular channels: connexin compatibility and functional consequences. J Bioenerg Biomembr 1996; 28:339-350.

24. Pepper MS, Montesano R, El Aoumari A, et al: Coupling and connexin 43 expression in microvascular and large vessel endothelial cells. Am J Physiol (Cell Physiol) 1992; 262:C1246-C1257.

25. Rennick RE, Connat J-L, Burnstock G, et al: Expression of connexin43 gap junctions between cultured vascular smooth muscle cells is dependent upon phenotype. Cell Tissue Res 1993; 271:323-332.

26. Andreeva ER, Serebryakov VN, Orekhov AN: Gap junctional communication in primary culture of cells derived from human aortic intima. Tissue Cell 1995; 27:591-597.

27. Kocher O, Gabbiani F, Gabbiani G, et al: Phenotypic features of smooth muscle cells during the evolution of experimgntal carotid artery intimal thickening. Biochemical and morphologic studies. Lab Invest 1991; 65:459-470.

28. Thyberg J, Blomgren K, Hedin U, et al: Phenotypic modulation of smooth muscle cells during the formation of neointimal thickenings in the rat carotid artery after balloon injury: an electron-microscopic and stereological study. Cell Tissue Res 1995; 281:421-433.

29. Haudenschild CC: Pathobiology of restenosis after angioplasty. Am J Med 1993; 94:40S-44S.

30. Lovqvist A, Emanuelsson H, Nilsson J, et al: Pathophysiological mechanisms for restenosis following coronary angioplasty: possible preventive alternatives. J Intern Med 1993; 233:215-226.
31. Yeh H-I, Lupu F, Dupont E, et al: Balloon catheter injury stimulates upregulation of connexin43 gap junctions in rat carotid artery. J Mol Cell Cardiol 1997; in press: (Abstract).
32. Mensink A, Brouwer A, Van den Burg EH, et al: Modulation of intercellular communication between smooth muscle cells by growth factors and cytokines. Eur J Pharmacol 1996; 310:73-81.
33. Yeh H-I, Kanthou C, Dupont E, et al: Differential effects of growth factors on gap junction expression in cultured human aortic smooth muscle cells. Eur Heart J 1996; 17:397. (Abstract)
34. Dupont E, Yeh H-I, Kanthou C, et al: Rapid modulation of gap junction expression by thrombin in cultured human smooth muscle cells. Eur Heart J 1996; 17:197. (Abstract)
35. Spach MS, Heidlage JF: The stochastic nature of cardiac propagation at a microscopic level: Electrical description of myocardial architecture and its application to conduction. Circ Res 1995; 76:366-380.
36. Severs NJ: Cardiac muscle cell interaction: from microanatomy to the molecular make-up of the gap junction. Histol Histopathol 1995; 10:481-501.
37. ten Velde I, De Jonge B, Verheijck EE, et al: Spatial distribution of connexin43, the major cardiac gap junction protein, visualizes the cellular network for impulse propagation from sinoatrial node to atrium. Circ Res 1995; 76:802-811.
38. Gourdie RG, Green CR, Severs NJ: Gap junction distribution in adult mammalian myocardium revealed by an antipeptide antibody and laser scanning confocal microscopy. J Cell Sci 1991; 99:41-55.
39. Hall J, Gourdie RG: Spatial organization and structure of cardiac gap junctions can affect access resistance. Microsc Res Tech 1995; 31:446-451.
40. Beyer EC, Kistler J, Paul DL, et al: Antisera directed against connexin43 peptides react with a 43-kd protein localized to gap junctions in myocardium and other tissues. J Cell Biol 1989; 108:595-605.
41. Gourdie RG, Severs NJ, Green CR, et al: The spatial distribution and relative abundance of gap-junctional connexin40 and connexin43 correlate to functional properties of the cardiac atrioventricular conduction system. J Cell Sci 1993; 105:985-991.
42. Kanter HL, Laing JG, Beau SL, et al: Distinct patterns of connexin expression in canine Purkinje fibers and ventricular muscle. Circ Res 1993; 72:1124-1131.
43. Davis LM, Kanter HL, Beyer EC, et al: Distinct gap junction protein phenotypes in cardiac tissues with disparate conduction properties. J Am Coll Cardiol 1994; 24:1124-1132.

44. Kanter HL, Saffitz JE, Beyer EC: Molecular cloning of two human cardiac gap junction proteins, connexin40 and connexin45. J Mol Cell Cardiol 1994; 26:861-868.

45. Van Kempen MJA, ten Velde I, Wessels A, et al: Differential connexin distribution accommodates cardiac function in different species. Microsc Res Tech 1995; 31:420-436.

46. Davis LM, Rodefeld ME, Green K, et al: Gap junction protein phenotypes of the human heart and conduction system. J Cardiovasc Electrophysiol 1995; 6:813-822.

47. Fishman GI, Hertzberg EL, Spray DC, et al: Expression of connexin43 in the developing rat heart. Circ Res 1991; 68:782-787.

48. Van Kempen MJA, Fromaget C, Gros D, et al: Spatial distribution of connexin43, the major cardiac gap junction protein, in the developing and adult rat heart. Circ Res 1991; 68:1638-1651.

49. Fromaget C, El Aoumari A, Gros D: Distribution pattern of connexin43, a gap-junctional protein, during the differentiation of mouse heart myocytes. Differentiation 1992; 51:9-20.

50. Gourdie RG, Green CR, Severs NJ, et al: Immunolabelling patterns of gap junction connexins in the developing and mature rat heart. Anat Embryol 1992; 185:363-378.

51. Bastide B, Neyses L, Ganten D, et al: Gap junction protein connexin40 is preferentially expressed in vascular endothelium and conductive bundles of rat myocardium and is increased under hypertensive conditions. Circ Res 1993; 73:1138-1149.

52. Gros D, Jarry-Guichard T, ten Velde I, et al: Restricted distribution of connexin40, a gap junctional protein, in mammalian heart. Circ Res 1994; 74:839-851.

53. Saffitz JE, Kanter HL, Green KG, et al: Tissue-specific determinants of anisotropic conduction velocity in canine atrial and ventricular myocardium. Circ Res 1994; 74:1065-1070.

54. Chen S-C, Davis LM, Westphale EM, et al: Expression of multiple gap junction proteins in human fetal and infant hearts. Pediatr Res 1994; 36:561-566.

55. Veenstra RD, Wang H-Z, Beyer EC, et al: Selective dye and ionic permeability of gap junction channels formed by connexin45. Circ Res 1994; 75:483-490.

56. Peters NS, Rowland E, Bennett JG, et al: The Wolff-Parkinson-White syndrome: the cellular substrate for conduction in the accessory atrioventricular pathway. Eur Heart J 1994; 15:981-987.

57. Fozzard HA, Arnsdorf MF. Cardiac Electrophysiology. In Fozzard HA, Haber E, Jennings RB, et al, eds: The Heart and Cardiovascular System. Raven Press Ltd., New York, 1992; 63-98.

58. Severs NJ: Pathophysiology of gap junctions in heart disease. J Cardiovasc Electrophysiol 1994; 5:462-475.

59. Kanter HL, Beyer EC, Saffitz JE: Structural and molecular determinants of intercellular coupling in cardiac myocytes. Microsc Res Tech 1995; 31:357-363.

60. Peters NS, Green CR, Poole-Wilson PA, et al: Cardiac arrhythmogenesis and the gap junction. J Mol Cell Cardiol 1995; 27:37-44.

61. Shaw RM, Rudy Y: The vulnerable window for unidirectional block in cardiac tissue: characterization and dependence on membrane excitability and intercellular coupling. J Cardiovasc Electrophysiol 1995; 6:115-131.

62. Luke RA, Saffitz JE: Remodeling of ventricular conduction pathways in healed canine infarct border zones. J Clin Invest 1991; 87:1594-1602.

63. Smith JH, Green CR, Peters NS, et al: Altered patterns of gap junction distribution in ischemic heart disease. An immunohistochemical study of human myocardium using laser scanning confocal microscopy. Am J Pathol 1991; 139:801-821.

64. Peters NS, Severs NJ, Coromilas J, et al: Disturbed connexin43 gap junction distribution correlates with the location of reentrant circuits in the epicardial border zone of healing canine infarcts that cause ventricular tachycardia. Circulation 1997; 95:988-996.

65. Matsushita T, Takahashi K, Yokoyama K, et al: Three dimensional and temporal expression of connexin43 in ischemic rat heart. Mol Biol Cell 1996;7 Suppl.:464a. (Abstract).

66. Sepp R, Severs NJ, Gourdie RG: Altered patterns of cardiac intercellular junction distribution in hypertrophic cardiomyopathy. Heart 1996; 76:412-417.

67. Luque EA, Veenstra RD, Beyer EC, et al: Localization and distribution of gap juncttions in normal and cardiomyopathic hamster heart. J Morphol 1994; 222:203-213.

68. Peters NS, Green CR, Poole-Wilson PA, et al: Reduced content of connexin43 gap junctions in ventricular myocardium from hypertrophied and ischaemic human hearts. Circulation 1993; 88:864-875.

69. Dupont E, Kaprielian RR, Yeh H-I, et al: Connexin messenger ribonucleic acid expression in the healthy and diseased human heart. Eur Heart J 1996; 17:600. (Abstract).

70. Kaprielian RR, Gunning M, Dupont E, et al: Down-regulation of immunodetectable connexin43 and decreased gap junction size in the pathogenesis of chronic hibernation in the human left ventricle. Circulation 1997; in press.

71. Rahimtoola SH: The hibernating myocardium. Am Heart J 1989; 117:211-221.

72. Campos De Carvalho AC, Masuda MO, Tanowitz HB, et al: Conduction defects and arrhythmias in Chagas' disease: possible role of gap junctions and humoral mechanisms. J Cardiovasc Electrophysiol 1994; 5:686-698.

73. Bastide B, Hu K, Gergs U, et al: Connexin expression in myocardial infarction. Eur Heart J 1994; 15 (Abst.Suppl.1702): 325.

74. Dupont E, Vozzi C, Coppen SR, et al: Connexin mRNA and protein expression is altered in human heart disease. J Mol Cell Cardiol 1997; in press, (Abstract).

75. Peters NS, Severs NJ, Rothery SM, et al: Spatiotemporal relation between gap junctions and fascia adherens junctions during postnatal development of human ventricular myocardium. Circulation 1994; 90:713-725.

76. Angst BD, Khan LUR, Severs NJ, et al: Dissociated spatial patterning of gap junctions and cell adhesion junctions during postnatal differentiation of ventricular myocardium. Circ Res 1997; 80:88-94.

77. Spach MS: Changes in the topology of gap junctions as an adaptive structural response of the myocardium. Circulation 1994; 90:1103-1106.

78. Soonpaa MH, Koh GY, Klug MG, et al: Formation of nascent intercalated disks between grafted fetal cardiomyocytes and host myocardium. Science 1994; 264:98-101.

79. Koh GY, Soonpaa MH, Klug MG, et al: Stable fetal cardiomyocyte grafts in the hearts of dystrophic mice and dogs. J Clin Invest 1995; 96:2034-2042.

9 CELLULAR ELECTRICAL UNCOUPLING DURING ISCHEMIA

Michiel J. Janse, Hanno L. Tan, Lukas R.C. Dekker and André G. Kléber

*Department of Clinical and Experimental Cardiology, Academic Medical Center, University of Amsterdam, and the Interuniversity Cardiology Institute, The Netherlands * Department of Physiology University of Bern, Switzerland*

1. INTRODUCTION

In 1875 T.W. Engelmann wrote: "Solche Zellen, die whrend des Lebens mit Verlust ihrer eigenen physiologischen Individualitt mit anderen zu einem Individuum höherer Ordnung verschmolzen sind, erhalten beim Absterben ihre Individualitt zurück ... Die Zellen leben zusammen, aber sterben einzeln". (1) In our translation: "Such cells, which during life, at the expense of their own identity, are joined with other cells to form an entity of higher order, regain their individuality when dying ... The cells live together, but die alone." Thus, Engelmann formulated on the one hand the concept that the normal heart functions as a syncytium, on the other hand that lethally injured cells become isolated from the rest of the heart, a phenomenon that later became known as "healing-over".

Important studies showing that healing-over is due to an increase in the resistance of gap junctions that normally provide low resistance pathways between cardiac cells are those of De Mello and associates (2,3) and of Délèze (4). These studies also emphasized the important role of calcium ions in causing cellular uncoupling. Later studies showed that both hypoxia and ischemia eventually result in an increase in coupling resistance (5,6,7,8). Apart from a rise in intracellular calcium concentration, other factors have been identified that may play a role in ischemia-induced uncoupling: an increase in intracellular protons (9,10,11,12,13) accumulation of long-chain acylcarnitines (14) and lysophosphatidylcholile (15), and a fall in ATP concentration (16).

In the present chapter we will 1) describe the time course of electrical uncoupling

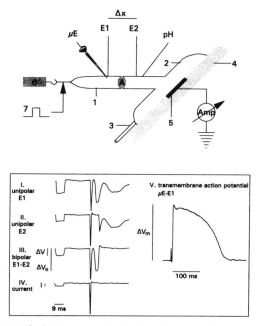

Figure 1. Upper panel shows schematic drawing of preparation and recording method. Papillary muscle (1) and interventricular septum (2) are perfused via a cannula (3) inserted in the septal artery and mounted on a silicone covered perspex plate (4) containing a large electrically grounded Ag/AgCl electrode (5). The papillary muscle is horizontally hooked to a force transducer (6). Subthreshold and excitatory current pulses are injected at the muscle apex (7). E1 and E2 = extracellular electrodes; μE = extracellular microelectrode; pH = extracellular pH electrode; Amp = current meter; Δx = distance between electrograms from E1 and E2, respectively; channel III = bipolar electrogram (E1 minus E2); IV = current signal from current meter; V = transmembrane action potential (μE minus E1); ΔV = drop of extracellular voltage between E1 and E2; ΔV_o = amplitude of bipolar electrogram; I = current strength of subthreshold pulse; ΔV_m = amplitude of transmembrane action potential. Records are plotted with a 2 kHz resolution. Note that the time scale of channel V is different from channels I to IV. (Reproduced with permission from ref. 21.)

during ischemia; 2) describe various interventions that can delay the moment of uncoupling, such as ischemic preconditioning, activation of the ATP sensitive K-channel, and reduction of cellular calcium overload; 3) discuss the central role of cellular calcium in uncoupling.

2. METHODS

In essence, the methods originally developed by Kléber and co-workers were used (7,17). Briefly, rabbits were anesthetized and heparinized, and the hearts were rapidly removed and submerged in cooled Tyrode's solution (4° C). The atria, free left ventricular wall and basal part of the ventricular septum were removed and the septal artery was cannulated and perfused. The delay between respiratory arrest and cannulation averaged 4 min. After removal of the free wall of the right ventricle, the preparation was positioned in a recording chamber and a right ventricular papillary muscle (length 4-6 mm, diameter 0.8-1.4 mm) with a single insertion of the tendon was horizontally hooked to a force transducer. The muscle was enclosed by a water-saturated gas mixture of 95% O_2 + 5% CO_2 at 37° C. Extracellular and intracellular electrodes for recording and stimulation were placed as indicated in Figure 1. Ischemia was induced by stopping perfusion and by changing the gas mixture inside the chamber to 95% N_2 + 5 CO_2.

2.1 Calculation of electrical resistance

The determination of tissue resistance is based on cable theory first applied to cardiac muscle by Weidmann (18). To determine total tissue resistance and its two components, intra- and extracellular resistance, two sequential measurements must be made (7,17). First, a subthreshold constant current pulse was applied between apex and septum (7 and 5 in Figure 1), and the voltage drop between extracellular electrodes E_1 and E_2 was measured. The subthreshold current will divide itself between intra- and extracellular compartments while spreading electrotonically along the long axis of the muscle. The transmembrane current approaches zero at three space constants of the membrane (i.e. approximately 1.5 mm) from the point of current injection. Beyond this point, extra- and intracellular voltages will decrease linearly. Therefore, longitudinal tissue resistance r_t, composed of intracellular (r_i) and extracellular (r_o) resistance in parallel, can be calculated as follows:

$$r_t = \frac{r_i \cdot r_o}{r_i + r_o} = \frac{\Delta V}{\Delta x. \, I}$$

where ΔV is the voltage drop between the two extracellular electrodes, Δx the distance between these two electrodes, and I the strength of the subthreshold current pulse.

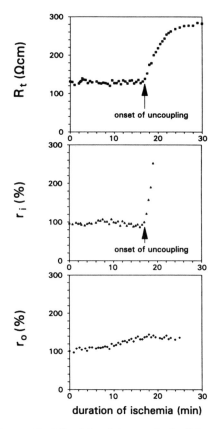

Figure 2. Graphs show method for determining onset of cellular electrical uncoupling in one representative experiment. Upper panel shows total specific resistance R_t during sustained ischemia, central and lower panels show relative values of intracellular resistance

For the second set of measurements, an excitatory current pulse was applied (30 msec after the subthreshold pulse), resulting in an action potential propagating from apex to septum. During propagation, the extracellular bipolar electrogram between E_1 and E_2 was measured and the transmembrane potential between an intracellular floating microelectrode and extracellular electrode E_i (Figure 1). The ratio of extra- to intracellular resistance was obtained from the amplitudes of the bipolar electrograms (ΔV_o) and the transmembrane action potential (ΔV_m):

$$\frac{r_o}{r_i} = \frac{\Delta V_o}{\Delta V_m - \Delta V_o}$$

From these two equations, r_i and r_o can be calculated.

2.2 Measurement of intracellular Ca^{2+}

The method to determine intracellular Ca^{2+} transients by means of indo 1 fluorescence has been described in detail elsewhere (19,20). Briefly, muscles were loaded with indo 1 during a 30 min period of perfusion. A circular area on the surface of the papillary muscle of 1.3 mm was illuminated by 340 nm excitation light and emitted light was simultaneously measured by two photomultipliers at 405 nm and 495 nm. The ratio R of the 405 nm and 495 nm signals, after subtraction of the autofluorescence at both wavelengths, was used as an indicator of $[Ca^{2+}]_i$.

3. RESULTS

3.1 Time course of electrical uncoupling during ischemia

Figure 2 shows the changes in total tissue resistance (R_t), and of intra- and extracellular resistances, in a representative experiment (21). Following the arrest of coronary flow, and changing the gaseous atmosphere to 95% N_2 and 5% CO_2, extracellular resistance rises by about 30% in the course of 15 to 20 min while intracellular resistance remains constant, in this experiment until 18 min. The rise in extracellular resistance is most likely due to osmotic cell swelling and the consequent

reduction of the extracellular space (22). The abrupt increase in both total and intracellular resistance marks the beginning of cellular uncoupling, which in this preparation occurs on average after 15 min of ischemia (17,21,23). This moment correlates well with the moments at which the first morphological changes at the intercalated disk are observed, such as a dissociation of the gap junctional membranes (24) and with the second phase of the increase in extracellular potassium concentration (25). All three phenomena can be regarded as markers for the onset of irreversible injury.

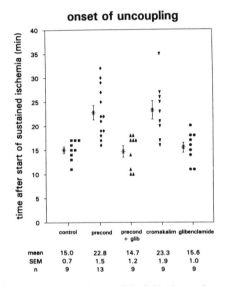

Figure 3. Onset of electrical uncoupling in all individual experiments is plotted along the Y-axis (in minutes after the start of sustained ischemia). Experiments are horizontally grouped according to the protocol. Every symbol represents one experiment. Asterisks at each group represent mean values. Bars are standard error bars. Mean values and SEM (minutes) are also shown below the graph. From left to right: control, squares; preconditioning, diamonds; preconditioning + 20 μM glibenclamide, triangles; 20 μM cromakalim, inverted triangles; circles, 20 μM glibenclamide. The graph shows a significant delay of onset of electrical uncoupling after preconditioning (p<0.001 vs. control). The delay is completely abolished when glibenclamide is added after the reconditioning occlusion. Cromakalim delays onset of uncoupling significantly in the absence of preconditioning (p<0.002 vs. control). Glibenclamide has no effect on the onset of uncoupling in the absence of preconditioning. (Reproduced with permission from ref. 23).

3.2 Delaying the onset of cellular uncoupling

Brief episodes of ischemia protect the heart from damage caused by a subsequent longer period of ischemia. Most often the effects of this so-called ischemic preconditioning is assessed by a reduction of infarct size following a certain period of ischemia, preceded by a brief episode of ischemia followed by reperfusion. The protection is not absolute, but consists of a delay in the onset of irreversible injury, as is apparent from the title of the first paper demonstrating ischemic preconditioning (26). The effects of ischemic preconditioning can therefore also be assessed by determining the delay in onset of electrical uncoupling (7,20,21). Figure 3 shows the results of five experimental protocols: 1) sustained ischemia; 2) sustained ischemia preceded by 10 min of ischemia and 10 min of reperfusion (preconditioning); 3) the same protocol as in 2), except for the addition of 20 μM glibenclamide (a blocker of the ATP-sensitive K^+ channel) at the start of reperfusion; 4) sustained ischemia induced 15 min after addition of 20 μM cromakalim (an activator of the ATP-sensitive K^+ channel) to the perfusate; 5) sustained ischemia induced 10 min after the addition of 20 μM glibenclamide to the perfusate. In all protocols the first intervention was made after an equilibration period of at least 60 min.

As can be seen, both preconditioning and the addition of cromakalim to the perfusate result in a significant delay in the onset of electrical uncoupling by 7 to 8 min. Glibenclamide, added to the perfusate during reperfusion after the first episode of ischemia, completely abolished the effect of preconditioning, but was without effect when added 10 min before sustained ischemia. From these data it was concluded that preconditioning delays the onset in electrical uncoupling and that this effect may be caused by activation of ATP-sensitive K^+ channels. This last conclusion should be viewed with caution because the use of so-called specific blockers and activators of the ATP-sensitive K^+ channels is fraught with pitfalls. Thus, glibenclamide has many other effects besides blocking the K_{ATP} channel: it blocks chloride channels, it blocks other K-channels, it affects calcium release from the sarcoplasmatic reticulum, it stimulates lactate production in normoxic conditions, it inhibits lactate production during hypoxia and ischemia, and finally, the efficacy of the drug to block the K_{ATP} channel may be lost during ischemia (for discussion and references see Wilde and Aksnes (27)).

Cromakalim in the concentration used causes extreme shortening of the action potential duration during ischemia and leads to inexcitability after about 5 min (23). Later, it was shown that both mechanical and electrical arrest significantly delay the onset of uncoupling (28).

The finding that the compound R 56865, which reduces cellular calcium overload secondary to reducing sodium overload (29), significantly delays cellular uncoupling (30), pointed to an important role of an increase in intracellular calcium in causing ischemia-induced uncoupling (17).

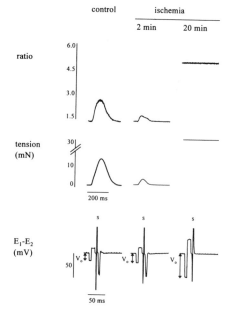

Figure 4. Simultaneous recordings from a papillary muscle during control conditions (left panels) and after 2 and 20 minutes of ischemia (middle and right panels). After 2 minutes of ischemia the Ca^{2+} transient and the developed tension have declined and subthreshold voltage drop has increased by 20%. After 20 minutes of ischemia Ca^{2+} transients and contractions have disappeared and diastolic Ca^{2+} and resting tension are high. Cellular uncoupling is indicated by the large increase of the subthreshold voltage drop. Note that the time scale for the electrograms is different from Indo-ratio and tension. (Reproduced with permission from ref. 19).

3.3 Calcium and ischemia-induced electrical uncoupling

Figure 4 shows simultaneous recordings of the indo 1 ratio, the developed tension and the bipolar electrogram during control perfusion and after 2 and 20 min of ischemia. After 2 min of ischemia the systolic ratio and the developed tension have substantially decreased, whereas the diastolic ratio and resting tension are unchanged. The subthreshold voltage drop between the two extracellular electrodes (V_o) has increased by 20%, corresponding to a rise in r_o. After 20 minutes R_t has increased to 230% of control and local electrical activation following the suprathreshold stimulus is absent. Diastolic ratio and resting tension are high. These changes indicate that after 20 min of ischemia the muscle has become inexcitable, myocytes have become uncoupled at a high intracellular Ca^{2+} concentration, and contracture has developed. The time course of the changes in indo 1 ratio, tissue resistance and tension are shown in Figure 5.

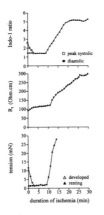

Figure 5. Plots showing diastolic and peak systolic indo 1 ratio (top panel), tissue resistance, R_t (middle panel), and resting and developed tension (bottom panel) during ischemia in one experiment. Values at t=0 are preischemic control values. Systolic Ca^{2+} levels and developed tension rapidly decline after the induction of ischemia. Small initial increase of R_t is caused by a rise in the extracellular longitudinal resistance. Diastolic Ca^{2+} and resting tension start to increase at 10 minutes of ischemia followed by an abrupt increase of R_t at 12 minutes of ischemia indicating the onset of uncoupling. (Reproduced with permission from ref. 19).

The relationship between the diastolic indo 1 ratio and tissue resistance is depicted in Figure 6. On average (n = 6) the diastolic indo 1 ratio started to increase after 12.6 ± 1.3 min, the onset of uncoupling occurred at 14.5 ± 1.2 min, and contracture at 12.6 ± 1.5 min.

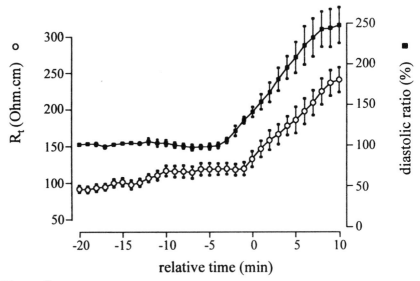

Figure 6. Average R_t and diastolic ratio of control preparations (n=6) during ischemia plotted on a relative time scale. Moment at which uncoupling started was assigned t=0 for each experiment. See text for further details. (Reproduced with permission from ref. 19.)

The effects of ischemic preconditioning are shown in Figure 7. On average (n = 6), in preconditioned muscles the rise in intracellular calcium started at 21.5 ± 4.0 min, uncoupling at 24.0 ± 4.1 min, and contracture at 23.0 ± 5.3 min of ischemia. Since both a rise in intracellular calcium and a decrease in intracellular pH have been implicated as factors that could cause uncoupling during ischemia, a set of experiments was performed in which ischemia was preceded by metabolic inhibition caused by pretreatment with 1 mmol/L iodoacetic acid. This substance

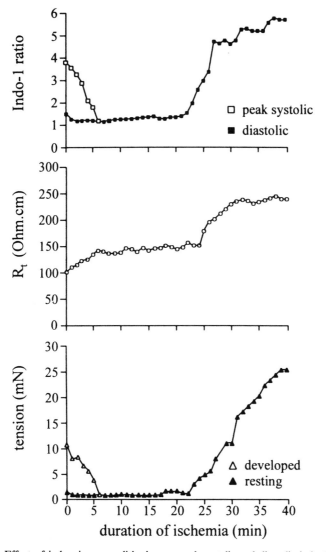

Figure 7. Effect of ischemic preconditioning on peak systolic and diastolic indo 1 ratio (top panel), tissue resistance R_t (middle panel), and resting and developed tension (bottom panel) during ischemia in a papillary muscle. Values at $t=0$ indicate values after preconditioning just before sustained ischemia. Systolic Ca^{2+} and developed tension rapidly decrease after induction of ischemia. Diastolic Ca^{2+} and resting tension start to increase after 23 minutes of ischemia. The rise in R_t after 25 minutes of ischemia marks the onset of uncoupling. (Reproduced with permission from ref. 19).

blocks glycolysis, causes a rapid depletion of ATP, and impairs anaerobic metabolism and acidification during ischemia (31). This was indirectly shown in our experiments by measuring extracellular pH. After 20 min of ischemia in untreated preparations, pH_o was on average 1.4 ± 0.05 pH units lower than during control perfusion. In metabolically inhibited muscles, pH_o maximally decreased by 0.15 pH units. As shown in Figure 8, the effect of pretreatment with iodoacetic acid leads to a very early rise in Ca^{2+} and a very early onset of uncoupling and con tracture.

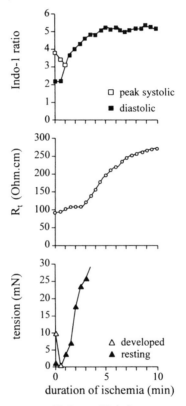

Figure 8. Effect of pretreatment with 1 mmol/L iodoacetate on peak systolic and diastolic fluorescence ratio (top panel), tissue resistance (middle panel) and resting and developed tension (bottom panel) during ischemia in a papillary muscle. Values at t=0 indicate preischemic values after pretreatment with iodoacetate. Decreasing systolic Ca^{2+} and developed tension merge into the terminal increase of diastolic Ca^{2+} and resting tension at 1.0 minute of ischemia. The increase of R_t at 3.0 minutes of ischemia indicates the onset of uncoupling. (Reproduced with permission from ref. 19).

In all three experimental groups (control ischemia, preconditioning and metabolic inhibition) the rise in intracellular calcium occurred significantly earlier than cellular uncoupling (paired t-test, p < 0.01), whereas the start of contracture was not significantly different from the moment of Ca^{2+} rise. This is shown in Figure 9, where the onset of rise in Ca^{2+} is plotted against the onset of uncoupling: all points are above the line of identity, indicating that uncoupling always followed the rise in Ca^{2+}. The average delay was 2.1 ± 0.2 min.

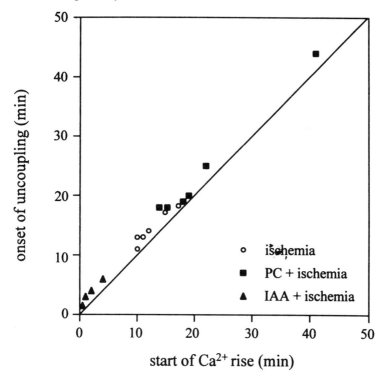

Figure 9. The relation between the moment of diastolic Ca^{2+} rise (on the abscissa) and the moment of the onset of uncoupling (on the ordinate) after the induction of ischemia for all experiments. Ischemia: sustained ischemia in control preparations; PC + ischemia: sustained ischemia in ischemically preconditioned preparations; IAA + ischemia: sustained ischemia in preparations pretreated with 1 mmol/L iodoacetate. The oblique line is the line of identity. Uncoupling always follows the increase of $[Ca^{2+}]_i$. The average interval is 2.1±0.2 minutes. (Reproduced with permission from ref. 19).

4. DISCUSSION

4.1 Calcium and ischemic injury

The first minutes of myocardial ischemia are characterized by increasing extracellular K^+ accumulation, acidification, depolarization of the cell membrane, development of inexcitability and contractile failure (32). The cardiac arrhythmias that occur during this early, reversible phase of ischemia, the so-called 1-A arrhythmias, are related to the changes in excitability, notably the decrease in conduction velocity and the inhomogeneities in refractory period (32,33,34).

After about 15 minutes of complete ischemia changes become irreversible. The transition to irreversible damage coincides with the secondary decline of the cytosolic phosphorylation potential (35), contracture and enzyme release (36), the secondary increase in extracellular K^+ accumulation and electrical cellular uncoupling (7,37). The second type of ischemia-induced arrhythmias, the 1-B arrhythmias, are associated with the onset of electrical uncoupling (38). Most hypotheses on the pathogenesis of irreversible ischemic injury center on intracellular calcium overload (36,39,40). Our findings also show that the increase of intracellular calcium is closely coupled to the onset of irreversible ischemic damage even in the absence of acidification (19,20).

Calcium overload in ischemia could in principle be caused by an enhanced influx of calcium from the extracellular space via the voltage sensitive Ca^{2+} channels or the Na^+/Ca^{2+} exchanger, or by release of calcium from the sarcoplasmatic reticulum.

A possible way leading to increased intracellular Ca^{2+} is via the Na^+/Ca^{2+} exchanger which is stimulated by an increase of intracellular Na^+, which in its turn is caused by an increase of Na^+/H^+ exchange secondary to acidosis. It is, however, unlikely that this is the main source of calcium influx. The rate of Na^+ dependent Ca^{2+} exchange is inhibited during ischemia (41), and in our experiments cytosolic calcium accumulation still occurred in the absence of acidification (19).

The calcium entry blocker verapamil postpones the onset of uncoupling, the secondary rise in extracellular K^+ accumulation and the rise in resting tension (37). However, this could be due to a variety of factors, such as a decrease in energy requirement with preservation of energy-rich phosphate compounds, and a decreased calcium concentration in the sarcoplasmatic reticulum. This would reduce the energy required to maintain a given level of cytosolic Ca^{2+} and, consequently, the cells would tolerate a lower ATP potential.

The most likely cause for the increase in cytosolic calcium during ischemia is a net release of calcium from the sarcoplasmatic reticulum (42,43). Normally, the Ca^{2+} pump of the sarcoplasmatic reticulum has to maintain a difference in calcium concentration of about a factor 100,000 over the sarcoplasmatic reticulum membrane. This is close to the thermodynamic limit imposed on a very efficient Ca^{2+} pump by the cytosolic phosphorylation potential (free energy change of ATP hydrolysis) (44). As the cytosolic phosphorylation potential decreases during ischemia (35), it will set the thermodynamic threshold value to a smaller maximal calcium gradient. This will result in a depletion of Ca^{2+} from the sarcoplasmatic reticulum and an increase in the cytosol, initiating the development of irreversible ischemic injury.

4.2 Cardioprotection by reduction of sarcoplasmatic reticulum calcium loading

Cardioprotection, by ischemic preconditioning or by pharmacological preconditioning by cromakalim, is related to postponement of the rise in cytosolic calcium and this may be due to a delay in release of calcium from the sarcoplasmatic reticulum (20). This is shown in a diagrammatic form in Figure 10.

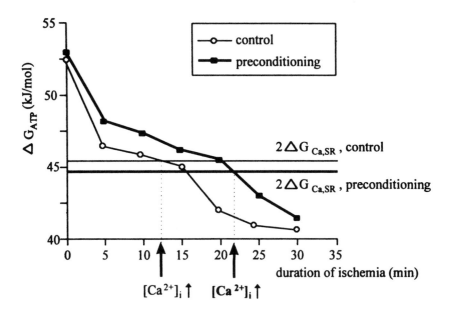

Figure 10. Theoretical diagram of relative decline of ΔG_{ATP} during ischemia in control (open circles and thin lines) and preconditioned (filled squares and thick lines) hearts. Horizontal lines represent proposed threshold ΔG_{ATP} (equivalent to 2 times $\Delta G_{Ca,SR}$) for control (thin line) and preconditioned (thick line) hearts. See text for further details. Dotted vertical lines represent moment of $[Ca^{2+}]_i$ rise during ischemia in control (thin) and preconditioned hearts (thick). (Reproduced with permission from ref. 20.)

There are three reasons why in preconditioned myocardium the release of calcium by the sarcoplasmatic reticulum may be delayed:

1) In preconditioned myocardium, creatine phosphate levels, and thus the cytosolic phosphorylation potential ΔG_{ATP}, are higher at the start of sus tained ischemia than in control hearts (35,45,46).

2) Both ischemic preconditioning and postponement of uncoupling by croma kalim are associated with a reduction in calcium loading of the sarcoplas matic reticulum (20). Moreover, reducing the sarcoplasmatic reticulum content with cyclopiazonic acid protects the heart during subsequent ischemia (20). Because of lowering of the calcium gradient across the sarco plasmatic reticulum membrane, energy consumption in preconditioned hearts is reduced, and the decline in ATP is decreased (35,45,46,47).

3) The lower calcium gradient across the sarcoplasmatic reticulum membrane can be maintained at a lower ΔG_{ATP}, i.e. the threshold beyond which the sarcoplasmatic reticulum will release calcium is lower. The threshold ΔG_{ATP} at which a net calcium efflux into the cytosol will occur equals $2 \Delta G_{Ca,SR}$ (the electrochemical gradient for calcium across the sarcoplasmatic reticulum membrane) (35).

In summary, the hypothesis based on the thermodynamic considerations described above, states that the reduction of calcium loading of the sarcoplasmatic reticulum attenuates the decline of ΔG_{ATP} and decreases the thermodynamic limit which determines the sarcoplasmatic calcium gradient during ischemia. As a result, during ischemia in hearts with prior reduced calcium content of the sarcoplasmatic reticulum, ΔG_{ATP} reaches the threshold for Ca^{2+} depletion at a later moment compared to hearts with a normal calcium content of the sarcoplasmatic reticulum (20).

A great many hypotheses have been put forward to explain the protective effects of preconditioning: activation of adenosine 1 receptors (A_1), alpha 1 adrenoreceptors ($_1$), muscarinic receptors (M_2), stimulation and translocation of protein kinase C (PKC), opening of ATP sensitive K channels and activation of heat shock proteins. Activation of A_1, $_1$ and M_2 receptors may lead to a G-protein-dependent activation of PKC, which reduces the field to two main candidates: activation of PKC and activation of ATP sensitive K channels. The ultimate mechanism underlying preconditioning is still unclear (48), but it is worthwhile to consider a low sarcoplasmatic reticulum calcium content as the final common pathway. PKC inhibits calcium accumulation in the sarcoplasmatic reticulum (49) and extracts calcium from the cytosol by stimulating the Na^+/Ca^{2+} exchanger and inhibiting sarcolemmal Ca^{2+} channels (50,51). It is more difficult to link activation of ATP-sensitive K^+ channels to sarcoplasmatic Ca^{2+} content. As already mentioned, glibenclamide and cromakalim have other effects besides blocking and activating ATP sensitive K^+ channels. Moreover, there is evidence that pharmacological preconditioning with openers of ATP-sensitive K^+ channels occurs independently from activation of sarcolemmal K_{ATP} channels. Pronounced alterations of calcium transients during exposure to cromakalim have been observed, indicative of calcium release from the sarcoplasmatic reticulum, without concomitant shortening of action potential duration (20). Also, the K_{ATP} channel opener bimakalim offered cardioprotection in the absence of action potential shortening (52).

Since only a tiny fraction of sarcolemmal K_{ATP} channels need to be activated to produce a substantial shortening of the action potential (53), these data indicate that these K channel openers have other actions besides activating sarcolemmal K_{ATP} channels. K channel openers directly decrease sarcoplasmatic reticulum calcium loading in smooth muscle cells (54,55) and probably do so as well in cardiac cells (20). Clearly, future research on the cardioprotective effect of reduced calcium loading of the sarcoplasmatic reticulum is needed to unravel the relationship between calcium transients, protein kinase C activity, activation of adenosine, alpha adrenergic and muscarinic receptors, the actions of K_{ATP} channel blockers and openers, the subcellular pathways involved and sarcoplasmatic calcium content.

REFERENCES

1. Engelmann TW. Ueber die Leitung der Erregung im Herzmuskel. Pfluegers Arch 1875; 11: 465-480.
2. De Mello WC, Motta GE, Chapeau M. A study on the healing-over of myocardial cells of toads. Circ Res 1969; 24:475-487.
3. De Mello WC. Effect of intracellular injection of calcium and stron tium on cell communication in heart. J Physiol 1975; 250:231-245.
4. Délèze J. The recovery of resting potential and input resistance in sheep heart injured by knife or laser. J Physiol 1970; 208:547-562.
5. Wojtczak J. Contractures and increase in internal longitudinal resis tance of cow ventricular muscle induced by hypoxia. Circ Res 1979; 44:88-95.
6. Ikeda K, Hiraoka M. Effects of hypoxia on passive electrical proper ties of canine ventricular muscle. Pfluegers Arch 1982; 393:45-50.

7. Kléber AG, Riegger CB, Janse MJ. Electrical uncoupling and increase of extracellular resistance after induction of ischemia in isolated, arterially perfused rabbit rapillary muscle. Circ Res 1987; 61:271-279.

8. Riegger CB, Alperovich G, Kléber AG. Effect of oxygen withdrawal on active and passive electrical properties of arterially perfused rabbit ventricular muscle. Circ Res 1989; 64:532-541.

9. Reber WR, Weingart R. Ungulate cardiac Purkinje fibres: the influence of intracellular pH on electrical cell-to-cell coupling. J Physiol 1982; 328:87-104.

10. Spray DC, Stern HJ, Harris AL, Bennett MVL. Gap junctional conductance: comparison of sensitivities to H and Ca ions. Proc Natl Acad Sci USA 1981; 79:441-445.

11. De Mello WC. The influence of pH on the healing-over of mammalian cardiac muscle. J Physiol 1983; 339:299-307.

12. Pressler ML. Effects of pCa_i and pH_i on cell-to-cell coupling. Experientia 1987; 43:1084-1092.

13. Noma A, Tsuboi N. Dependence of junctional conductance on proton, calcium and magnesium ions in cardiac paired cells of guinea-pig. J Physiol 1987; 382:193-211.

14. Wu J, McHowat J, Saffitz JE, Yamada KA, Corr PB. Inhibition of gap junctional conduction by long-chain acetylcarnitines and their preferential accumulation in junctional sarcolemma during hypoxia. Circ Res 1993; 72:879-889.

15. Daleau P. Effects of lysophosphatidylcholine on intercellular resistance of guinea pig ventricular cell pairs (abstract). Circulation 1996; 94:I-9.

16. Sugiura H, Toyama J, Tsuboi N, Kamiya K, Kodama I. ATP directly affects junctional conductance between paired ventricular myocytes isolated from guinea pig heart. Circ Res 1990; 66:1095-1102.

17. Kléber AG, Riegger CB. Electrical constants of arterially perfused rabbit papillary muscle. J Physiol 1987; 385:307-324.

18. Weidmann S. Electrical constants of trabecular muscle from mammalian heart. J Physiol 1970; 210:1041-1054.

19. Dekker LRC, Fiolet JWT, Van Bavel E, Coronel R, Opthof T, Spaan JAE, Janse MJ. Intra cellular Ca^{2+}, intercellular coupling resistance, and mechanical activity in ischemic rabbit papillary muscle. Effects of preconditioning and metabolic blockade. Circ Res 1996; 79:237-246.

20. Dekker LRC. Role of intracellular calcium in ischemic damage and precondi tioning in cardiac muscle. Thesis, University of Amsterdam (ISBN 90-9009992-1), 1996.

21. Tan HL. Cellular electrical uncoupling and protection of ischemic myocardium. Thesis, University of Amsterdam (ISBN 90-9006433-8), 1993.

22. Tranum-Jensen J, Janse MJ, Fiolet JWT, Krieger WJG, Naumann d'Alnon court C, Durrer D. Tissue osmolality, cell swelling, and reperfusion in acute regional myocardial ischemia in the isolated porcine heart. Circ Res 1981; 49:364-381.

23. Tan HL, Mazón P, Verberne HJ, Sleeswijk ME, Coronel R, Opthof T, Janse MJ. Ischaemic preconditioning delays ischaemia-induced cellular electrical uncoupling in rabbit myocardium by activation of ATP-sensitive K^+ channels. Cardiovasc Res 1993; 27:644-651.

24. McCallister LP, Trapudki S, Neely JR. Morphometric observation on the effects of ischemia in the isolated perfused rat heart. J Mol Cell Cardiol 1979; 11:619-630.

25. Hill JL, Gettes LS. Effects of acute coronary artery occlusion on local myocardial extracellular K^+ activity in swine. Circulation 1980; 61:768-778.

26. Murry CE, Jennings RB, Reimer KA. Preconditioning with ischemia: a delay of lethal cell injury in ischemic myocardium. Circulation 1986; 74:1124-1136.

27. Wilde AAM, Aksnes G. Myocardial potassium loss and cell depolarization in ischaemia and hypoxia. Cardiovasc Res 1995; 29:1-15.

28. Tan HL, Janse MJ. Contribution of mechanical activity and electrical activity to cellular uncoupling in ischemic rabbit papillary muscle. J Mol Cell Cardiol 1994; 26:733-742.

29. Ver Donck L, Borgers M, Verdonck F. Inhibition of Na^+ and Ca^{2+} overload in the myocardium: a new cytoprotective principle. Cardiovasc Res 1993; 37:349-357.

30. Tan HL, Netea AO, Sleeswijk ME, Mazón P, Coronel R, Opthof T, Janse MJ. R56865 delays cellular electrical uncoupling in ischemic rabbit papillary muscle. J Mol Cell Cardiol 1993; 25:1059-1066.

31. Jennings RB, Reimer KA, Steenbergen Jr C, Schaper J. Total ischemia III: effect of inhibition of anaerobic metabolism. J Mol Cell Cardiol 1989; 21 (Suppl I): 37-54.

32. Janse MJ, Wit AL. Electrophysiological mechanisms of ventricular arrhyth mias resulting from myocardial ischemia and infarction. Physiol Rev 1989; 69:1049-1169.

33. Coronel R, Wilms-Schopman FJG, Dekker LRC, Janse MJ. Heterogeneitis in $[K^+]_o$ and TQ potential and the inducibility of ventricular fibrillation during acute regional ischemia in the isolated porcine heart. Circulation 1995; 92:120-19.

34. Kléber AG, Janse MJ, Wilms-Schopman FJG, Wilde AAM, Coronel R. Changes in conduction velocity during acute ischemia in ventricular myocar dium in the isolated porcine heart. Circulation 1986; 73:189-198.

35. Fiolet JWT, Baartscheer A, Schumacher CA, Coronel R, Ter Welle HF. The change of the free energy of ATP hydrolysis during global ischemia and anoxia in the rat heart. J Mol Cell Cardiol 1984; 16:1023-1036.

36. Steenbergen C, Murphy E, Waths JA, London RE. Correlation between cytosolic free calcium, contracture, ATP, and irreversible ischemic injury in perfused rat heart. Circ Res 1990; 66:135-146.
37. Cascio WE, Yan G, Kléber AG. Passive electrical properties, mechanical activity, and extracellular potassium in arterially perfused and ischemic rabbit ventricular muscle. Effects of calcium entry blockade or hypocalcemia. Circ Res 1990; 66:1461-1473.
38. Smith WT, Fleet WF, Johnson TA, Engle CL, Cascio WE. The 1b phase of ventricular arrhythmias in ischemic in situ porcine heart is related to changes in cell-to-cell coupling. Circulation 1995; 92:3051-3060.
39. Poole-Wilson PA, Harding DP, Bourdillon PDV, Tones MA. Calcium out of control. J Mol Cell Cardiol 1984; 16:175-187.
40. Katz AM, Reuter H. Cellular calcium and cardiac cell death. Am J Cardiol 1979; 44:188-190.
41. Dixon IM, Eyolfson DA, Dhalla NS. Sarcolemmal Na^+/Ca^{2+} exchanger activity in hearts subjected to hypoxia reoxygenation. Am J Physiol 1987; 253:H1026-H1034.
42. Kléber AG, Oetliker H. Cellular aspects of early contractile failure in ischemia, in Fozzard HA, Haber E, Jennings RB, Katz AM, Morgan HE (eds): The heart and cardiovascular system, 2nd edition, New York, Raven Press, 1992 pp 1975-1996.
43. Marban E, Koretsune Y, Corretti M, Chacko VP, Kusuoka H. Calcium and its role in myocardial cell injury during ischemia and reperfusion. Circulation 1989; 80 (Suppl IV): 17-22.
44. Hasselbach W, Oetliker H. Energetics and electrogenicity of the sarcoplas matic reticulum calcium pump. Annu Rev Physiol 1983; 45:325-339.
45. Steenbergen C, Perlman ME, London RE, Murphy E. Mechanism of preconditioning: ionic alteration. Circ Res 1993; 72:112-125.
46. Kida M, Fujiwara H, Ishida M, Kawai C, Ohura M, Miura I, Yabuuchi Y. Ischemic precon ditioning preserves creatine phosphate and intracellular pH. Circulation 1991; 84:2495-2503.
47. Murry CE, Richard VJ, Reimer KA, Jennings RB. Ischemic precon ditioning slows energy metabolism and delays ultrastructural damage during a sustained ischemic episode. Circ Res 1990; 913-931.
48. Lawson CS, Downey JM. Preconditioning: state of the art of myocardial protection. Cardiovasc Res 1993; 27:542-550.
49. Rogers RB, Gaa ST, Massey C, Dösemeci A. Protein kinase C inhibits Ca^{2+} accumulation in cardiac sarcoplasmatic reticulum. J Biol Chem 1990; 265:4302-4308.

50. Brechler V, Pavoine C. Lotersztajn S, Garbare E, Pecker F. Activation of the Na/Ca exchanger by adenosine in the ewe heart sarcolemma is mediated by a pertussis toxin sensitive G protein. J Biol Chem 1990; 265:16851-16855.
51. Lacerda AE, Romyze D, Brown AM. Effects of protein kinase C activators on cardiac Ca^{2+} channels. Nature 1988; 333:249-251.
52. Yao Z, Garrett JG. Effects of the K.ATP channel opener bimakalim in coronary blood flow, monophasic action potential duration, and infarct size in dogs. Circulation 1994; 89:1769-1775.
53. Weiss JN. ATP-sensitive K channels in myocardial ischemia, in Vereecke J, Van Bogaert PP (eds): Potassium channels in normal and pathological conditions, Leuven, Leuven University Press, 1996; pp 119-132.
54. Chopra LC, Twort CHC, Ward JPT. Direct action of BRL 38227 and glibenclamide on intracellular calcium stores in cultured airway smooth muscle cells of rabbit. Br J Pharmacol 1992; 105:259-260.
55. Bray KM, Weston AH, Duty S, Nargreen DT, Longmore J, Edwards G, Brown TJ. Differences between the effects of cromakalim and nifedipine on agonist-induced responses in rabbit aorta. Br J Pharmacol 1991; 102:337-344.

10 Gap Junctions, Cardiac Excitability and Clinical Arrhythmias

Morton F. Arnsdorf and Samuel C. Dudley

Cardiology Section, Department of Medicine, Pritzker School of Medicine, University of Chicago

1. INTRODUCTION

The explosive growth in our understanding of cellular electrophysiology and the relationship to clinical arrhythmias continues. Much of the basic science that concerns the role of gap junctions in arrhythmias has been reviewed in other chapters in this book. The purpose of this chapter is to create an intellectual framework for the clinician that is based on biophysical theory and to allow the researcher who is not a physician insight into clinical thought processes. The emphasis will be on the known and probable role of gap junctions in normal and abnormal cardiac excitability with an emphasis on arrhythmogenesis due to anisotropic conduction.

The concept of cardiac excitability is vague to most clinicians. Intuitively, cardiac excitability brings to mind the ability of heart cells regeneratively to depolarize and repolarize during the action potential and to activate the heart in a sequence that assures a proper cardiac output. The next level of understanding includes cellular characteristics such as ionic channels, the manner in which cells communicate with each other through gap junctions, and anisotropy of conduction that results from a difference in physical properties of the heart that preferentially favors conduction in one direction over another. There are indications that this inhomogeneity is important in the initiation and maintenance of clinical arrhythmias.

The interplay of biophysical theory, prediction, experiment and refined theory has been a successful paradigm for the advancement of our understanding. In an earlier and more technical publication, we stressed that the practical use of biophysical theory is to support predictions of how a system under study might respond to new contingencies {1}. Examples were that these predictions could be long term, for instance, of the risk for sudden cardiac death, or short term, as in the reconstruction of the action potential from currents identified and manipulated by voltage-clamping. The results derived from these predictions themselves become new hypotheses for experimental testing. Computers have allowed the development, testing, modification and application of increasingly more refined theoretical models, as in the fascinating application of nonlinear dynamics {2} and the development of cell models, such as that provided by Dr. Rudy in his chapter in this book. Increasingly, such models will be used to create and test hypotheses.

Physicians, who often lack the background to develop and even understand such models, are the experts in developing questions that deal with clinical problems and, therefore, are a necessary link to the researcher. The relationship between gap junctions and cardiac arrhythmias is *terra incognita* for most physicians. The physician, then, needs an intellectual framework for discussing complex topics that can be translated by the latter into hypotheses, experiments, and finally clinical application. The non-physician researcher, in turn, needs a bridge to the bedside.

2. ELECTROPHYSIOLOGIC MATRICAL CONCEPT OF CARDIAC EXCITABILITY

2.1 Nonlinearities of Biologycal Systems and the Relation to Arrhythmia

Biophysical systems have inputs (stimuli) and outputs (responses) which exist in time and are organized in space and are subject to controlling or influencing feedback systems. The relationship between inputs and outputs may be linear or nonlinear, continuous or discontinuous. The relationship is linear when a stimulus produces a proportional output; for example, proportional current output to a step change in voltage across a resistor as described by Ohm's Law ($V = IR$) where V is voltage, I is current and R is resistance so continuous one volt changes over a one ohm resister produces a continuous set of one ampere responses. Even a more complex function such as decremental conduction can be described using linear differential equations. The response of a linear system to periodic inputs always has the same periodicities as the input.

Most biological systems, however, are *nonlinear* in that a stimulus produces a disproportional response. An example of nonlinear behavior is the regenerative response of the action potential on the attainment of threshold. Subthreshold responses in transmembrane voltage to intracellular current injection may be fairly continuous until threshold is attained. At this point, there is a sudden *discontinuous* response to the same magnitude stimulus. This type of nonlinear behavior leads to responses that are inconsistent with the idea of proportional responses to stimuli {3} including, for example, bifurcations {4}, bistability {5} and hysteresis {6}. In bifurcations, the character of the response evolves in time, or as a parameter is changed, in a specific sequence; and one of us has suggested that bifurcations, particularly those assisted by conditions, occur commonly in clinical electrophysiology, and that this is an important principle in arrhythmogenesis and in the actions of antiarrhythmic drugs {1, 7-16, among others, and see below}. Bistable systems are characterized by a given stimulus leading to two or more kinds of response; for example, a propagated response and the initiation of triggered activity. In hysteresis, the response after a stimulus has reached some fixed amplitude differs, depending on how fast and/or in what direction the stimulus had been changed previously in the course of reaching that amplitude. The response of a nonlinear system to a periodic input the response may include harmonic and/or subharmonic frequencies, or can fall in arbitrary ratios (N:M) of integers, with respect to the input period. These integer ratios can be affected by gap junctions.

2.2 Gap Junctions, The Electrophysiologic Matrix, and Assisted Bifurcations

As mentioned, cardiac excitability has a certain intuitive meaning suggesting the ease with which cardiac cells undergo individual and sequential regenerative depolarization and repolarization, communicate with each other, and propagate electrical activity in a normal and abnormal manner. The heart beat arises from a highly organized control of ionic flow through channels in the cardiac membrane, the myoplasm, the gap junctions between cells and the extracellular space. These bioelectric events are regulated within very tight limits to allow the coordinated propagation of excitation and contraction of the heart that is necessary for an efficient cardiac output. Abnormalities in the regulatory mechanisms often accompany cardiac disease.

Conceptually, cardiac excitability can be thought of as resulting from the action and interactions of an electrophysiologic matrix of cellular properties. The normal matrix must be altered by arrhythmogenic influences which affect one or more components of excitability to produce abnormal excitability, and the interaction between the matrix altered by an arrhythmogenic influence and an antiarrhythmic drug creates yet another matrix that hopefully is antiarrhythmic or antifibrillatory, but which may be proarrhythmic. The matrical concept we have proposed previously {1, 7-16} describes the essentially nonlinear character of cardiac excitability and propagation in a way that is intuitive to the physiologist and hopefully the clinician without requiring explicit mathematical equations, but since they are system parameters, also have mathematical relationships.

Figure 1 is a bifurcation diagram of the electrophysiologic matrices obtained from data in a recent cellular electrophysiologic study on the interactions between changes in extracellular potassium concentration, $[K^+]_o$, and flecainide {16}. The matrix, labeled Normal , is at a physiologic $[K^+]_o$ and has a regular hexagonal shape indicative of a normal state. Abnormal states, presumably the arrhythmogenic matrical configurations, are represented by matrices of irregular polygonal shape. The bonds between the matrix elements indicate the interactions and mutual dependencies. This matrix includes the resting potential (V_r), threshold voltage (V_{th}), Na^+ conductance (g_{Na}), membrane resistance (R_m), the length constant ( ), and, as a measure of overall excitability, the liminal length (LL), all of which will be defined below. There are many other determinants that could have been included in this depiction, but these have been chosen for simplicity. The matrix is a shorthand way of delineating complex interactions. The interactions, however, are dynamic. The interactions, then, are not constant, but vary between homeostatic limits.

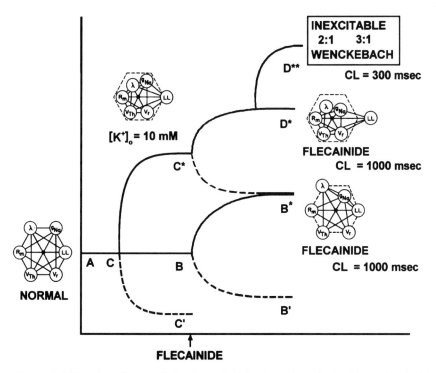

Figure 1. Bifurcation diagram of the electrophysiologic matrices obtained from data in this study. The major points made in the text are that electrophysiologic changes occur as a system, such change may be antiarrhythmic or proarrhythmic, often there is little difference in the antiarrhythmic and proarrhythmic matrix, and the predominant effect of a drug depends on the matrix encountered. See text for discussion. Reproduced with permission from Arnsdorf and Sawicki {16}.

The interaction between the antiarrhythmic drug flecainide and the normal matrix at point B results in a new matrix at B*, which in this experiment was largely unchanged except for a slight decrease in sodium conductance indicated by g_{Na} moving towards the center of the hexagon. Hyperkalemia alone, in contrast, caused multiple electrophysiologic changes in both active and passive properties and drove the equilibrium from C to a new equilibrium at point C* characterized by decreases in R_m, , V_{th}, V_r, and g_{Na}. Hyperkalemia consistently produced this type of matrical configuration and was responsible for what is termed an *assisted bifurcation* that consistently moved the system from point A to point C*.

If the tissue with the electrophysiologic matrix created by hyperkalemia at C* was exposed to flecainide, a second bifurcation occured leading to the equilibrium at D*. Further bifurcations occur that depended on the rate of stimulation resulting in a situation at point D** in which the liminal length requirements were either not met resulting in inexcitability or were met intermittently resulting in a 2:1 or some other excitable response. Note how similar the matrical configurations are after the "arrhythmogenic" intervention of increasing $[K^+]_o$ and after the application of flecainide, suggesting a narrow toxic to therapeutic ratio. The dashed lines represent paths that might be taken were another drug used (B'), were $[K^+]_o$ lowered below 5.4 mM (C'), or were $[K^+]_o$ returned from 10 mM to 5.4 mM in the presence of flecainide (C* to B*).

The matrix has many more dimensions than are shown here, as there are many more ionic channels including gap junctions and each element, in turn, is determined by underlying properties, such as ion channel conductances. Hence, there is a need for models, particularly nonlinear models. The active (source) and passive (sink) properties, that form the elements of the matrix, are not independent of each other. For example, gap junctional conductance determines in large part all these depicted parameters. For the sake of discussion, let us focus on two of these parameters, the length or space constant( ) and the liminal length (LL).

The *length* or *space* constant ( ) is a measure that expresses the distance over which the   influence of the electrotonic wavefront that precedes the action potential.   Figure 2A shows the experimental arrangement for cable analysis. The stimulus consists of a sudden injection of intracellular current (S) through a microelectrode near the ligated end of a cardiac Purkinje fiber, and the response to the change in transmembrane voltage (V_m) is recorded at several points along the preparation. The stimulating current, I_m, is monitored via the bath ground. An electrical analog for a cable-like preparation, showing membrane resistance (r_m), membrane capacitance (c_m), internal longitudinal resistance (r_i) due to the myoplasm and gap junctions, and external resistance (r_o) due to the extracellular space, is shown in the upper portion of Figure 2B. Panel C is an analog which represents membrane behavior more accurately by inclusion of series elements r_s and c_s in addition to r_m and c_m. Returning to panel B, below the electrical analog is plotted V_m as a function of distance between the stimulating and the recording microelectrodes (x) in steady state after intracellular current application. The arrow marks length constant, which is defined as $V_o e-1$, where V_o is the voltage at the point of stimulation and can be expressed as: $\lambda = \sqrt{r_m / (r_i + r_o)}$ or, when r_o can be neglected, $\lambda = \sqrt{r_m / r_i}$ R_m depends on the integrity of the cell membrane, and r_i depends primarily on the state of the gap junctions linking the cell. An increase in r_i, then, as may occur with the closing of gap junctions secondary to injury will decrease. It should be mentioned that r_o may be important with fibrosis or cellular swelling. Note again, the exponential fall of the voltage. It is this electrotonic voltage that fulfils or fails to fulfil the requirements for the next patch of membrane to attain threshold and produce a regenerative action potential.

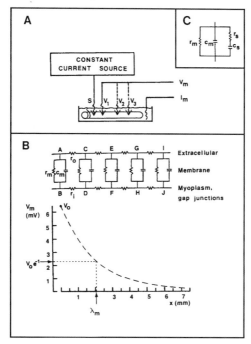

Figure 2. Experimental measurement of cable properties in a long sheep Purkinje fiber. Top trace: record of rectangular current step (I_m); amplitude during step was 45.5 nA. Middle trace: record of transmembrane voltage response (V_m); final amplitude was 5.44 mV. Bottom trace: record of V_m at a greater distance from the stimulating electrode than that of the middle trace; final amplitude was 4.05 mV. After the rectangular step change in I_m, V_m changes gradually as membrane capacitance c_m charges. In the middle trace, the arrow marks the time (26.8 msec) at which the change in V_m after current onset had reached 4.56 mV, 84% of its final value (arrow). The resting potential of this fiber was -79 mV.

Liminal length (LL) is the amount of tissue that must be raised above threshold so that the inward depolarizing current from that patch of membrane exceeds the repolarizing influences of adjacent tissues and results in an action potential. If the local electrotonic currents are sufficient to fulfill the liminal length requirements of the neighboring patch or patches of membrane, these patches will also produce action potentials. These events repeat and the sequential depolarization of patches of membrane results. If the liminal length of a patch is not fulfilled, this patch will not be activated, and propagation will not occur. The concept of liminal length was first proposed by Hodgkin and Rushton in nerve {17}, and subsequently by Fozzard and his coworkers in cardiac Purkinje fibers {18, 19}. Liminal length can be well-approximated by the relation:

$$\frac{0.855 Q_{th}}{2\,(\pi)^{3/2} a\,C_m\,\lambda\,V_{th}}$$

where Q_{th} is the charge threshold, a is the radius, C_m is the membrane capacitance, is the length constant and V_{th} is the voltage threshold. As discussed in the previous paragraph, an increase in r_i will decrease which, in turn, will increase the liminal length thereby decreasing cardiac excitability. A decrease in r_i will have the opposite effect on liminal length and cardiac excitability. As we have discussed in some detail recently, the action potential can be considered a local membrane event and the fulfillment of the liminal length requirement by the local circuit currents can be considered the propagated event {16}.

A schematic representation of the liminal length concept and the interplay between the current generators and the electronic influence is shown in Figure 3. In panel A, the black circles represent active generator sites (e.g., sodium channels), the circle surrounding each is the electrotonic influence of the generator, the stippled area is the amount of tissue required to be raised above threshold to provide activation current sufficient to overcome the repolarizing currents of neighboring cells, and the white areas represent the excess in source over sink. In panel B, the strength of the active generator site (grey circles) and the distance of the electrotonic currents (smaller circles) are decreased. More active generator sites must be recruited to attain the liminal length requirements (stippled area), and the excess of source to sink is less than in panel A. A further increase in the liminal length from whatever cause will render the tissue inexcitable (panel C).

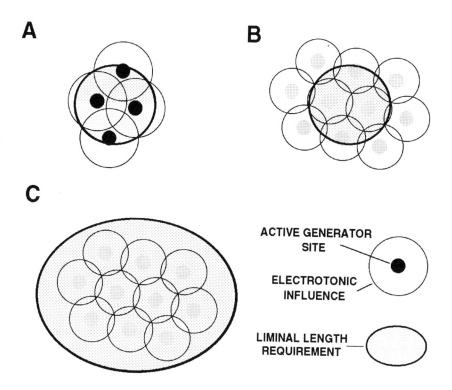

Figure 3. Schematic representation of the liminal length concept. Panel A: The black circles represent active generator sites, the circle surrounding each is the electrotonic influence of the generator, the stippled area is the amount of tissue required to be raised above threshold to provide activation current sufficient to overcome the repolarizing currents of neighboring cells, and the white areas represent the excess in source of sink. B. The strength of the active generator site (grey circles) and the distance of the electrotonic currents (smaller circles) are decreased. More active generator sites must be recruited to attain the liminal length requirements (white area), and the excess of source to sink is less than in panel A. A further increase in the liminal length from whatever cause will render the tissue inexcitable. See text for discussion. Reproduced with permission from Arnsdorf and Sawicki {16}.

Returning again to Figure 1, the idea of the bifurcation diagram is that it shows the transition from one equilibrium to another. If conditions favor taking one path to a new equilibrium rather than another, this is called an *assisted* bifurcation. The bifurcations depicted reflect a set of experiments in which $[K]_0$ was varied in controls and after exposure of cardiac Purkinje fibers to flecainide {16}. Point A is the normal dynamic equilibrium shown as a normal matrix. The interaction between flecainide and the normal matrix at point B resulted in a new matrix at B*, which in this experiment was largely unchanged except for a slight decrease in sodium conductance. Hyperkalemia alone drove the equilibrium primarily upward from C to a new equilibrium at point C*. Hyperkalemia, then, was responsible for an *assisted bifurcation* that consistently drove the system from point A to point C*.

If the tissue with the electrophysiologic matrix created by hyperkalemia at C* was exposed to flecainide, a second bifurcation occurred and led to the equilibrium at D*. Further bifurcations occurred that depended on the rate of stimulation resulting in a situation at point D** in which the liminal length requirements were not met resulting in inexcitability or were met intermittently resulting in a 2:1 or some other response. Note how similar the matrical configurations were after the "arrhythmogenic" intervention of increasing $[K^+]_0$ and after the application of flecainide, suggesting a narrow toxic to therapeutic ratio. The dashed lines represent paths that might be taken were another drug used (B'), were $[K^+]_0$ lowered below 5.4 mM (C'), or were $[K^+]_0$ returned from 10 mM to 5.4 mM in the presence of flecainide (C* to B*).

Changes in gap junctional conductance that would increase liminal length and decrease   as discussed above would result in a matrical configuration similar to that seen at D* in Figure 1, except that g_{Na} would not be reduced and V_r would likely remain unaffected. Although not experimentally tested, our presumption is that a decrease in gap junctional conductance would produce an assisted bifurcation that routinely would result in a characteristic and reproducible matrical configuration. Complete closure of the gap junctions would tend to render the tissue inexcitable unless some other type of cell-cell communication were present (e.g., some type of capacitative coupling).

3. THE CONTROL OF GAP JUNCTIONS

The control of gap junctions has been an important part of many Chapters in this book. A few points, however, are particularly important to provide the bridge between basic science and the clinical domain. The work of Heidenheim around the turn of the century {20} led to the idea that the heart was an anatomical and electrical syncytium. This conflicted with the earlier physiologic observations of Engelmann {21, 22} who noted a decline in injury current and a sealing off of cells after injury to the frog heart. When Engelmann cut the heart with scissors, the cells at the cut surface became inexcitable while those at a short distance remained excitable. Moreover, the injury current after the cut decreased with time. Small myocardial segments, connected by bridges of intact tissue, could be stimulated at any point, and stimulation at any point caused contraction throughout the entire preparation. Microscopically, Engelmann could not detect nerves connecting the cells and concluded that the impulse was conducted from one cell to the next. Cells in healthy tissue were connected electrically with each others, but cell injury and death resulted in a sealing off of the normal from the injured or dead cells. This led to Engelmann's famous dictum that "Cells live together but die singly".

The electron microscopic studies of Sjöstrand and Anderson in 1954 {23} described the intercalated disk and showed that cardiac cells were bound by membranes without any direct cytoplasmic connection between cells. The structure responsible for intercellular communication is the gap junction. Connexins group to form a hexameric structure containing a central pore. This structure is termed a connexon or hemichannel. A working gap junctional channel is formed when a connexon in one cell becomes localized in a cell membrane and matches sterically with a connexon from a neighboring cell. How this coupling of hemichannels is driven to occur is unknown.

Aspects of gap junctional control were summarized in our recent review {1} and are considered in depth in this book. To briefly summarize, gap junctional conductance may be nearly ohmic or, under some conditions, can be voltage-dependent. We have suggested that voltage-dependency may be important in poorly coupled cells, and perhaps this voltage-dependency fine tunes cell-cell communication in injury {24}. Gap junctional conductance can be modified by transients in internal calcium concentration and/or pH, the presence of lipophiles, arachidonic acid pathway intermediates, hypoxia, strophanthidin, hypertonicity and other changes that may be part of the ischemic process or therapeutic intervention. The specific distribution of gap junctions becomes less organized in injury. There may also be tissue specific differences in the density and distribution of gap junctions. The distribution in SA nodal tissue, atria, the AV node, Purkinje fibers, and ventricular muscle differs and may well play an important role in physiologic regulation.

4. CLINICAL EXTRAPOLATIONS

Gap junctions play a number of roles in health and disease. Although often characterized as a passive cellular property, as discussed, gap junctions gate or close in response to a number of stimuli, environmental changes and, in poorly communicating cells, to voltage. We will consider clinical extrapolations of gap junctional function in three areas related to arrhythmogenesis and the actions of certain drugs: (1) integrative functions, (2) anisotropy, and (3) the isolation of injured cells.

5. INTEGRATIVE FUNCTIONS

5.1 Excitability

The concept of liminal length has been introduced earlier as has the contribution of gap junctions to the determinants of the liminal length. Liminal length and excitability is critically important in the design and use of cardiac pacemakers and implantable cardioverter-defibrillaors. Only one publication has attempted to relate current thresholds and liminal length using disc electrodes of various sizes, the experimental findings corresponded closely to the theoretical calculations {25}.

If our argument is correct that the action potential is the local event and the fulfillment of the liminal length requirements is the propagated event {16}, the clinical importance of this concept becomes apparent. Quite possibly the dysfunction or failure of normal pacemakers (e.g., SA nodal arrest or SA nodal block), deviations from preferential conduction, abnormalities of impulse propagation and other electrophysiologic events that relate to excitability are determined, in part, by abnormalities of the gap junctions.

5.2 Automaticity

The mechanism of automaticity in the SA node is not fully understood, but it seems to arise from a changing balance between positive inward currents which favor depolarization and positive outward currents which favor repolarization: the depolarizing inward current being primarily a calcium current and the outward repolarizing currents primarily calcium currents.

Entrainment can be defined as the coupling of a self-sustaining oscillatory system to an external forcing oscillation with the result that either both oscillations have the same frequency or the frequencies are related in a harmonic fashion {26}. The concept of electrotonic interactions and entrainment among cells is difficult, but will is very important to our thinking about clinical arrhythmias.

Cardiac pacemaker rhythms may be synchronized to a variety of external periodicities including cellular and vagal stimulation {27-30}. Brief perturbations of cardiac pacemaker activity indicates that the sensitivity to the perturbation varies periodically {see review 26}. A periodic perturbing input, such as a pacemaker cell of electrical stimulation, can influence a second pacemaker to discharge at rates that are faster or slower than its intrinsic rate.

Bleeker et al {31} used correlative morphologic and electrophysiologic approaches to assess the functional and morphological organization of the rabbit SA node. They found that there is a dominant pacemaker region rather than a dominant cell that is responsible for the automatic activity of the SA node. The compact portion of the SA node contains several thousand cells that depolarize and production action potentials almost synchronously. All these cells seem to be influencing each other through cell-to-cell coupling, a process that has been called *mutual entrainment* {32}. The entrainment may be 1:1 or some harmonic of the underlying, basic frequency. Jalife and Michaels {33} list the requisites for mutual entrainment as follows: (1) there must be some form of communication that allows for mutual interaction between pacemakers; (2) the response of any given pacemaker to perturbations by its neighbor(s) must be phase-dependent; and (3) this phase-dependent response must have an advancing or delaying influence on its neighbor(s) so equality of periods can results. Jalife and his coworkers {34} further suggested that the synchronization of cells is due not to the influence of a "dominant" pacemaker cell, but from the mutual interaction of many individual pacemaker cells that represented a "democratic consensus" as to when the cells should discharge.

The interactions between the vagus and the SA node have been reviewed recently {33}. Brown and Eccles in 1934 observed that the effects of brief bursts of vagal stimuli on the rate of the sinus pacemaker depended on the intensity and timing of the train {35}. Experimental and simulation studies suggest that the vagal control of the SA nodal rate can be explained by vagal input entraining the already mutually entrained pacemaker cells that are responsible for SA nodal pacemaker {34, 36-38}. In these studies and simulations, phase-locking, period-doubling bifurcations, and other characteristics were observed that suggested nonlinear or chaotic dynamics.

Normally, the integrated activity of pacemaker cells in the compact region of the SA node has the fastest rate and the most consistent pacemaker. This initiates the sequential depolarization of the atria, AV node, His-bundle branch-terminal Purkinje system, and ventricular muscle. The propagating impulse will activate the latent pacemaker cells before they can spontaneously depolarize sufficiently to produce an action potential. The latent pacemaker is then reset, and repetitive excitation of the pacemaker cell will actually inhibit spontaneous phase 4 depolarization. So long as the SA node remains the fastest pacemaker and conduction throughout the heart is intact, subsidiary pacemakers will be suppressed and the SA node will control the overall heart beat.

The electrotonic interaction between pacemaker and nonpacemaker cells because of current flow among cells through gap junctions favors the suppression of subsidiary or abnormal pacemakers. Wit and Rosen {39} suggest that this mechanism may be important in suppressing automaticity in the AV node where atrial cells, which normally do not have pacemaker activity and which have resting potentials that are more negative than those of the AV nodal cells, creates a circuit with current flow between AV nodal and atrial cells that suppresses nodal automaticity. The whole issue of how the AV node is clamped by the mass of atrial tissue and how it becomes unclamped is poorly understood and is of great interest. Similar interactions may occur where latent pacemaker cells are next to non-pacemaker cells such as in the atria or perhaps in areas where the terminal Purkinje fibers, which normally possess pacemaker activity, may be modulated by the greater mass of well-coupled ventricular tissue that normally does not have pacemaker activity. It is interesting to speculate that normal non-pacemaker cells may suppress areas of abnormal automaticity as well.

Chronic or inappropriate nonparoxysmal sinus tachycardia occurs is an unusual condition that occurs in individuals without apparent heart disease or other causes for sinus tachycardia such as thyrotoxicosis, heart failure, anemia, fever, and infection {40, 41}. Its cause is unknown, but it is thought to reflect a disorder of autonomic control. Some individuals, however, are quite resistant to pharmacologic interventions, and one might speculate that perhaps part of the democratic entrainment and subsequent modulation of the sinus rate is lost, the result being that more rapid pacemakers control the heart rate. The sinus node is a long complex distributed along the crista terminalis. Intracardiac echocardiography was used in dogs to define the crista terminalis and to localize the position of an ablation catheter relative to the sinus node, following which radiofrequency ablation could modify or shift the site of sinus pacemaker function {42}. The same approach was used to modify sinus node function in individuals with inappropriate sinus tachycardia {43}. The region ablated was that showing the earliest atrial activation which, presumably, is the area of the SA node containing the fastest pacemakers. The result was a 25% reduction in the sinus heart rate, and it seems likely that the fastest pacemaker cells were either ablated or otherwise physically separated from the remainder of the pacemaker complex and the atria. The remaining SA nodal cells then mutually entrained at a slower rate.

The classical definition of parasystole is a rhythm arising from an automatic focus that is surrounded by an area that protects it from being influenced by any other non-parasystolic beat. We now know that parasystole can be modulated or at times annihilated by electronic interactions through gap junctions {see review 44}. The rate of the parasystolic pacemaker will be slowed by entrainment with early non-parasystolic beats, while the rate of the pacemaker will be increased by entrainment with late non-parasystolic beats. Phase-response curves can be generated in some individuals. The modifying beats may result from a normal sinus rhythm or from any other type of rhythm. If there is an area of partial conduction block around the parasystolic focus, self-modulation can occur depending on the degree of block. Self-entrainment can also occur which may be responsible for alternating short-long cycles sometimes seen in ectopic ventricular tachycardia. In the laboratory, critically timed subthreshold depolarizations can annihilate an automatic focus, and possibly this type of pacemaker annihilation occurs clinically.

5.3 Integrated and Fragmented Wavefronts in Impulse Propagation

Normally, gap junctions integrate the wave front through electrotonic interactions. Given two neighboring cell columns in which one column conducts more rapidly than the other, the faster fiber through electrotonic interaction will speed up the slower fiber, and the slower fiber will slow down the faster fiber. The result is a unit of two columns, traveling at a uniform, intermediate speed. In the heart, many such interactions produce a smooth, integrated wavefront of activation that is responsible for the highly controlled and efficient contraction of the heart needed to maximize cardiac output. An integrated wavefront is unlikely to produce reentry.

In the 8 week canine infarct, fractionated electrograms can be recorded from the surface of the infarct zone, yet action potentials recorded from myocytes within these zones are normal {45, 46}. Pathological studies showed that the muscle fibers were widely separated and disoriented by connective tissues. The slow, fragmented activation that gave rise to the fractionated electrograms, therefore, was not due to changes in the active generator, but rather to disruption in the integrative electrotonic interaction between cells caused by fibrosis that physically disconnected the cells. This type of fragmented conduction is thought to be an important substrate for reentrant arrhythmias. It is these signals that are recorded by the signal-averaged electrocardiogram and are sought during ablation studies, so they are very important markers diagnostically and clinically.

5.4 Anisotropy in Arrhythmogenesis

The concept of anisotropy has been considered in substantial detail in other Chapters in this book as well as in reviews {1, 47-51}. In essence, anisotropy is a measured difference of a physical property related to the direction in which the measurement is made. Structural anisotropy is intrinsic to the structure of the myocardial tissue. This anisotropy can be a normal characteristic of tissues depending on the fiber axis and the distribution and functionality of gap junctions linking cells longitudinally and transversely. Anisotropy can be the result of disease; or, at times, it can be created with a therapeutic intention. Functional anisotropy can result from the establishment of lines of functional block. Since gap junctions probably play little role in functional anisotropy, this will not be discussed in any detail. Much of what follows is speculation since it is difficult to study cellular coupling in man.

A few comments on what underlies anisotropy are in order. As a general statement, the velocity of impulse propagation is faster parallel to fiber orientation than perpendicular, and these velocities are termed longitudinal and transverse, respectively. Passive resistivity within and between cells depends on geometry and gap junctional connections including tapering, shape and bifurcations, and several of these influences have been elegantly modeled. Some studies have found a rough relationship between diameter and conduction velocity {52}, but others have found conduction velocity to be quite constant regardless of diameter, as in Purkinje fibers {53}. Anisotropy within a fiber may explain in part the failure of conduction velocity to correlate with diameter in the Purkinje fiber {54}. In this situation, the local circuit currents at the edge of the propagating wave front preferentially flow longitudinally within a column of cells, and conduction velocity, then, would be independent of diameter if the fiber size was determined not by the size of the individual cells, but rather by the number of cells. The extracellular space also may influence conduction, particularly in the presence of edema, cellular swelling or fibrosis. Another possible interpretation of the failure of conduction velocity to correlate with diameter in Purkinje fibers assumes that the extracellular clefts are more important in larger cells so that the effects of $r_o + r_i$ may be counter the influence of diameter. Goldstein and Rall {55} modeled the change in conduction velocity in situations of changing fiber and geometry and found that with a step reduction in diameter, conduction velocity increases, with a step increase in diameter, conduction velocity decreases. This follows from the amount of current lost downstream in the sink. When branching was considered, the impulse approaching the branching site first decreased in velocity since the branches provided a larger sink, and, once beyond the junction and into a smaller branch, the conduction velocity increased. Interestingly, extracellular space anisotropy may be discordant directionally with intracellular anisotropy {56}.

Propagation through three-dimensional tissues is far more complex than one-dimensional propagation along cable-like fibers such as Purkinje fibers. To describe anisotropic propagation empirically on a macroscopic scale, Madison Spach and his colleagues proposed measurement of the effective axial resistivity which is the value of internal resistivity which would account for the observed speed of propagation in any direction, not just along the long axis of muscle fibers {48, 57, 58}. Unlike R_i in linear continuous cable theory, which incorporates only axial cytoplasmic resistivity and end-to-end gap junctional conductivity, axial resistivity also includes implicitly the influences of cellular geometry and packing, extracellular resistivities, side-to-side couplings, and other features. Equations based on axial resistivity have successfully predicted propagation on a macroscopic scale (several mm or more), even along pathways of complex or heterogeneous structure. Excitation in young hearts spreads along smooth contours in directions off the long axis, indicating uniform anisotropy (somewhat of an oxymoron), but, in older preparations, the fast longitudinal path was narrow and had abrupt borders {59-61}. Off the long axis, excitation spread very slowly and in irregular or zigzag fashion and often reached a transverse site multiphasically. This dissociation or fractionation indicates propagation by multiple paths, which could not occur in uniformly anisotropic tissue. Propagation with these features has been called discontinuous, dissociated microscopic, or fractionated {59, 62} and is seen frequently in the electrophysiology laboratory where fractionated potentials serve as a marker for ablation. Figures 4-6 summarize some of these concepts. Figure 4 show the characteristics of tissues when viewed as a conductive media supporting propagation. Figure 5 shows anisotropy of the action potential waveform and propagation velocity in the crista terminalis. Figure 6 shows nonuniform anisotropic propagation in atrial tissue in human tissues of different ages.

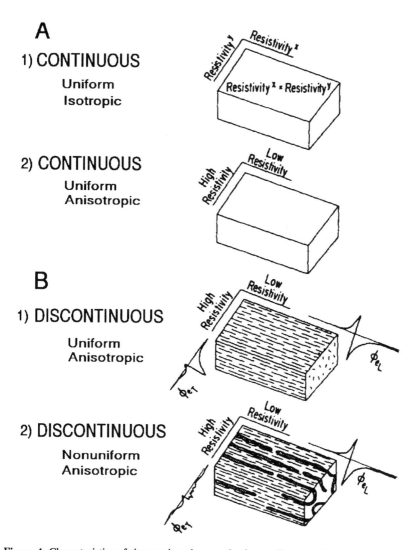

Figure 4. Characteristics of tissues viewed as conductive media supporting propagation. A1: Medium whose resistivity is constant and the same in all directions. A2: Medium whose resistivity is constant in a given direction but differs in different directions. B1: Medium with discrete impedances, such as high-resistance junctions, in the transverse direction. The resistivity is not constant, but the distribution of these impedances is similar throughout the medium. B2: Medium with irregularly arranged discrete transverse barriers. Transverse propagation can occur simultaneously via multiple paths. ϕ_e symbolizes extracellularly recorded potentials.

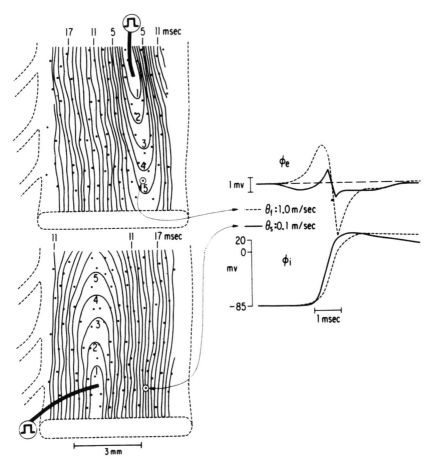

Figure 5. Anisotropy of AP waveform and propagation velocity in the crista terminalis. Left: Points of stimulation are indicated by square pulses; dots indicate sites of extracellular recording. Right: Extracellular (ϕ_e) and intracellular (ϕ_i) potentials at the right were recorded at points (circled and arrowed) longitudinal (dotted traces) and transverse (solid traces) to a point of stimulation. dV/dt$_{max}$ was higher and τ_{foot} was longer in the transverse direction. Isochrone maps (left), constructed from the extracellular recordings, indicate uniform anisotropy; conduction velocity, calculated as the distance travelled normal to an isochrone per unit time, was lower transversely, despite higher dV$_m$/dt$_{max}$.

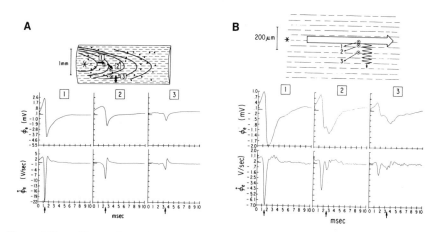

Figure 6. Nonuniform anisotropic propagation in atrial tissue. A: Preparation from 2-year-old male. Excitation spread smoothly from site of initiation (*), as shown by the continuous isochrones (top). Smooth extracellular voltage waveforms (ϕ_e) and their time derivatives, recorded from circled points numbered (1,2,3), indicate monophasic excitation (bottom). The thin dashed lines show the orientation of the fibers. Arrows at the bottom of each panel mark the times of dV_m/dt_{max} of the underlying action potentials, which were used to construct the isochrones. Isochrones are separated by 1 msec. B: Preparation from 42-year-old male. The prominent open arrow on the preparation (top) indicates that in a narrow longitudinal region, propagation was fast and uniform as shown in trace (1) at bottom. The sawtooth indicates that, in directions not collinear with the fiber axis, excitation spread along an irregular zigzag course. The corresponding extracellular waveforms and derivatives, seen in traces (2) and (3) at bottom, are multiply peaked, indicating that excitation spread nonuniformly by multiple paths.

Anisotropic activation and propagation originate in large part with structural features of cardiac muscle. The fine structure of normal cardiac muscle suggest that myocytes form "unit" bundles of 2-15 cells that have connections every 0.1 mm to 0.2 mm which are arranged into separate fascicles that connect with each other at longer distances, possibly related to diameter {63}. The fascicles group into macroscopic bundles that have complex and varying interconnections. The localization of gap junctions, particularly in adult tissues, is dominantly in end-to-end connections, leaving transverse electrical coupling with a smaller magnitude and less uniformity than longitudinal coupling, consistent with slower and more indirect propagation off the long axis {64-68). The density of immunostained Cx43 per cell is less in the AV node than in either atrial or ventricular myocardium with a punctate distribution within and along the borders of the nodal cells as well as variation in intensity of Cx43 staining in different portions of the AV node {68}. The predominantly end-to-end distribution in atrial, Purkinje and ventricular tissues favors longitudinal and, therefore, anisotropic conduction, while the punctate distribution in the AV node would favor current distribution in all directions.

Anisotropies are also relevant to pathology, and some of the underlying pathology has been discussed above in the section on integrative function. Anisotropic structural changes in the chronic phase after injury. For example, it has been observed in experimental animals that damaged longitudinal pathways can be supplanted by intact transverse-longitudinal-transverse alternates which may be very long and have less than the normal strength of coupling {39, 51, 69}. Propagation through such restructured tissue should become substantially slower and more variable than normal, and electrotonic coupling may become more prominent {70, 71}. These are features that can support stable arrhythmogenic patterns of propagation {51, 72}.

Anisotropic conduction, then, can cause the slow conduction, the area of unidirectional conduction block, or both involved in reentry. Anatomical pathways may be involved, but anisotropy can also occur without an anatomical pathway. Wit et al {51} distinguish between functional and anisotropic reentry. They suggest that the functional characteristic that causes the leading circle type of reentry is a difference in refractory periods in adjacent areas caused by inhomogeneous conduction. In reentry caused by anisotropy, the essential feature is a difference in effective axial resistance to impulse propagation dependent on fiber direction. Clearly, the two overlap.

5.5 Safety Factor

Another concept that should be understood by the clinician is the concept of the safety factor. As discussed above, liminal length (LL) is the amount of tissue that must be raised above threshold so that the inward depolarizing current from that patch of membrane exceeds the repolarizing influences of adjacent tissues and results in an action potential. If the local electrotonic currents are sufficient to fulfill the liminal length requirements of the neighboring patch or patches of membrane, these patches will also produce action potentials. These events repeat and the sequential depolarization of patches of membrane results. The term safety factor is the excess in the activating current or charge over that just required to produce a regenerative propagated response, or, more succinctly, the excess of source over sink.

Clinicians are well aware that propagation can fail more readily in certain tissues such as the AV node, while propagation rarely fails in the His-Purkinje system or in atrial and ventricular muscle. Fast response tissues that depend on the rapid inward sodium current for regenerative depolarization (atria, bundle of His, fascicles and bundle branches, terminal Purkinje fibers, ventricular muscle, and accessory pathways) have a higher safety factor than slow response tissues that depend on the kinetically slow inward calcium current for regenerative depolarization (AV node). Fast response tissues that are depolarized during injury have a lower safety factor than normal because of partial inactivation of the sodium current or, at times, because the tissue now becomes dependent on the calcium current for phase 0 depolarization.

Passive properties of the sink also determine the safety factor. Failure of conduction can occur at points where passive properties change discontinuously, for example at points of branching. If the cross-sectional area and length of a segment are constant, membrane surface area will increase and R_m will decrease at a branch point. As mentioned, conduction velocity will change when fibers change their diameter or branch {55}. In general, increased diameter or more branching led to a slower conduction velocity as the sinking of current downstream is greater. Critically slowed conduction at times resulted in the failure of propagation and, at other times, in an echo beat, reflections, and other signs of mismatch (see also {73-75}). Extensive branching, as found in the AV node, is associated with lower safety.

Gap junctions also play an important role in determining the safety factor, and we have previously considered this in some technical detail {1}. Although longitudinal propagation is faster than transverse propagation, it may not be safer. Heptanol uncoupling of gap junctions {76-78} and injury {79, 80} blocked slow transverse propagation earlier than fast longitudinal propagation. Increasingly premature extrastimuli which encroaches upon the relative refractory period of the myocardial tissue has been observed to block longitudinal propagation earlier than transverse {57, 58, 61}. In these studies, fast longitudinal propagation became first decremental and then ceased, while transverse propagation, though fractionated, continued. The underlying reason for disparate observations with respect to safety or failure of propagation is most likely differences in the microscopic nonuniform anisotropy of tissue structure {61}.

Gap junctional conductances have been studied using voltage clamping, and the same type of source over sink relationship applies. Most simply, the safety factor of the transfer of current from one cell to another can be considered in terms of the number of open gap junctions which in turn translates as the conductance (reciprocal of resistance) between cells. When the input resistance is high, as in the SA node, junctional conductance can be sufficient to allow synchronization of cells when there are only a few gap junction channels {81, 82}. When input resistance is low, as in ventricular muscle, rapid conduction requires tens or hundreds of active channels {82, 83}. Injury affects the spatial distribution and overall density of gap junctions {70, 84}. Further, injury decreases cellular coupling and, therefore, makes properties that are dependent on coupling, such as conduction velocity, more susceptible to modification by rate-dependent factors such as intracellular calcium concentration and pH {68, 85-87} or transjunctional voltage {24, 88, 89} than in normal tissue {89, 90}. These influences may be exquisitely sensitive to beat to beat changes in rate.

5.6 Excitable Gap and Entrainment

An *excitable gap* in a reentrant circuit is a region of the circuit where the cardiac cells have had sufficient time to reactive and recover their excitability before the return of the reentrant wave. In general, the excitable gap is larger in areas of slow conduction and smaller or nonexistent in areas of rapid conduction. Once again, anisotropy in which transverse conduction is slower than longitudinal conduction would be expected to produce excitable gaps with differing spatial extents.

A fully excitable gap in an anisotropic reentrant circuit allows termination of a reentrant arrhythmia. A spontaneous extrasystole or an electrically paced beat can enter the circuit in the excitable gap and influence the reentrant circuit in a number of ways. The termination of a reentrant tachycardia by a single extrasystole or a burst of extrasystoles is thought to result from the entry of an impulse into the excitable gap which, in turn, renders a critical portion of the circuit inexcitable.

A fully excitable gap also allows *entrainment*, which, as described earlier, concerns the interaction of two oscillators. Entrainment clinically refers to special interactions between stimulation of the tissue and the reentrant circuit. Waldo and his coworkers in a classic paper published in 1977 described the transient entrainment of type I atrial flutter {91}. They observed that if the atrium was paced somewhat faster than the rate of the type I atrial flutter, the rate of the tachycardia increased to match that of the faster pacing rate; that is, it was entrained; and, with cessation of the pacing or slowing of the pacing rate, the original rate of the atrial flutter returned or, frequently, the arrhythmia terminated. Studies by Waldo and his colleagues and others followed on transient entrainment in atrial flutter {92-94}, ventricular tachycardia {93, 95-98}, AV nodal reentrant tachycardia or AV reentrant tachycardia using an accessory AV bypass tract {93}, intraatrial reentrant atrial tachycardia {93, 99} and even atrial fibrillation {100}.

Waldo and his colleagues propose four criteria to establish the presence of transient entrainment {92, 101, 102}. Constant fusion beats must be recorded in the ECG during constant pacing at a rate somewhat faster than the rate of the spontaneous atrial flutter, except for the last paced beat which is entrained but not fused. The last beat, then, will have the morphology of the spontaneous atrial flutter. The fusion beats during rapid pacing will result in morphologically constant atrial deflection on the ECG. At different rates of constant pacing, however, the fusion differs, and the morphology of the atrial recording will also differ. But the morphology will be constant for the new rate. Interruption of the tachycardia is associated with localized conduction block to one or more sites for one beat, followed by subsequent activation of that site or sites from a different direction. The morphology of the atrial electrogram at the blocked site or sites will change, and the conduction time will be shorter. Evidence for progressive fusion on the electrogram with a demonstration of a change in conduction time and electrogram morphology at one recording site when paced from another site at two different constant pacing rates that are faster than the spontaneous rate of the tachycardia but which do not interrupt the arrhythmia.

Sometimes, pacing at a rate somewhat faster than that of the spontaneous atrial flutter results in capturing the tachycardia without interrupting the tachycardia and without demonstrating any of the criteria for entrainment. This may be due to concealed entrainment in which the antidromic wave of the paced beat blocks in an area of slow conduction due to collision with the wavefront of the preceding beat. The orthodromic wavefront conducts completely around the circuit, traverses the area of slow conduction which allows previously excited tissue to become reactivated, finds no wavefront with which to collide, and so continues in the circuit restoring the atrial flutter. The circuit, however, may be interrupted if the antidromic beat and the orthodromic wave front from the previous beat block in the area of slow conduction. None of the transient entrainment criteria are met, yet the arrhythmia may be terminated. As Waldo and his colleagues point out, concealed entrainment can be established only if transient entrainment can be demonstrated by pacing at another site, and they suggest that pacing from sites high in the right atrium should always permit the demonstration of transient entrainment.

The issues involved in entrainment concern all reentrant arrhythmias. Because of the importance in determining the site of reentry and ablation in ventricular tachycardia, most of the discussion of entrainment will be part of the discussion of sustained monomorphic ventricular tachycardia.

6. ISOLATION OF INJURED CELLS

Teleologically, the shutdown of gap junctions by increased $[Ca^{++}]i$, lowered pH or other determinants may isolate cells that have undergone injury from normal cells. The analogy would be the closing watertight doors in a submarine when the integrity of one compartments has been compromised. In cells, this isolation means that normal cells will not lose their cytoplasmic contents by leakage through the injured cell to the outside cell. This isolation will prevent toxic metabolites, high concentrations of calcium and hydrogen ions from entering normal cells, thereby creating a chain reaction of cell injury and death. This isolation will also prevent the flow of current between cells having different transmembrane potentials (e.g., normal transmembrane voltage in normal cells and a less negative than usual transmembrane voltage in injured, depolarized cells). Clinically, such mechanisms may be protective of the injured heart. Such mechanisms, however, may also be arrhythmogenic since the cells taken out of the circuit may cause zig-zag activation conducive to reentry.

7. SELECTED ARRHYTHMIAS

Gap junctional function cannot be studied easily in the human heart. Much of what follows about the relationship between anisotropy and arrhythmias in man is inferred from the study of conduction.

7.1 Atrial Flutter

Atrial flutter is a reentrant arrhythmia that excites an area of the atrium and then travels sufficiently slowly in a pathway that is sufficiently long that the initially excited area recovers its excitability and can be reactivated {91, 103-110}. A single premature extrastimulus or rapid atrial pacing can both initiate atrial flutter and, because there is generally an excitable gap, terminate the arrhythmia. As discussed above, the excitable gap is the portion of a reentrant circuit during any one cycle length that has recovered its excitability and can again be depolarized. The excitable gap allows entrainment with overdrive pacing during atrial flutter {91, 92, 94, among others}.

As noted by Lesh et al. {47}, who reinterpreted the early observations by Watson and Josephson in 1980 {103}, the site of dependency of the induction of the arrhythmia suggests that anisotropy is an important mechanism in atrial flutter. Induction of the arrhythmia in the high right atrium was consistent and reproducible, suggesting that it is within the reentrant pathway. Stimulation in the region of the coronary sinus, however, rarely induced the arrhythmia and presumably is outside the reentrant pathway. Moreover, Watson and Josephson noted fragmented electrograms in the atrium near the His Bundle suggesting slow, discontinuous propagation transverse to fiber orientation. Whether such slow conduction is necessary for atrial flutter, however, has been debated.

Electrophysiologic mapping has been performed in patients with atrial flutter in the catheterization laboratory and at surgery. A large macroreentrant circuit in the right atrium is involved in counterclockwise type I atrial flutter. If one begins the cycle at the end of the negative deflection of the F wave in lead II, the impulse at that point exists in the low right atrial septum between the inferior vena cava and the tricuspid valve; it then travels anteriorly through the region of the low septum, then superiorly and anteriorly up the medial surface of the right atrium, and returns over the lateral and posterior free wall. It has been suggested that a narrow portion of right atrial septal myocardium, located between the orifice of the tricuspid valve and the coronary sinus, is a required part of the reentrant circuit in most types of atrial flutter {106, 108, 109, 111, 112}. Figure 7 depicts the postulated reentrant loop involved in common atrial flutter.

There is an anatomical as well as a pathophysiologic basis for this commonly utilized pathway in atrial flutter. It has long been known that transverse conduction velocity across the crista terminalis is much slower than the longitudinal conduction velocity, being 0.09 m/sec and 1.05 m/sec in the 1981 investigation by Spach and his colleagues {113} (see Fig. 5). In a recent compilation, the weighted average in a number of studies was a conduction velocity of 1.23 m/sec for longitudinal and 0.09 m/sec for transverse conduction {68, 114-116}. The distribution and density of gap junctions is most likely responsible for the difficulty of an impulse to cross the crista terminalis and the eustachian ridge and valve, thus favoring anisotropic propagation around rather than through these structures. The eustachian valve and ridge or the inferior vena cava form one border of the isthmus and the tricuspid valve annulus the other (see Fig. 7).

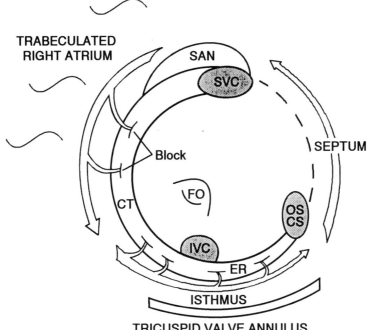

Figure 7. Diagrammatic representation of the circuit used in the common form of atrial flutter. The wavefront courses in the trabeculated right atrium and usually fails to cross the crista terminalis (CT) due to poor cell-cell connections in the crista itself (indicated by "block"). The Eustachian ridge (ER) is an extension of this anatomical barrier. The impulse passes through an area called the "isthmus" that is bound on each side by the Eustachian ridge (ER) and the tricuspid valve annulus. The isthmus is an anatomic target for ablation, usually between the inferior vena cava (IVC) and the tricuspid annulus but also between the Eustachian ridge and the tricuspid annulus. The small isthmus between the tricuspid valve annulus and the coronary sinus ostium (OS CS) has also been the target of ablation with some success. Activation continues in the intraatrial septum. SAN, sinoatrial node; SVC, superior vena cava; IVC, inferior vena cava; CT, crista terminalis; ER, Eustachian ridge; FO, foramen ovale; OS CS, os of the coronary sinus.

Nomenclature for the types of atrial flutter has been confusing. It has been suggested that the classification of atrial flutter be based on the location of these anatomical barriers {117}. Typical atrial flutter would be rotation around the tricuspid annulus with the crista terminalis and the Eustachian ridge as posterior barriers. Subclassification of typical atrial flutter would depend on the direction of rotation of the wavefront. The common form of atrial flutter uses the circuit described above which can be described as counterclockwise flutter if one looks from the left ventricle through the tricuspid valve into the right atrium. Atrial flutter may use the same circuit defined by the same anatomical barrier in a clockwise manner. In this scheme, clockwise flutter would be a subclassification of common flutter. The experience of some suggests that although clockwise flutter is the presenting clinical arrhythmia in only a few patients, it can be induced by EPS study in most {117}. In this classification, a true atypical form of atrial flutter uses circuits and barriers other than those of clockwise and counterclockwise flutter {117}.

Atypical flutter is heterogeneous, tends to be unstable, often converts into atrial fibrillation, and may terminate spontaneously or become a typical clockwise or clockwise atrial flutter {117}. The mechanisms of atypical atrial flutter are speculative. On the one hand, the transitions between atypical atrial flutter, atrial fibrillation, and common atrial flutter suggest that lines of functional block are involved; while on the other hand, patients tend to develop the same morphology of atypical flutter suggesting that the lines of block may have an anatomic basis {117}.

7.3 Other Atrial Arrhythmias

Spach and his coworkers studied the electrophysiologic properties in human atrial pectinate bundles that had been removed at surgery from aged individuals {62}. Premature beats were introduced in these non-uniformly anisotropic bundles resulting in dissociated zig-zag conduction and anisotropic reentry within regions as small as 50 mm^2. Electrograms were fragmented, analogous to those recorded at the time of open heart surgery. It is quite likely that this type of non-uniformly anisotropic substrate underlies virtually all reentrant atrial arrhythmias by contributing to the formation of the areas of slow conduction and unidirectional block essential for reentry. These atrial rhythms and even atrial flutter can be entrained from reproducible locations in a given individual, thereby supporting the idea that anisotropy is important in these reentry circuits {92, 93, 99, 100}.

7.4 Atrioventricular Nodal Reentrant Tachycardia

Atrioventricular nodal reentrant tachycardia (AVNRT) is a common arrhythmia, accounting for approximately two-thirds of cases of paroxysmal supraventricular tachycardia. AVNRT is a reentrant rhythm that utilizes the AV node and, usually, perinodal atrial tissue {118, 119}. The term "atrioventricular junctional reentrant tachycardia" is being used increasingly, because more than just the AV node is often involved in the reentrant circuit. The bundle of His is probably not a necessary part of the reentrant circuit, since the arrhythmia is at times associated with 2:1 AV block (ie, the completion of two complete circuits is evidenced by two retrograde P waves while only one of the impulses traverses the His bundle on the way to the ventricles indicating that the bundle of His is not a necessary component of the circuit). In addition, His bundle electrograms indicate that reentry is proximal to the recording site {120, 121}. The topic has been comprehensively reviewed recently {122}.

The AV node depends upon the inward calcium current for the regenerative phase of the action potential which, in large part along with anatomical factors, accounts for the slow, but not necessarily safe, conduction through the AV node. The simplest concept of AV nodal physiology that allows AV nodal reentry has long been based on the postulated existence of two functionally different AV nodal pathways, now thought likely to be primarily in the perinodal atrial tissue with AV nodal connections, with differing conduction velocities and refractory periods {123}. The so-called fast or - pathway conducts rapidly and most commonly has a relatively long refractory period; while the slow or - pathway conducts relatively slowly and most commonly has a shorter refractory period. These pathways join and enter a final common pathway in the AV node.

These early studies suggested functional dissociation into a fast and slow pathway {124}, and functional dissociation, in turn, implies anisotropy due to relative isolation from the influence of neighboring tissue mediated by the nature of gap junctional communication. Two forms of AVNRT based this model were identified: the common slow-fast AVNRT in which antegrade conduction was through the slow pathway and retrograde conduction through the fast pathway and uncommon fast-slow AVNRT in which antegrade conduction occurred through the fast pathway and retrograde conduction through the slow pathway. A third form of AVNRT utilizes a slow pathway for antegrade conduction and another slow pathway for retrograde conduction.

For a number of years, it was postulated that there was a proximal common pathway within the AV node, but, as mentioned, it is now thought that the proximal fast and slow pathways are in perinodal atrial tissue in virtually all patients. The functional dissociation results in a rather reproducible sequence of events. The proposed sequence in the common form of AVNRT, which affects 80 percent or more of patients, is as follows. The normal sinus beat enters the AV node and the impulse travels down both the fast and slow pathways. The impulse traveling down the fast pathway reaches the His bundle first creating a refractory wake, and the impulse in the slow pathway runs into the refractory wake of the impulse that had traveled down the fast pathway. The impulse traveling down the slow pathway is extinguished when, in the area of the final common pathway, it runs into the refractory wake of the impulse that had traveled down the fast pathway. The fast pathway has a longer refractory period than the slow pathway, so a critically timed premature atrial beat (or less commonly, a premature junctional or ventricular beat with retrograde conduction) may enter the AV node, find the fast pathway refractory, but still be able to conduct via the slow pathway through the final common pathway to the bundle of His. If the fast pathway has recovered its excitability by the time the slow pathway impulse reaches the distal junction of the two pathways, the impulse may be able to conduct retrogradely up the fast pathway. The circuit may then become repetitive with antegrade conduction down the slow pathway and retrograde conduction up the fast pathway resulting in a sustained tachycardia, the so-called slow-fast pathway type of AVNRT. The electrocardiogram in this setting shows a supraventricular tachycardia in which the P wave is buried in the QRS complex or occurs slightly before or slightly after the QRS complex, often in fusion with the QRS complex. In about 10 percent of patients, the reentrant circuit involves antegrade conduction down the fast pathway and retrograde conduction down the slow pathway. This is called the uncommon or fast-slow pathway type of AVNRT. The P wave that appears shortly before the QRS complex. In another 9 or 10% of individuals, both antegrade and retrograde conduction occur over slow pathways.

The exact anatomic distribution of these pathways is uncertain. As illustrated in Figure 8, Koch's triangle is bounded by the tricuspid ring and the tendon of Todoro which bracket the coronary sinus at the base of the triangle and are in close proximity forming the apex near the His bundle at the membranous septum. As an approximation, Koch's triangle can be divided into thirds: the anterior which contains the compact AV node and the fast pathways; the middle; and the posterior which is associated with the coronary sinus. High resolution electrophysiologic mapping indicates that retrograde fast pathway conduction during the common form of AVNRT causes the earliest atrial activation at the apex of Koch's triangle in the vicinity of the junction between the AV node and the bundle of His {118}. Retrograde slow pathway conduction during the uncommon form of AVNRT activates the atrium earliest in the lower (most frequent) or middle portion of Koch's triangle near the os of the coronary sinus. This localization has allowed the successful ablation of fast and slow pathways to cure recurrent AVNRT. Figure 8 shows the landmarks related to Koch's triangle.

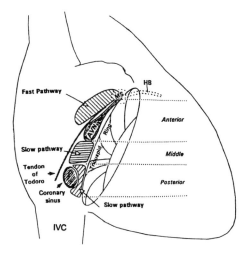

Figure 8. Schematic representation of Koch's triangle which is bounded by the tricuspid ring and the tendon of Todoro. The tendon of Todoro and the tricuspid ring are in close proximity forming the apex of the triangle near the His bundle at the membranous septum. Koch's triangle can be divided into thirds: the anterior contains the compact AV node; the posterior contains the coronary sinus; and the middle or mid-septal third is between the anterior and posterior portions. The anterior third is associated with fast pathways, and the middle and posterior thirds with slow pathways.

The microscopic anatomy of the AV node and the perinodal atrial tissues is complex, and the relationship of anatomy to electrophysiology is only poorly understood {125-127}. The AV node appears to be non-uniformly anisotropic from the macroscopic to the microscopic scales. The small unorganized cells are poorly coupled as indicated by the short space constant recorded by DeMello {128}. The paucity of gap junctions in the AV node is, in part, responsible for the slowing of conduction velocity within the AV node and at its interface with the atria {68, 129-131}. The density and distribution of Cx43 in the AV node is of interest {68}. The density of immunostained Cx43 per cell is less in the AV node than in either atrial or ventricular myocardium, the distribution of Cx43 is punctate within and along the borders of the nodal cells, and the intensity of Cx43 staining varies in different parts of the AV node {68}. It is interesting to speculate that these characteristics of Cx43 density and distribution would disperse currents in many directions rather than in a preferred direction. Gordon Moe and his colleagues in their landmark 1957 study thought longitudinal dissociation as likely underlying the observed dual AV nodal physiology {123}, an assumption that has been confirmed subsequently in studies that demonstrated longitudinal dissociation without anatomical evidence of separate pathways {125, 132}. Indeed, the existence of both horizontal and longitudinal dissociation have been demonstrated in man {133}. The reentrant circuit has an excitable gap and, therefore, can be terminated by a single extrasystole and can be entrained; evidence that favors an anisotropic basis for reentry.

7.5 Atrioventricular Reentrant Tachycardia

Approximately 30% of cases of paroxysmal supraventricular tachycardia arise from reentry that utilizes both the AV node and an atrioventricular accessory pathway in the reentrant circuit. The features of the AV node of importance to anisotropy have been discussed above. Atrioventricular accessory pathways can conduct antegradely or orthodromically (atrium to ventricle) in which case the ventricles are excited earlier than they would be through normal AV nodal conduction, and this is called preexcitation. The ventricles are also activated eccentrically as compared to the AV node. Atrioventricular accessory pathways can also conduct retrogradely or antidromically (ventricle to atrium). For reasons that are not clear, these accessory pathways result from incomplete isolation of the atria from the ventricles during cardiogenesis.

The characteristics of the active generator properties and cell-cell conduction as well as the electrotonic influence of the ventricles and, to a lesser extent, of the atria determine the functional characteristics of these accessory pathways. The speed of conduction and refractoriness of the accessory pathway vary greatly. Some allow conduction at rates of 300 beats/min and even faster; others conduct very slowly, have long action potentials; and yet others even have some nodal qualities. Some allow bidirectional conduction, while others allow conduction one way but not the other. Overall, about 95% of atrioventricular accessory pathways conduct rapidly and have the characteristics of sodium dependent phase 0 action potentials that occur in normal "fast response" myocardium. Five percent show decremental conduction, the mechanism of which is uncertain. Possible explanations include geometric factors including those involved in anisotropy, partial inactivation of the sodium channel and perhaps dependence on a calcium channel.

Usually there is no evidence of preexcitation during normal sinus rhythm, but AVRT is a common arrhythmia (perhaps 5%) in individuals with preexcitation, most commonly involving atrioventricular and atrionodal or atriofascicular pathways. AVRT tends to have a faster rate than atrioventricular nodal reentrant tachycardia (AVNRT) and often exceeds 200 beats/min, but there is a great deal of overlap in the rates of the two arrhythmias. The arrhythmia may occur in the absence or presence of other structural heart disease, and the symptoms and importance often depend on the underlying heart disease. Accessory pathways may be multiple {134-136}, and individuals with AVRT may not infrequently have AVNRT {137, 138}.

The reentrant circuit responsible for the AVRT can be of two types: *orthodromic* in that the impulse travels through the AV node, down the infranodal specialized conduction system, to the ventricles, and returns to the atrium through an accessory pathway; or *antidromic* in that it conducts from the atrium to the ventricle through the accessory pathway and returns through the AV node.

In orthrodromic AVRT antegrade conduction is through the AV node and retrograde conduction through an accessory pathway, usually of the atrioventricular type. There is usually no evidence on the routine ECG of an accessory pathway during normal sinus rhythm, that is, there is no evidence of ventricular preexcitation, since these accessory pathways cannot conduct antegradely from the atrium to the ventricles, but they can conduct unidirectionally from the ventricle to the atrium {139-142}. These pathways are said to be "concealed" since their existence cannot be ascertained from the ECG during normal sinus rhythm, but demonstrate an electrophysiologic effect during the orthodromic AVRT. Possibly, some pathways are not "concealed" but cause little preexcitation on antegrade conduction due to location or electrophysiologic properties.

The reasons for this unidirectional conduction are uncertain, but perhaps safety factor is of importance. It seems reasonable to hypothesize that the electrical mass of the ventricle is sufficient to generate electrotonic currents that can activate the accessory pathway, while the mass of the atrium is insufficient to active the ventricular myocardium. Other possibilities include geometric differences or perhaps rectification. Whatever the mechanism, the atrial impulse seems to enter the accessory pathway and blocks near the ventricular insertion site {143}. Anisotropic reentry is suggested further by the existence of an excitable gap permits termination by one or more extrastimuli and entrainment.

The rate may exceed 200 beats/min. Since antegrade AV conduction is over the normal pathway, the QRS complexes are normal, may show functional aberrant conduction, or, reflect preexisting bundle branch or fascicular block. The reentrant circuit is relatively large, as compared to AV nodal reentrant tachycardia, so the P wave follows the QRS complex and usually appears in the ST segment or the T wave. The RP interval will be less than half the RR interval. Most pathways are eccentric and left-sided, so atrial activation commonly begins in the left atrium resulting in inverted P waves in lead I. Septal pathways and right-sided pathways near the AV node may give rise to the usual type of retrograde atrial activation.

Antidromic AVRT is responsible for perhaps 10% of paroxysmal supraventricular tachycardias in patients with accessory pathways and is a wide complex tachycardia due to antegrade conduction through the accessory pathway and retrograde conduction through the AV node. These patients frequently have several accessory pathways that can support antidromic AVRT {134-136}. Because of the eccentric antegrade activation of the ventricles and lack of AV nodal conduction, full preexcitation will be displayed with a large delta wave and broadened QRS complex. Because the circuit is relatively long, the retrograde P wave will appear in the ST segment or the T wave. Since retrograde atrial activation arises from the impulse emerging from the AV node, the usual retrograde activation pattern will be observed with the RP interval less than half the RR interval. Functional bundle branch block on the ipsilateral side of the accessory pathway results in a longer circuit length which in turn slows the rate of the tachycardia; lengthening in cycle length by more than 35 msec strongly suggests AVRT. Conversely, the disappearance of bundle branch block may decrease the cycle length. Septal pathways, however, may not result in such changes.

Orthodromic AVRT and AVNRT together form most cases of paroxysmal supraventricular tachycardia. The common form of AVNRT has a shorter circuit than AVRT, so the retrograde P wave in AVNRT is usually buried in the QRS complex (may be slightly before or after the QRS complex) while, as mentioned, the retrograde P wave in AVRT usually appears in the ST segment or the T wave. AVNRTs occur in patients with the Wolff-Parkinson-White syndrome {137, 138, 144}.

AVRT often precedes atrial fibrillation in individuals with {145-147} or without {148} preexcitation. Most patients who have been resuscitated from ventricular fibrillation secondary to preexcitation have inducible AVRT or a previous history of this arrhythmia. In one laboratory, 35% of episodes of atrial fibrillation were preceded by AVRT {147}. AVRT seems to be a trigger for atrial fibrillation only in the susceptible patient with preexcitation, and there is some suspicion that there are intrinsic electrophysiologic abnormalities in the right atrium {147} which most likely would be related to conditions that cause anisotropic reentry. Operative ablation of accessory pathways often results in the cure of both AVRT and atrial fibrillation in individuals who have both arrhythmias {149}. There has also been some success with intracardiac ablation {150}, and perhaps the accessory pathway is not necessary for atrial fibrillation but it may help perpetuate atrial fibrillation in individuals who have a predisposition to such an arrhythmia {151}.

7.6 Atrioventricular reentrant tachycardia associated with a long RP' interval

The term "incessant" supraventricular tachycardia is applied to a supraventricular tachycardia when it is present for at least 90% of the time a patient is monitored {152}. The underlying mechanism may be reentry or enhanced automaticity, and here we will consider only the former. Coumel et al. in 1967 reported on a "permanent" form of reciprocating supraventricular tachycardia that they considered due to AV nodal reentry that involved antegrade conduction through a functionally fast pathway and retrograde conduction through a functionally slow pathway {153}, and this was subsequently confirmed by others {154}. Later investigations indicated that such incessant or permanent forms of junctional reciprocating tachycardia utilized accessory pathways {154, 155}. There has been some debate as to whether the intranodal mechanism exists, but it is accepted now that both types of mechanisms can produce incessant tachycardia.

Antegrade conduction through the accessory pathway does not occur. Electrophysiologic testing indicates that these pathways are almost always posteroseptal, decrease their ability to conduct as a function of rate, and result in eccentric atrial activation until block occurs in the accessory pathway. The decremental conduction properties have led to speculation that the return pathway may be accessory AV nodal structures {156}, but such decremental conduction has been documented in a case of verapamil-sensitive incessant tachycardia utilizing a left lateral accessory pathway {157}. A complex, tortuous paraseptal pathway has been describe in one patient which may explain, in part, the decremental conduction {158}. Most commonly, the return pathway is a posteroseptal accessory pathway. Atrial activation, then, begins in the low right atrium or near the coronary sinus. It is intriguing to attribute conduction slowing and unidirectional block to anisotropy, perhaps with a marginal safety factor, to these cases, particularly in the report by Okumura and his colleagues {158).

There is no evidence of preexcitation on the ECG during sinus rhythm or atrial pacing since antegrade conduction does not occur over the accessory pathway. Because of slow conduction through the retrograde limb of the circuit, the interval between the QRS aomplex and the retrograde P wave (the R-P' interval) is long. The retrograde P wave occurs late in the cardiac cycle and the RP' interval is longer than the PR interval. Since atrial activation begins in the low right atrium or near the coronary sinus in the most common form, the P waves are inverted in II, III and aVF. The appearance of ventricular preexcitation has noted in some patients who have undergone ablation therapy, usually with first-degree AV block but at times with a very short PR interval {158}.

7.7 Atrioventricular Accessory Pathways

As mentioned, ninety-five percent of atrioventricular accessory pathways conduct rapidly and have the characteristics of sodium-dependent phase 0 action potentials of normal "fast response" myocardium. Five percent show decremental conduction that may be due to geometric factors including those involved in anisotropy, partial inactivation of the sodium channel and perhaps dependence on a calcium channel, or some combination. The last two would decrease the safety factor.

A few comments on the controversial nature of the so-called James and Mahaim fibers are in order as part of the discussion of anisotropy. The Lown-Ganong-Levine syndrome is characterized by palpitations in patients with an ECG that shows a short PR interval and a normal QRS duration {159}. For many years, this disorder was thought to be due to tracts that connected the atrium with the low AV node or the His bundle via the so-called James fibers {160}. An alternative concept is that the short PR interval with a normal QRS pattern results, in most cases, from enhanced or accelerated AV nodal conduction and less often from an accessory pathway {161-163}. A short PR interval appears to be more frequent in patients with concealed accessory pathways {162}, but has also been associated with dual pathway physiology and AV nodal reentrant tachycardia. However, only patients with symptomatic tachyarrhythmias are studied electrophysio-logically; as a result, it is uncertain whether all individuals with a short PR interval and normal QRS complex have enhanced AV nodal conduction or accessory pathways near the AV node. The loss of normal integrative function within the AV node could explain the observation in that a very rapidly conducting bundle, unmodified by the electrotonic interactions from more slowly conducting neighboring tissues, would result in more rapid conduction through the AV node.

The issue of the Mahaim pathways, which arise from the AV node or one of the bundle branches and insert into ventricular tissue, has been reviewed in detail {164}. It was presumed that these pathways could explain patients in whom the PR interval was normal (because the AV node was normally traversed) but the QRS was widened (presumably due to eccentric activation of the ventricles) {165}. Some patients also had a prolonged PR interval with eccentric ventricular activation. This could be explained by slowed AV nodal conduction and anomalous connections at the level of or below the AV node. Surgical {166, 167} and more recent catheter ablation studies {168-171}, however, suggest that electrophysiologic characteristics attributed to nodoventricular Mahaim fibers are due to atriofascicular accessory connections with decremental conduction. One report, for example, suggests the presence of an atrioventricular connection in the tricuspid ring which has slow and rate-dependent conduction, blocks with adenosine, has intrinsic automaticity, and links to a rapidly conducting insulated pathway that generates a "His-like" potential {168}. For the reasons discussed earlier, anisotropy and a decreased safety factor could produce the appropriate electrophysiologic environment.

7.8 Ventricular Tachycardia

Most ventricular arrhythmias are due to reentry. Reentry, as illustrated in the discussion of supraventricular arrhythmias, requires an area of conduction sufficiently slow that the tissue to be reentered can be reactivated. The area of unidirectional block plays the role initially of determining the direction of the initiating wavefront and then provides an area for the returning wavefront to conduct. The details of the underlying electrophysiology in anisotropic reentry as a cause of ventricular arrhythmias have been reviewed recently in detail {51}.

Coronary artery disease is the most important cause of sustained monomorphic ventricular tachycardia. The important mechanisms have already been discussed. Several are likely related to gap junctional function. This includes the slowing of conduction due to increased resistance to the axial flow of current which, if thought of in terms of Spach's effective axial resistivity includes the influences of cellular geometry and packing, extracellular resistivities, and side-to-side couplings, and other features (see above). In ventricular tissue as in atrial tissue, non-uniform anisotropy due to preserved longitudinal conduction but disturbed lateral cell-cell connections (resulting from fibrosis or other causes) results in irregular activation, disruption of an integrated wavefront and zigzag conduction which, in turn, results in slow activation {see, for example, 45, 58, 59, 172}. Themes discussed in the supraventricular arrhythmias repeat in the ventricular arrhythmias. Again, in the setting of anisotropic conduction, the safety factor may actually be lower for longitudinal than for transverse conduction. As mentioned earlier, the underlying reason for disparate observations with respect to safety or failure of propagation is most likely differences in the microscopic nonuniform anisotropy of tissue structure {61} as well as alterations in the active generator source during injury. The decreased safety factor in the longitudinal as compared to the transverse direction discussed above may also be important in establishing the characteristics of unidirectional conduction in tissues. The important studies from Andrew Wit s laboratory have been mentioned, but deserve reemphasis because they indicate the importance of altered structural properties without significant change in the active generator properties. In these studies, dogs were studied 8 weeks after the induction of a myocardial infarction. Fractionated electrograms were recorded from the surface of the infarct zone, yet action potentials recorded from myocytes within these zones are normal {45, 46}. Under the microscope, connective tissue widely separated and distorted the muscle fibers. The conclusion was that the slow, fragmented activation that gave rise to the fractionated electrograms was not due to changes in the active generator which indeed had normal action potentials, but rather to disruption in the integrative electrotonic interaction between cells caused by fibrosis that physically disconnected the cells. These signals that are recorded by the signal-averaged electrocardiogram and are sought during ablation studies, so they are very important markers diagnostically and clinically. The sustained monomorphic tachycardia in these as well as in other similar studies most likely has anisotropic reentry as the primary underlying mechanism although damage to the source may contribute {173-176, among others}.

Figure 9 is a simple model of the functional components of the reentrant circuits in chronic post-infarction tissue as conceptualized by Stevenson {97}. The propagating wave fronts are shown as black arrows, the inexcitable areas are shaded, and the numbers are catheter mapping sites. The wavefront enters the slow conduction zone (SCZ) at point 10 in the scar, passes through a zone of slow conduction near point 15 and exits at point 1, producing the onset of the QRS complex near site 38. The impulse may pass through one of two reentrant circuits. The clockwise outer loop extends from point 1 through points 22 and 25 to point 30 in myocardium at the border of the scar and contributes to the QRS complex. An inner loop extends from point 1 through points 3 and 6 to site 10. Depolarization in the inner loop does not contribute to the surface ECG. The inner and out loops meet at point 10, the entrance to the slow conduction zone. If the conduction time through the two loops is similar, the circuit has a figure-of-eight configuration and the region from point 10 to point 1 is a common pathway. If the conduction time in the two loops is not equal, the faster loop determines the cycle length of the tachycardia and is called the dominant loop with the slower, non-dominant loop behaving as a bystander. There may be dead ends (sites C, E, and H), multiple reentrant circuits and more than one entrance or exit site. If there are two areas of exit, the same slow conduction zone may result in two different QRS morphologies. Sometimes, the scar may create a single outer loop with no common pathway, or, the reentrant circuit may be entirely within the scar.

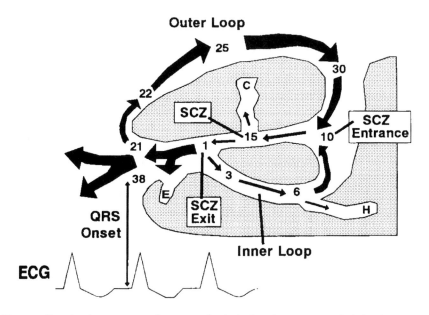

Figure 9. Functional components of reentrant circuits in chronic post-myocardial infarction. The shaded areas are inaccessible. The black arrows are propagating wavefronts. The numbers refer to the points or sites at which recordings were obtained during mapping. The electrocardiogram (ECG) is that of the sustained monomorphic ventricular tachycardia. The slow conduction zone (SCZ) and its entrance and exit are indicated. Two reentrant loops are depicted: an outer loop that includes the myocardium bordering the scarred zone and an inner loop that is determined and defined by the scarring and electrical uncoupling. Sites C, E and H represent dead ends. From Stevenson with permission {97}.

Pacing at or near some reentrant circuit sites may entrain the circuit without altering the QRS complexes of the tachycardia. For example, pacing at point 15 may produce an orthodromic wave front that propagates to the exit as in the spontaneous tachycardia. The stimulated antidromic wave fronts, that is, the wave front from point 15 to point 10, are extinguished by collision with a returning orthodromic wavefront. This is an example of entrainment with concealed fusion. With the cessation of pacing, the last stimulated orthodromic wavefront passes through the circuit and returns once again to depolarize the pacing site after one complete circuit. As a result, the interval from the last paced stimulus to the next depolarization at the pacing site approximate the ventricular cycle length. This is called the postpacing interval.

Pacing at a site distant from the reentrant circuit, say at the border of the infarct scar in the outer loop, may entrain or reset the tachycardia, but the QRS complexes differ from the spontaneous arrhythmia due to fusion of the stimulated excitation wavefronts with the tachycardia wave fronts in the myocardium. This would be an example of classic entrainment. The postpacing interval in this case would also match the ventricular tachycardia cycle length.

Pacing at bystander sites adjacent to the reentrant circuit, for example site C, may entrain with concealed fusion. The postpacing interval in this case, however, would be the circuit time plus the time it takes to travel from C to point 15, and the cycle length is longer than the cycle length of the tachycardia.

Sustained monomorphic ventricular tachycardia can be initiated electrophysiologically in most patients with ischemic heart disease who have sustained the arrhythmia spontaneously {177 and many others}. Sustained monomorphic ventricular tachycardia associated with MI most commonly occurs during the chronic phase {178-180, among others}. The first episode of sustained monomorphic ventricular tachycardia is often seen within the first year post-MI. However, the median is three years and the onset of the arrhythmia may occur as late as 10 to 15 years, a possible reflection of a ventricular aneurysm {181}. a left ventricular aneurysm develops in up to 15 percent of patients who experience a myocardial infarction. An aneurysm, of course, is a classical substrate for reentrant arrhythmias.

The relationship between sustained monomorphic ventricular tachycardia and ventricular fibrillation is uncertain. Sustained monomorphic ventricular tachycardia may simply be the company kept by ventricular fibrillation in a number of patients or, in the appropriate setting such as recurrent ischemia, it may provide a rapid wavefront that becomes fractionated, leading to ventricular fibrillation.

Nonischemic dilated cardiomyopathy is often accompanied by poor R-wave progression in the precordial leads, reflecting a decrease in anterior forces due either to replacement of muscle with fibrous tissue or perhaps to a change in the activation sequence due to fibrosis affecting the subendocardial Purkinje system {182}, conditions favorable to anisotropic reentry. Intraventricular conduction abnormalities, particularly left bundle branch block, and ST-T wave abnormalities are also common. Premature ventricular beats and couplets occur in over 90 percent of patients and nonsustained ventricular tachycardia in up to 60 percent; however, sustained monomorphic ventricular tachycardia is unusual, occurring in five percent or less {183, 184}.

Hypertrophic cardiomyopathy is characterized by massive myocardial hypertrophy. At a microscopic level, there is extensive myocardial array with bundles crossing each other in different directions, whorls of muscle cells, perpendicular branchings, and fibrosis. It is likely that anisotropic reentry underlies many of these reentrant arrhythmias as a result of the increased ventricular thickness, disorganized cardiac muscle architecture, fibrosis and microvascular abnormalities. The muscular disarray and fibrosis often results in a pseudoinfarct pattern with poor R wave progression across the precordium, and up to one-half have Q-wave abnormalities in the inferior and/or lateral leads. Frequent ventricular arrhythmias and an increase in sudden death has been reported for hypertrophic cardiomyopathy {185-190, among others}. Hypertrophic cardiomyopathy may or may not be obstructive, and both forms have a similar natural history. Ventricular tachycardia has been found in about 25 percent of patients studied with Holter monitoring, and some believe that ventricular tachycardia is associated with a higher risk of sudden death. The incidence of sustained monomorphic ventricular tachycardia varies with the population observed. In a general population with HCM, 20 percent had nonsustained ventricular tachycardia but sustained monomorphic ventricular tachycardia was rare {191}. On the other hand, inducible sustained monomorphic ventricular tachycardia is present in almost 50 percent of patients who have had either cardiac arrest or syncope and who undergo programmed electrical stimulation {192-194}.

Bundle branch reentrant ventricular tachycardia is a somewhat special category of sustained monomorphic ventricular tachycardia in that its mechanism involves abnormal conduction through structures that are normally present {195, 196}. The bundle branches consist of bundles of Purkinje fibers which are inherently anisotropic to favor rapid conduction. Bundle branch reentrant ventricular tachycardia occurs with both ischemic and nonischemic heart disease. Usually the disease is advanced with cardiomegaly and a history of congestive heart failure. The associated fibrosis may affect conduction and unidirectional block in a way favorable to the induction of this arrhythmia. Antegrade conduction may be down the right bundle branch with delayed depolarization of the left ventricle resulting in a ventricular tachycardia with a typical left bundle branch block appearance. In some patients, the reverse sequence of conduction occurs, leading to a right bundle branch block appearance. The PR interval may be normal or prolonged. The mean electrical axis is usually about +30 degrees, but a conduction defect in the left anterior fascicle will produce a marked leftward (superior) axis deviation.

Although sustained monomorphic ventricular tachycardia is most commonly due to organic heart disease, particularly chronic ischemic heart disease, both sustained and nonsustained monomorphic ventricular tachycardia can occur in the absence of any demonstrable heart disease. Most fall into three descriptive categories, namely, repetitive monomorphic ventricular tachycardia, paroxysmal sustained ventricular tachycardia and left ventricular idiopathic ventricular tachycardia. As will be discussed, although triggered activity has been suggested as the underlying mechanism for most of these arrhythmias, anisotropy at a microscopic scale may underlie the arrhythmias as well.

Repetitive monomorphic ventricular tachycardia is characterized by frequent short bursts of monomorphic nonsustained ventricular tachycardia and is also called right ventricular tachycardia, catecholamine sensitive ventricular tachycardia and exercise-induced ventricular tachycardia {197-200, among others}. The arrhythmia usually arises at the septal aspect of the right ventricular outflow tract, but may arise from the right ventricular inflow tract, the free wall of the right ventricular outflow track and the left ventricle. The electrocardiogram in some 70% of patients shows left bundle branch block and an inferior axis {197}. A right bundle branch pattern with a monophasic R wave in V_1 with an inferior axis suggests the origin at the left ventricular outflow tract.

On the basis of electrophysiologic testing, the sensitivity to catecholamines and the response to calcium antagonists, -adrenoreceptor blockers and adenosine has led to the supposition that triggered activity rather than reentry has been thought to be the mechanism. While it is true that the signal averaged ECG in the time domain is usually normal, high frequency components are often recorded within the QRS complex using fast Fourier transformation {201}, components not recorded in normals or in patients with arrhythmogenic right ventricular dysplasia. These high frequency components perhaps represent anisotropic reentry on a microscopic scale.

Paroxysmal sustained ventricular tachycardia is considered by some to be a distinct clinical syndrome {202}, but not all investigators agree {203}. It seems to be more commonly induced by electrophysiologic provocation suggesting a reentrant mechanism. Triggered arrhythmias at time may also be induced by extrastimuli, and other evidences favor abnormal automaticity as an underlying mechanism. For example, adenosine and edrophonium rather consistently terminate the arrhythmia, suggesting that cAMP-mediated triggered activity is the underlying mechanism {204}.

Zipes and his colleagues described idiopathic left ventricular tachycardia in 1979 {205}, and Belhassen and his colleagues described the termination of this ventricular tachycardia with intravenous verapamil {206}. Electrophysiologic mapping localizes the site of origin to the inferior aspect of the midseptal region. The electrocardiogram characteristically shows a right bundle branch block, a left superior axis, and a QRS duration usually of 120 to 140 msec. A few show right axis deviation. Frequency analysis using fast Fourier transform has shown an abnormal high-frequency component of the terminal portion of the QRS complex that may distinguish these patients from normals {201} which, with the ability of electrophysiolgic stimulation to provoke, entrain and terminate the arrhythmia, suggests a reentrant mechanism {207} despite the verapamil-sensitivity. The arrhythmia has also been called fascicular since a distinct Purkinje spike usually precedes the onset of the QRS, but the retrograde His bundle spike can be dissociated from the QRS complex by premature stimulation in the ventricle, atrium, or bundle of His suggesting that the posterior fascicle of the left bundle branch may be involved in or at least in close proximity to the reentrant circuit {208}.

8. CREATION OF ANISOTROPY WITH THERAPEUTIC INTENTION

As mentioned, anisotropy can be created with a therapeutic intention. In this case, surgery or radiofrequency ablation is used to dissociate and uncouple cells through trauma and subsequent scarring. A few examples will be considered.

8.1 Atrial Flutter

As discussed earlier, typical atrial flutter is clockwise or counterclockwise rotation around the tricuspid annulus with the crista terminalis and the Eustachian ridge as posterior barriers. The isthmus is a reasonable anatomic target for ablation, usually between the inferior vena cava and the tricuspid annulus but also between the Eustachian ridge and the tricuspid annulus {106, 107, 112, 209-219}. A smaller isthmus is present between the tricuspid valve annulus and the coronary sinus ostium, and there has been some success in abolishing atrial flutter by ablating this isthmus. The initial success rate for the ablation of atrial flutter, as defined by the termination of the arrhythmia and/or the inability to induce atrial flutter has ranged from 65% to 100%. The recurrence rate is between 7% and 44%. Factors which increase the risk for recurrence include a history of atrial fibrillation, increased right atrial size and perhaps anatomic features {216}. The data suggests that the criteria for successful ablation need to more stringent including, for example, the demonstration of block in the isthmus during proximal coronary sinus and low right atrial pacing {214}. Ablation guided by intracardiac echocardiography may be useful with one study showing that the best site for ablation may be between the tricuspid annulus and the Eustachian ridge rather than the more commonly used area between the tricuspid annulus and the orifice of the inferior vena cava {112}. Ablation of this site is more difficult, however, and new types of ablation catheters may need to be developed to ablate this area efficiently. Intracardiac echocardiography may also be useful in identifying anatomic variability among patients.

8.2 Atrial Fibrillation

Atrial fibrillation is another arrhythmia in which anisotropy may be produced with therapeutic intention. Because of the morbidity and mortality associated with atrial fibrillation and the disappointing results of pharmacologic therapy in maintaining sinus rhythm after cardioversion, there has been increasing interest in nonpharmacologic strategies, and both surgical and nonsurgical interruption of old pathways with the creation of new pathways of conduction are interesting strategies.

The goals of the ideal procedure for atrial fibrillation have been summarized by Ferguson and Cox {220} are abolition of atrial fibrillation, restoration of sinus rhythm, reestablishment or maintenance of atrioventricular synchrony, restoration of atrial transport and reduction or elimination of the risk of thromboembolism by eliminating passive stasis of blood in either or both atria.

The first attempts were surgical. One such technique is the "corridor" operation in which the sinus node, a strip of atrial tissue, and the atrioventricular node were isolated from the rest of the atria, thereby allowing sinus rhythm to be sustained. In an initial report, seven of nine patients treated with this procedure maintained sinus rhythm with a mean follow-up of three to 41 months, but four patients required a pacemaker due to postoperative sinus node dysfunction {221}. In a larger study, the biatrial isolation procedure was found to leave the free wall tissue of the right and left atria fibrillating, while the ventricles were being activated by the SA node through the corridor {222}. The corridor procedure, therefore, fails attaining the criteria since long term anticoagulation is required and normal atrial-ventricular synchrony is not restored.

An alternative is the "maze" operation in which several small incisions are made in the atrium to interrupt the potential reentrant pathways required for atrial fibrillation {223}. Atrial fibrillation cannot be sustained after this procedure because the impulse is not able to reenter upon itself. The maze procedure meets the five criteria for an ideal treatment of atrial fibrillation outlined above. The five-year experience in one center with 65 patients has recently been described . The procedure cured AF, restored atrioventricular synchrony, and preserved atrial transport function in 98 percent of patients, with only nine percent requiring antiarrhythmic medications {224}. Postoperative atrial pacemakers were implanted in 40 percent of cases, mostly for preoperative sick sinus syndrome but occasionally for iatrogenic sinus node injury. Encouraging results have also been obtained in a study from Japan {225}. A modified maze procedure, designed to limit myocardial damage, reports in patients undergoing surgery for mitral valve disease or an atrial septal defect reported that the technique was effective in restoring sinus rhythm (85 percent) and atrial contractility (71 percent) {226}.

The surgical experience inspired interventional electrophysiologists who are using radiofrequency catheter ablation for atrial fibrillation. Preliminary results of an initial experience using radiofrequency catheter ablation in an attempt to cure atrial fibrillation has been reported {227}. Anatomically conforming introducers were used to guide the radiofrequency catheter along predesignated courses that would roughly reproduce the surgical "maze" procedure described above. A transseptal approach was used for left atrial ablation. Swartz's informally reported experience in over 20 patients is quite encouraging but the procedure is very long and the radiation exposure is substantial. There has also been a report of the abolition of episodes of AF in a patient who developed AF following radiofrequency ablation at the IVC-tricuspid isthmus for common atrial flutter {228}.

8.3 Atrioventricular Nodal Reentrant Tachycardia

As mentioned above, the most common circuit (over 90 percent) is antegrade down a relatively slowing conducting pathway and retrograde up a more rapidly conducting pathway. Less commonly, the antegrade circuit utilizes the more rapidly conducting pathway with return along the slower pathway. The delineators of Koch's triangle have been discussed, and the triangle itself can be divided into thirds. The anterior third contains the fast pathways and is in close proximity to the compact AV node. The posterior third is associated with the coronary sinus, and the middle third is between the two. The slow pathways are in the middle and posterior thirds.

Radiofrequency ablation can be aimed either at the fast pathway (anterior) or the slow pathway (posterior) (see Fig. 8). The anterior approach to ablation delivers the RF energy in the anterior third of Koch's triangle somewhat anterior and proximal to the His Bundle. The target site is determined either anatomically or by the amplitude of the local atrial electrogram. In about 30 percent of patients with successful ablation, there is still an antegrade gap and retrograde conduction despite elimination of the reentrant arrhythmia. This observation demonstrates that small alterations in the reentrant circuit are often sufficient to prevent the arrhythmia. Perhaps ablation injury is in itself creating zig-zag preferential conduction that cannot sustain the arrhythmia. Complete AV block, as would be expected, is a not uncommon complication of the anterior approach with an incidence of about six percent (range 0 to 21 percent).

The posterior approach delivers the RF energy in the middle or posterior septal region near the coronary sinus ostium with the slow pathway as the target. The target site is determined either by anatomic position or by the morphology of the electrogram. Some electrophysiologists begin ablation in the mid-septal portion, but most begin in the posterior third of Koch's triangle where the risk of AV block is the least. With anatomic targeting, the ablation catheter is placed posterior to the coronary sinus ostium and is then progressively moved anteriorly towards the His bundle. RF energy is applied in each position and provocative electrophysiologic stimulation is used to determine efficacy. With electrogram targeting, the ablation catheter is positioned at the His bundle and then withdrawn posteriorly along the mitral annulus searching for putative slow pathway potentials. Again, the RF energy is titrated. Approximately 80 percent of successful ablation sites are found between the coronary os and the tricuspid valve. The dual pathway physiology is eliminated about one-half to two-thirds of cases. In the remainder, the dual pathway physiology persists even though reentrant arrhythmia is abolished. It is not necessary to eliminate all slow pathway conduction, since it may be possible to induce single atrial echoes even though the sustained arrhythmia has been eliminated. As a technical note, the wide distribution of sites and the fact that slow pathway conduction can be affected by energy application at several sites in the same patient suggests that there may be multiple slow pathways or multiple atrial insertions.

8.4 Ventricular Arrhythmias

Catheter ablation has been primarily used in three types of ventricular tachycardia: microreentrant, bundle branch block reentrant and idiopathic ventricular tachycardia in which the arrhythmia is not associated with underlying structural heart disease. The vast majority of microreentrant ventricular tachycardias that have been treated with ablation are of the sustained monomorphic form. A number of recent reports have reviewed the methods that have been advocated to locate the site of ventricular tachycardia {95, 97, 229-233}. During reentrant types of ventricular tachycardia accompanying ischemic heart disease, low amplitude signals detected by electrophysiology testing usually allow the identification of the orthodromic and antidromic areas of conduction and indicate the area of interest for ablation. The slow conduction and areas of unidirectional block of anisotropic conduction are often detected by locating areas with isolated mid-diastolic potentials which cannot be dissociated from the tachycardia by pacing and often represent a vulnerable portion of the reentrant circuit and predict a good response to ablation {234}. Entrainment has been discussed in detail above, and the best ablation site can, in about 50 percent of cases, be further defined by entrainment, without evidence for fusion, in an area of slow conduction {234-237}. This results in a QRS complex that is identical to that of the spontaneous ventricular tachycardia (entrainment with concealed fusion) and that has a long stimulus to QRS duration. If the anisotropic pathways that underlie reentry are constant, pacing from near the site of arrhythmogenesis should have a QRS morphology similar to the spontaneous arrhythmia. This is called pace mapping in which left and right endocardial ventricular pacing is performed during sinus rhythm in an attempt to mimic the QRS complex of the spontaneous arrhythmia. The correlation between the site of stimulation and the resultant point of epicardial emergence of activation may be poor, however, and there is concern about the frequency of both false negative and false positive results {238-240}. The long term success of ablation remains to be determined. The experience with catheter ablation remains small, and has been primarily performed with DC shock ablation. It is difficult to summarize the data because of differences in patient populations, details of the mapping and ablation, and number of patients {see review, 233}. The Percutaneous Catheter Mapping and Ablation Registry reported that only about one-third of subjects remained free of arrhythmia while the mortality rate, including mortality related to the procedure itself, was 25 percent {241}. Less information is at present available with radiofrequency current ablation, although this procedure is being used with increasing frequency. Gonska and his colleagues published two reports on the use of radiofrequency ablation for ventricular arrhythmias {242, 243}. In the larger study, 136 patients with coronary disease who had one configuration of sustained monomorphic ventricular tachycardia underwent either radiofrequency ablation (72 patients) or DC current ablation (64 patients) {242}. The mapping procedure included pace mapping during sinus rhythm, endocardial activation mapping, identification of isolated mid-diastolic potentials, and pacing interventions during ventricular tachycardia. The success rate (74 versus 77 percent) and complication rate (10 versus 14 percent) were similar with the two procedures.

Bundle branch reentry has been successfully treated using ablation. The site of ablation for ventricular tachycardia due to bundle branch reentry with the most common left bundle branch block pattern is the right bundle branch. Catheter ablation has been very successful in bundle branch reentrant tachycardia that characteristically has a left (rarely a right) bundle branch morphology. In one report, for example, DC current ablation of the right bundle branch in seven patients resulted in abolition of the arrhythmia in all patients; there were no recurrences on follow-up {244}. Similar findings were noted in a larger study of ablation in 28 patients {196}. These results suggest that ablation therapy is the treatment of choice for this type of ventricular tachycardia.

Idiopathic ventricular tachycardia, thought not associated with structural organic heart disease, usually arises in the right ventricular outflow tract. In the discussion of these arrhythmias above, it was suggested that anisotropic microreentry might underlie at least some of these tachycardias. Triggered activity may also be a mechanism, arising from a very localized area of myocardium. Pace mapping is a useful means to identify the best sites for ablations in idiopathic ventricular tachycardia arising from the right ventricular outflow tract {245}. On the other hand, the target for ablation in idiopathic left ventricular tachycardia (which originates in the apicoseptal portion of the left ventricle) is often best defined as site with the earliest local electrogram and identification of a Purkinje potential {246, 247}. a number of ablation studies of modest size have now been reported in idiopathic ventricular tachycardia with initial success rates ranging from 75 to 100 percent for tachycardias that originate in the right ventricular outflow tract, and 50 to 90 percent for those that originate at other sites. There is limited information on long-term follow-up. In one study of 20 patients with idiopathic left ventricular tachycardia, for example, the initial success rate was 85 percent and there were no recurrences at 7± 8 months {248}. Six patients underwent a repeat electrophysiologic study; none were inducible.

The data is very limited for other forms of ventricular tachycardia that may have anisotropic reentry as a basis. The role of ablation in arrhythmogenic right ventricular dysplasia and tetralogy of Fallot remains to be defined. Preliminary evidence suggests that radiofrequency catheter ablation may be successful in some patients with sustained ventricular tachycardia and dilated cardiomyopathy {233, 249}.

Surgery is another way of eliminating pathways by creating barriers and redirecting the wavefront of activation, and the topic has been reviewed recently {250}. The most commonly employed surgical techniques are endocardial resection, myocardial excision and cryoablation. The need for surgery for ventricular tachycardia has decreased given the improvements in acute care of myocardial infarction to prevent the formation of aneurysms and extensive fibrosis, catheter ablation and the use of tiered implantable devices that including pacing and d.c. electroversion. Other types of nonischemic ventricular tachycardia amenable to some form of surgery include cardiomyopathies (dilated and hypertrophic), arrhythmogenic right ventricular dysplasia, cardiac tumors, long QT syndrome, postoperative tetralogy of Fallot, valvular heart disease and a smattering of other etiologies. The results currently are quite good in the highly selected cases that come to surgery.

9. SUMMARY AND THE FUTURE

The intention of this Chapter was to create an intellectual framework for the clinician based on biophysical theory, and to allow the researcher who is not a physician an insight into clinical thought processes. The role of gap junctions in normal excitability, the synchronization of pacemakers, anisotropic conduction and the maintenance of an integrated wave front through electrotonic interactions among fiber bundles was central to the discussion. Aspects of abnormal cardiac excitability, emphasizing anisotropic reentry, were discussed. Many experimental observations discussed in this and other Chapters as well as a few clinical studies suggest that gap junctional dysfunction resulting in abnormal anisotropic conduction and reentry likely underlies in various degrees many, if not most, supraventricular and ventricular arrhythmias, particularly in chronic organic heart disease. Experimental studies in chronic infarction in which fibrosis has separated the myocytes while the myocytes themselves have normal action potentials show that non-uniform anisotropic conduction provides a substrate sufficient for reentrant tachycardias. To make the discussion seemingly less esoteric for the clinician, the results of surgical procedures and catheter ablation have been considered techniques to create anisotropic conduction with therapeutic intention. Possibly, antiarrhythmic drugs will be developed that improve coupling or induce uncoupling specifically in injured cells, or pacing from multiple sites may normalize non-uniform anisotropy.

Much work remains to be done mapping clinical arrhythmias with high density electrodes.

ACKNOWLEDGEMENTS

Supported in part by HL-21788 (MERIT).

REFERENCES

1. Ginsburg K and Arnsdorf MF (1995). Cardiac excitability, gap junctions, cable properties and impulse propagation. In: Sperelakis N (ed). Physiology and Pathophysiology of the Heart (ed 3rd). Boston: M. Nijhoff, pp. 153-199.
2. Kovacs SJ (1991). A Clinical Perspective on Theory of Heart. In: Glass L, Hunter P and McCulloch A (eds). Theory of Heart: Biomechanics, Biophysics, and Nonlinear Dynamics of Cardiac Function. New York: Springer, pp. 609-611.
3. Goldberger AL and Rigney DR (1991). Nonlinear Dynamics at the Bedside. In: Glass L, Hunter P and McCulloch A (eds). Theory of Heart: Biomechanics, Biophysics, and Nonlinear Dynamics of Cardiac Function. New York: Springer, pp. 584-605.
4. Denton TA, Diamond GA, Helfant RH, Khan S, and Karagueuzian H: Fascinating rhythm (1990). A primer on chaos theory and its application to cardiology. Am Heart J, 120: 1419-1440.
5. Landau M, Lorente P, Michaels D, and Jalife J (1990). Bistabilities and annihilation phenomena in electrophysiological cardiac models. Circ Res, 66: 1658-1672.
6. Lorente P and Davidenko J (1990). Hysteresis phenomena in excitable cardiac tissues. Ann NY Acad Sci, 591: 109-127.
7. Arnsdorf MF, Schmidt GA, and Sawicki G (1985). The effects of encainide on the determinants of cardiac excitability in sheep Purkinje fibers. J Pharmacol Exp Ther, 223: 40-48.

8. Sawicki GJ and Arnsdorf MF (1985). Electrophysiologic actions and interactions between lysophosphatidylcholine and lidocaine in the non-steady state: The match between multiphasic arrhythmogenic mechanisms and multiple drug effects in cardiac Purkinje fibers. J Pharmacol Exp Ther, 235: 829-838.

9. Arnsdorf MF and Wasserstrom JA (1987). A matrical approach to the basic and clinical pharmacology of antiarrhythmic drugs. Reviews in Clinical and Basic Pharmacology, 6: 131-188.

10. Arnsdorf MF (1987). Intracardiac electrophysiologic studies for drug selection in ventricular tachycardia: The need for new approaches based on perturbations of the electrophysiologic matrix. Circulation, 75: III-137-139.

11. Arnsdorf MF and Sawicki GJ (1987). The effects of quinidine sulfate on the balance among active and passive cellular properties which comprise the electrophysiologic matrix and determine excitability in sheep Purkinje fibers. Circ Res, 61: 244-255.

12. Arnsdorf MF (1989). Cardiac excitability and antiarrhythmic drugs: A different perspective. J Clin Pharmacol, 29: 395-404.

13. Arnsdorf MF (1990). Arnsdorf's Paradox. J Cardiovas Electrophys, 1: 42-52.

14. Arnsdorf MF (1990). The cellular basis of cardiac arrhythmias: A matrical prespective. Ann NY Acad Sci, 601: 263-280.

15. Arnsdorf MF (1990). Electrophysiologic matrices, cardiac arrhythmias, and antiarrhythmic drugs. In: Rosen MR, Janse MJ and Wit AL (eds). Cardiac Electrophysiology: A Textbook. Mount Kisco: Futura Publishing Company, pp. 3-28.

16. Arnsdorf MF and Sawicki GJ (1996). Flecainide and the electrophysiologic matrix: The effects of flecainide acetate on the determinants of cardiac excitability in sheep Purkinje fibers. J Cardiovasc Electrophysiol, 7: 1172-1182.

17. Hodgkin AL and Rushton WAH (1946). The electrical constants of a crustacean nerve fibre. Proc Roy Soc B, 133: 444-479.

18. Dominguez G and Fozzard HA (1970). Influence of extracellular K+ concentration on cable properties and excitability of sheep cardiac Purkinje fibers. Circ Res, 26: 565-574.

19. Fozzard HA and Schoenberg M (1972). Strength-duration curves in cardiac Purkinje fibres: Effects of liminal length and charge distribution. J Physiol (Lond), 226: 593-618.

20. Heidenheim M (1901). Über die Structur des menschlichen Herzmuskels. Anat Anz, 20: 3-79.

21. Engelmann TW (1875). Über die Leitung der Erregung im Herzmuskel. Pflügers Arch, 11: 465-480.

22. Engelmann TW (1877). Vergleichende Untersuchungen zur Lehre von der Muskel-und Nervenelectricitat. Pfluegers Arch Physiol, 15: 116-148.

23. Sjostrand FS and Andersson E (1954). Electron microscopy of the intercalated discs of cardiac muscle tissue. Experientia, 10: 369-372.

24. Lal R and Arnsdorf MF (1992). Voltage-dependent gating and single channel conductance of adult mammalian atrial gap junctions. Circ Res, 71: 737-743.
25. Lindemans FW and Denier Van der Gon JJ (1978). Current thresholds and liminal size in excitation of heart muscle. Cardiovasc Res, 12: 477-485.
26. Michaels DC, Slenter VA, Salata JJ, and Jalife J (1983). A model of dynamic vagus-sinoatrial node interactions. Am J Physiol, 245: H1043-1053.
27. Guevara MR, Glass L, and Shrier A (1981). Phase locking, period-doubling bifurcations, and irregular dynamics in periodically stimulated cardiac cells. Science, 214: 1350-1353.
28. Jalife J and Moe GK (1979). A biologic model of parasystole. Am J Cardiol, 43: 761-772.
29. Jalife J, Slenter VAJ, Salata JJ, and Michaels DC (1983). Dynamic vagal control of pacemaker activity in the mammalian sinoatrial node. Circ Res, 52: 642-656.
30. Levy MN, Martin PJ, Lano TH, and Zieske H (1969). Paradoxical effect of vagus nerve stimulation on heart rate in dogs. Circ Res, 25: 303-314.
31. Bleeker WK, MacKay AJC, Masson-Pevet M, Bouman LN, and Becker AE (1980). Functional and morphological organization of the rabbit sinus node. Circ Res, 46: 11-22.
32. Winfree AT (1980). The Geometry of Biological Time. New York, Springer-Verlag.
33. Jalife J and Michaels DC (1985). Phase dependent interactions of cardiac pacemakers as machanisms of control and sychronization in the heart. In: Zipes DP and Jalife J (eds). Cardiac Electrophysiology and Arrhythmias. Orlando, FL: Grune and Stratton, pp. 109-119.
34. Jalife J (1984). Mutual entrainment and electrical coupling as mechanisms for synchronous firing of rabbit sino-atrial pacemaker cells. J Physiol (London), 221-243: 1984.
35. Brown G and Eccles J (1934). The action of a single vagal volley on the rhythm of the heart beat. J Physiol (Lond), 82: 211-241.
36. Michaels DC, Matyas EP, and Jalife J (1984). A mathematical model of the vagal control of sinoatrial pacemaker activity. Circ Res, 55: 89-101.
37. Mobley BA and Page E (1972). The surface area of sheep cardiac Purkinje fibers. J Physiol, 220: 547-563.
38. Michaels DC, Matyas EP al, and Jalife J (1989). Experimental and mathematical observations on pacemaker interactions as a mechanisms of synchronization in the sinoatrial node. In: Zipes DP and Jalife J (eds). Cardiac Electrophysiology: From Cell to Bedside. Philadelphia: W.B. Saunders Co., pp. 182-214.
39. Wit AL and Rosen MR (1989). Cellular electrophysiological mechanisms of cardiac arrhythmias. In: MacFarlane PW, Veitch TD and Lawrie (eds). Comprehensive Electrocardiology:Theory and Practice in Health and Disease (vol 2). New York: Pergamon Press, pp. 801-841.

40. Bauernfeind RA, Amat-y-Leon F, Dhingra RC, et al. (1979). Chronic nonparoxysmal sinus tachycardia in otherwise health persons. Ann Intern Med, 91: 702-710.
41. Yee R, Guiraudon GM, Gardner MJ, Gulamhusein SS, and Klein GJ (1984). Refractory paroxysmal sinus tachycardia: Management by subtotal right atrial exclusion. JACC, 3: 400-404.
42. Kalman JM, Lee RJ, Fisher WG, Chin MC, Ursell P, Stillson CA, Lesh MD, and Scheinman MM (1995). Radiofrequency catheter modification of sinus pacemaker function guided by intracardiac echocardiography. Circulation, 92: 3070-3081.
43. Lee RJ, Kalman JM, Fitzpatrick AP, Epstein LM, Fisher WG, Olgin JE, Lesh MD, and Scheinman MM (1995). Radiofrequency catheter modification of the sinus node for "inappropriate" sinus tachycardia. Circulation, 92: 2919-2928.
44. Castellanos A, Moleiro F, Saoudi NC, and Myerburg RJ (1990). Parasystole. In: Zipes DP and Jalife J (eds). Cardiac Electrophysiology from Cell to Bedside. Philadelphia: W. B. Saunders Company, pp. 619-627.
45. Gardner PI, Ursell PC, Fenoglio JJ Jr, and Wit AL (1985). Electrophysiologic and anatomic basis for fractionated electrograms recorded from healed myocardial infarcts. Circulation, 72: 596-611.
46. Ursell PC, Gardner PI, Albala A, Fenoglio JJ Jr, and Wit AL (1985). Structural and electrophysiological changes in the epicardial border zone of canine myocardial infarcts during infarct healing. Circ Res, 56: 436-451.
47. Lesh MD, Spear JF, and Moore EN (1990). Myocardial anisotropy: Basic electrophysiology and role in cardiac arrhythmias. In: Zipes DP and Jalife J (eds). Cardiac Electrophysiology: From Cell to Bedside. Philadelphia: W. B. Saunders Company, pp. 364-376.
48. Spach MS (1995). Microscopic basis of anisotropic propagation in the heart: The nature of current flow at a cellular level. In: Zipes DP and Jalife J (eds). Cardiac Electrophysiology: From Cell to Bedside (ed Second). Philadelphia: W. B. Saunders Company, pp. 204-215.
49. Keener JP and Panfilov AV (1995). Three-dimensional propagation in the heart: The effects of geometry and fiber orientation on propagation in myocardium. In: Zipes DP and Jalife J (eds). Cardiac Electrophysiology: From Cell to Bedside (ed Second). Philadelphia: W. B. Saunders Company, pp. 335-347.
50. Wikswo JP (1995). Tissue anisotropy, the cardiac biodomain, and the virtual cathode effect. In: Zipes DP and Jalife J (eds). Cardiac Electrophysiology: From Cell to Bedside (ed Second). Philadelphia: W. B. Saunders Company, pp. 348-362.
51. Wit AL, Dillon SM, and Coromilas J (1995). Anisotropic reentry as a cause of ventricular tachycarrhythmias. In: Zipes DP and Jalife J (eds). Cardiac Electrophysiology: From Cell to Bedside (ed Second). Philadelphia: W. B. Saunders Company, pp. 511-526.
52. Draper MH and Mya-Tu M (1959). A comparison of the conduction velocity in cardiac tissues of various mammals. Quar J Exp Physiol, 44: 91-109.

53. Schoenberg M, Dominguez G, and Fozzard HA (1975). Effect of diameter on membrane capacity and conductance of sheep cardiac Purkinje fibers. J Gen Physiol, 65: 441-458.
54. Pressler ML (1984). Cable analysis in quiescent and active sheep Purkinje fibres. J Physiol (Lond), 352: 739-757.
55. Goldstein SS and Rall W (1974). Changes in action potential shape and velocity for changing core conductor geometry. Biophys J, 14: 731-757.
56. Sepulveda NG, Walker CF, and Heath RG (1983). Finite element analysis of current pathways with implanted electrodes. J Biomed Eng, 5: 41-48.
57. Spach MS, Miller WT, Geselowitz DB, Barr RC, Kootsey JM, and Johnson EA (1981). The discontinuous nature of propagation in normal canine cardiac muscle. Evidence for recurrent discontinuities of intracellular resistance that affect membrane currents. Circ Res, 48: 39-54.
58. Spach MS, Miller WT, Dolber PC, Kootsey JM, Sommer JR, and Mosher CE Jr (1982). The functional role of structural complexities in the propagation of depolarization in the atrium of the dog. Cardiac conduction disturbances due to discontinuities of effective axial resistivity. Circ Res, 50: 175-191.
59. Spach MS and Dolber PC: Relating extracellular potentials (1986). Evidence for electrical uncoupling of side-to-side fiber connections with increasing age. Circ Res, 58: 356-371.
60. Spach MS and Dolber PC (1990). Discontinuous anisotropic propagation. In: Rosen M, Janse MJ and Wit AL (eds). Cardiac Electrophysiology: A Textbook. Mt Kisco: Futura Publishing Company, pp. 517-534.
61. Spach MS, Dolber PC, and Heidlage JF (1990). Properties of Discontinuous Anisotropic Propagation at a Microscopic Level. Ann NY Acad Sci, 591: 62-74.
62. Spach MS, Dolber PC, and Heidlage JF (1988). Influence of the passive anisotropic properties on directional differences in propagation following modification of the sodium conductance in human atrial muscle. A model of reentry based on anisotropic discontinuous propagation. Circ Res, 62: 811-832.
63. Sommer JR and Johnson EA (1979). Ultrastructure of cardiac muscle. In: Berne RM (ed). The Handbook of Physiology, I: The Cardiovascular System. Baltimore: The American Physiological Society, Williams and Wilkins, pp. 113-186.
64. Gourdie RG, Green CR, and Severs NJ (1991). Gap junction distribution in adult mammalian myocardium revealed by an anti-peptide antibody and laser scanning confocal microscopy. J Cell Sci, 99: 41-55.
65. Gourdie RG, Green CR, Severs NJ, and Thompson RP (1992). Immunolabeling patterns of gap junction connexins in the developing and mature rat heart. Anat Embryol (Berlin), 185: 363-378.
66. Hoyt RH, Cohen ML, and Saffitz JE (1989). Distribution and three-dimensional structure of intercellular junctions in canine myocardium. Circ Res, 64: 563-574.
67. Sommer JR and Scherer B (1985). The geometry of intercellular communication in cardiac muscle with emphasis on cell and bundle appositions. Am J Physiol, 17: H792-H803.

68. Pressler ML, Munster PN, and Huang X (1995). Gap junction distribution in the heart: Functional Relevance. In: Zipes DP and Jalife J (eds). Cardiac Electrophysiology: From Cell to Bedside (ed Second). Philadelphia: W. B. Saunders Company, pp. 144-181.
69. Kootsey JM (1991). Electrical Propagation in Distributed Cardiac Tissue. In: Glass L, Hunter P and McCulloch A (eds). Theory of Heart: Biomechanics, Biophysics, and Nonlinear Dynamics of Cardiac Function. New York: Springer, pp. 391-403.
70. Luke RA and Safitz JE (1991). Remodeling of Ventricular Conduction Pathways in Healed Canine Infarct Border Zones. J Clin Invest, 87: 1594-1602.
71. Smith JH, Green CR, Peters NS, Rothery S, and Severs NJ (1991). Altered patterns of gap junction distribution in ischemic heart disease. Am J Pathol, 139: 801-821.
72. Spach MS (1991). Anisotropic Structural Complexities in the Genesis of Reentrant Arrhythmias (Editorial Comment). Circulation, 84: 1447-1450.
73. Lewis MA and P Grindrod: One-way blocks in cardiac tissue (1991). A mechanism for propagation failure in Purkinje fibers. Bull Math Biol, 53: 881-899.
74. Mendez C, Mueller WJ, and Urquiaga X (1970). Propagation of impulses across the Purkinje fiber-muscle junctions in the dog heart. Circulation, 26: 135-150.
75. Veenstra RD, Joyner RW, and Rawling DA (1984). Purkinje and ventricular activation sequences of canine papillary muscle. Circ Res, 54: 500-515.
76. Balke CW, Lesh MD, Spear JF, Kadish A, Levine JH, and Moore EN (1988). Effects of cellular uncoupling on conduction in anisotropic canine ventricular myocardium. Circ Res, 63: 879-892.
77. Delgado C, Steinhaus B, Delmar M, Chialvo DR, and Jalife J (1990). Directional differences in excitability and margin of safety for propagation in sheep ventricular epicardial muscle. Circ Res, 67: 97-110.
78. Delmar M, Michaels DC, Johnson T, and Jalife J (1987). Effects of Increasing Intercellular Resistance on Transverse and Longitudinal Propagation in Sheep Epicardial Muscle. Circ Res, 60: 780-785.
79. Kleber AG and Janse MJ (1990). Impulse Propagation in Myocardial Ischemia. In: Zipes DP and Jalife J (eds). Cardiac Electrophysiology: From Cell to Bedside (ed 1st). Philadelphia: W. B. Saunders, pp. 156-161.
80. Kleber AG, Fleischhauer J, and Cascio WE (1995). Ischemia-induced propagation failure in the heart. In: Zipes DP and Jalife J (eds). Cardiac Electrophysiology: From Cell to Bedside (ed Second). Philadelphia: W. B. Saunders Company, pp. 174-181.
81. Anumonwo JMB, Delmar M, Vinet A, Michaels DC, and Jalife J (1991). Phase resetting and entrainment of pacemaker activity in single sinus nodal cells. Circ Res, 68: 1138-1153.
82. Weingart R and Maurer P (1988). Action potential transfer in cell pairs isolated from adult rat and guinea pig ventricles. Circ Res, 63: 72-80.

83. Weingart R, Rüdisüli A, and Maurer P (1990). Cell to cell communication. In: Zipes DP and Jalife J (eds). Cardiac Electrophysiology: From Cell to Bedside (ed 1st). Philadelphia: W. B. Saunders, pp. 122-127.
84. Smith JM and Cohen RJ (1984). Simple finite-element model accounts for wide range of cardiac dysrhythmias. Proc Natl Acad Sci USA, 81: 233-237.
85. Buchanan JW and Gettes LS (1990). Ionic Environment and Propagation. In: Zipes DP and Jalife J (eds). Cardiac Electrophysiology: From Cell to Bedside. Philadelphia: Saunders, pp. 149-156.
86. Hiramatsu Y, Buchanan JW, Knisley SB, and Gettes LS (1988). Rate-dependent effects of hypoxia on internal longitudinal resistance in guinea pig papillary muscles. Circ Res, 63: 923-929.
87. Maurer P and Weingart R: Cell pairs isolated from adult guinea pig (1987). effects of [Ca++]i on nexal membrane resistance. Pflugers Arch, 409: 394-402.
88. Jongsma HJ, Wilders R, van Ginneken ACG, and Rook MB (1991). Modulatory effect of the transcellular electrical field on gap junction conductance. In: Peracchia C (ed). Biophysics of Gap Junction Channels. Boca Raton: CRC Press, pp. 163-172.
89. Veenstra RD (1991). Physiological modulation of cardiac gap junction channels. J Cardiovasc Electrophysiol, 2: 168-189.
90. Spach MS, Kootsey JM, and Sloan JD (1982). Active modulation of electrical coupling between cardiac cells of the dog. A mechanism for transient and steady state variations in conduction velocity. Circ Res, 51: 347-362.
91. Waldo AL, Maclean WAH, Karp RB, Kochoukos NT, and James T (1977). Entrainment and interruption of atrial flutter with pacing; Studies in man following open heart surgery. Circulation, 56: 737-745.
92. Waldo AL (1995). Atrial flutter: Mechanisms, clinical feture and management. In: Zipes DP and Jalife J (eds). Cardiac Electrophysiology: From Cell to Bedside (ed 2nd). Philadelp;hia: W. B. Saunders Company, pp. 666-681.
93. Stevenson WG, Sager PT, and Friedman PL (1995). Entrainment techniques for mapping atrial and ventricular tachycardias. [Review]. J Cardiovas Electrophys, 6: 201-216.
94. Cosio FG, Arribas F, Lopez-Gil M, and Palacios J (1996). Atrial flutter mapping and ablation. I. Studying atrial flutter mechanisms by mapping and entrainment. [Review] [39 refs]. PACE, 19: 841-853.
95. Blanck Z, Dhala A, Deshpande S, Sra J, Jazayeri M, and Akhtar M (1994). Catheter ablation of ventricular tachycardia. [Review]. Am Heart J, 127: 1126-1133.
96. Jazayeri MR, Deshpande S, Dhala A, Blanck Z, Sra J, and Akhtar M (1994). Transcatheter mapping and radiofrequency ablation of cardiac arrhythmias. [Review]. Current Problems in Cardiology, 19: 287-395.
97. Stevenson WG (1995). Catheter mapping of ventricular tachycardia. In: Zipes DP and Jalife J (eds). Cardiac Electrophysiology: From Cell to Bedside (ed 2nd). Philadelphia: W. B. Saunders Company, pp. 1093-1112.

98. Klein LS and Miles WM (1995). Ablative therapy for ventricular arrhythmias. [Review] [51 refs]. Progr Cardiovasc Dis, 37: 225-242.
99. Poty H, Saoudi N, Haissaguerre M, Daou A, Clementy J, and Letac B (1996). Radiofrequency catheter ablation of atrial tachycardias. Am Heart J, 131: 481-489.
100. Kalman JM, Olgin JE, Karch MR, and Lesh MD (1996). Regional entrainment of atrial fibrillation in man. J Cardiovas Electrophys, 7: 867-876.
101. Okumura K, Olshansky B, Henthorn RW, Epstein AE, Plumb VJ, and Waldo AL (1987). Demonstration of the presence of slow conduction during sustained ventricular tachycrdia in man: Use of transient entrainment of the tachycardia. Circulation, 75: 369-378.
102. Henthorn RW, Okumura K, Olshansky B, Plumb VJ, Hess PG, and Waldo AL (1988). A fourth criteria for transient entrainment: The electrogram equivalent of progressive fusion. Circulation, 77: 1003-1012.
103. Watson RM and Josephson ME (1980). Atrial flutter. I. Electrophysiologic substrates and modes of initiation and termination. Am J Cardiol, 45: 732-741.
104. Inoue H, Matsuo H, Takayanagi K, and Murao S (1981). Clinical and experimental studies of the effects of atrial extrastimulation and rapid pacing on the atrial flutter cycle. Evidence of macro-reentry with an excitable gap. Am J Cardiol, 48: 623-631.
105. Disertori M, Inama G, Vergara G, Guarniero M, Del Favero A, and Furlanello F (1983). Evidence of a reentry circuit in the common type of atrial flutter in man. Circulation, 67: 434-440.
106. Klein GJ, Guiraudon GM, Sharma AD, and Milstein S (1986). Demonstration of macroreentry and feasibility of operative therapy in the common type of atrial flutter. Am J Cardiol, 57: 587-591.
107. Cosio FG, Arribas F, and Barbero MJ (1988). Validation of double-spike electrograms as markers of conduction delay or block in atrial flutter. Am J Cardiol, 61: 775-780.
108. Kalman JM, Olgin JE, Saxon LA, Fisher WG, Lee RJ, and Lesh MD (1996). Activation and entrainment mapping defines the tricuspid annulus as the anterior barrier in typical atrial flutter [see comments]. Circulation, 94: 398-406.
109. Nakagawa H, Lazzara R, Khastgir T, Beckman KJ, McClelland JH, Imai S, Pitha JV, Becker AE, Arruda M, Gonzalez MD, Widman LE, Rome M, Neuhauser J, Wang X, Calame JD, Goudeau MD, and Jackman WM (1996). Role of the tricuspid annulus and the eustachian valve/ridge on atrial flutter. Relevance to catheter ablation of the septal isthmus and a new technique for rapid identification of ablation success [see comments]. Circulation, 94: 407-424.
110. Lesh MD, Kalman JM, and Olgin JE (1996). New approaches to treatment of atrial flutter and tachycardia. [Review]. J Cardiovas Electrophys, 7: 368-381.

111. Chu E, Kalman JM, Kwasman MA, Jue JC, Fitzgerald PJ, Epstein LM, Schiller NB, Yock PG, and Lesh MD (1994). Intracardiac echocardiography during radiofrequency catheter ablation of cardiac arrhythmias in humans. JACC, 24: 1351-1357.

112. Olgin JE, Kalman JM, Fitzpatrick AP, and Lesh MD (1995). Role of right atrial endocardial structures as barriers to conduction during human type I atrial flutter. Activation and entrainment mapping guided by intracardiac echocardiography. Circulation, 92: 1839-1848.

113. Spach MS, Miller WT, Geselowitz DB, Barr RC, Kootsey JM, and Johnson EA (1981). The discontinuous nature of propagation in normal canine cardiac muscle. Evidence for recurrent discontinuities of intracellular resistance that affect membrane currents. Circ Res, 48: 39-54.

114. Armen RN and Frank TV (1949). Electrocardiographic patterns in pneumothorax. Diseases of the Chest, 15: 709-.

115. Simonson E (1961). Differentiation Between Normal and Abnormal in Electrocardiography. St. Louis, C.V. Mosby.

116. Morady F, Scheinman MM, Kou WH, Griffin JC, Dick M 2d, Herre J, Kadish AH, and Langberg J (1989). Long-term results of catheter ablation of a posteroseptal accessory atrioventricular connection in 48 patients. Circulation, 79: 1160-1170.

117. Kalman JM, Olgin JE, Saxin LA, Lee RJ, Scheinman MM, and Lesh MD (1997). Electrocardiographic and electrophysiologic characterization of atypical atrial flutter in man: Use of activation and entrainment mapping and implications for catheter ablation. J Cardiovas Electrophys, 8: 121-144.

118. McGuire MA, Bourke JP, Robotin MC, Johnson DC, Meldrum-Hanna W, Nunn GR, Uther JB, and Ross DL (1993). High resolution mapping of Koch's triangle using sixty electrodes in humans with atrioventricular junctional (AV nodal) reentrant tachycardia. Circulation, 88: 2315-2328.

119. McGuire MA, Janse MJ, and Ross DL (1993). "AV nodal" reentry: Part II: AV nodal, AV junctional, or atrionodal reentry? J Cardiovas Electrophys, 4: 573-586.

120. Schmitt C, Miller JM, and Josephson ME (1988). Atrioventricular nodal supraventricular tachycardia with 2:1 block above the the bundle of His. PACE, 11: 1018-1023.

121. Weh S-J, Yamamoto T, Lin F-C, and Wu D (1990). Atrioventricular block in the atypical form of junctional reciprocating tachycardia: Evidence supporting the atrioventricular node as the site of reentry. JACC, 15: 385-392.

122. Jackman WM, Nakagawa H, Heidbuchel H, Beckman K, McClelland J, and Lazzara R (1995). Three forms of atrioventricular nodal (junctional) reentrant tachycardia: Differential diagnosis, electrophysiological characteristics and implications for anatomy of the reentrant circuit. In: Zipes DP and Jalife J (eds). Cardiac Electrophysiology: From Cell to Bedside (ed Second). Philadelphia: W. B. Saunders Company, pp. 620-637.

123. Moe GK, Preston JB, and Burlington HJ (1956). Physiologic evidence for a dual A-V transmission system. Circ Res, 4: 357-375.
124. Denes P, Wu D, Dhringra RD, Chuquimia R, and Rosen KM (1973). Demonstration of dual A-V nodal pathways in patients with paroxysmal supraventricular tachycardia. Circulation, 48: 549.
125. Janse MJ, van Capelle FJL, Freud GE, and Durrer D (1971). Circus movement within the AV node as a basis for supraventricular as shown by microelectrode recording in the isolated rabbit heart. Circ Res, 28: 403-414.
126. Ho SY, Kilpatrick L, Kanai T, Germroth PG, Thompson RP, and Anderson RH (1995). The architecture of the atrioventricular conduction axis in dog compared to man: its significance to ablation of the atrioventricular nodal approaches. J Cardiovas Electrophys, 6: 26-39.
127. Anderson RH, Ho SY, Wharton J, and Becker AE (1995). Gross anatomy and microscopy of the conducting system. In: Mandel WJ (ed). Cardiac Arrhythmias (ed 3rd). Philadelphia: J. B. Lippincott Company, pp. 13-54.
128. DeMello (1977). Passive electrical properties of the atrio-ventricular node. Pfluegers Arch, 371: 135-139.
129. DeFelice LJ and Challice CE (1969). Anatomical and ultrastructural study of the electrophysiological atrioventricular node of the rabbit. Circ Res, 24: 457-474.
130. Kawamura K and James TN (1971). Comparative ultrastructure of cellular junctions in working myocardium and the conduction system under normal and pathologic conditions. J Mol Cell Cardiol, 3: 31-60.
131. Marino TA (1979). The atrioventricular node and bundle in the ferret heart: A light and quantitative electron microscopic study. Am J Anat, 154: 365-392.
132. Mendez C and Moe GK (1966). Some characteristics of transmembrane potentials of AV nodal cells during propagation of premature beats. Circ Res, 19: 993-1010.
133. Roy D, Waxman HL, Boxton AE, and Josephson ME (1983). Horizontal and longitudinal dissociation of the A-V node during atrial tachycardia. PACE, 6: 569-576.
134. Gallagher JJ, Sealy WC, Kasell J, and Wallace AG (1984). Multiple accessory pathways in patients with the pre-excitation syndrome. Circulation, 54: 571-591.
135. Bardy GH, Packer DL, German LD, and Gallagher JJ (1984). Preexcited reciprocating tachycardia in patients with Wollf-Parkinson-White syndrome: Incidence and mechanisms. Circulation, 70: 377-391.
136. Ward DE, Bennett DH, and Camm J (1984). Mechanisms of junctional tachycardia showing ventricular pre-excitation. Br Heart J, 52: 369-376.
137. Pritchett ELC, Prystowsky EN, Benditt DG, and Gallagher (1980). "Dual atrioventricular nodal pathways" in patients with Wolff-Parkinson-White syndrome. Br Heart J, 43: 7-13.
138. Smith WM, Broughton A, Reiter MJ, Benson DW Jr, Grant AO, and Gallagher JJ (1983). Bystander accessory pathway during AV node reentrant tachycardia. PACE, 6: 537-547.

139. Coumel P and Attuel P (1974). Reciprocating tachycardia in overt and latent preexcitation: Influence of bundle branch block on the rate of the tachycardia. Eur J Cardiol, 1: 423-436.

140. Barold SS and Coumel P (1977). Mechanisms of atrioventricular junctional tachycardia: Role of reentry and concealed accessory bypass tracts. Am J Cardiol, 39: 97-106.

141. Neus H, Schlepper M, and Thormann J (1975). Analysis of re-entry mechanisms in three patients with concealed Wolff-Parkinson-White syndrome. Circulation, 51: 75-81.

142. Pritchett ELC, Gallagher JJ, Sealy WC, Anderson R, Campbell RW, Seller TD Jr, and Wallace AG (1978). Supraventricular tachycardia dependent upon accessory pathways in the absence of ventricular preexcitation. Am J Med, 64: 214-220.

143. Kuck KH, Friday KJ, and Kunze KP (1990). Sites of conduction block in accessory pathway conduction during the induction of orthodromic reciprocating tachycardias. Circulation, 82: 407-417.

144. Wellens HJJ and Durrer D (1973). Combined conduction distrubances in two AV pathways in patients with Wolff-Parkinson-White syndrome. Eur J Cardiol, 1: 23-28.

145. Campbell RW, Smith RA, Gallagher JJ, Pritchett EL, and Wallace AG (1977). Atrial fibrillation in the preexcitation syndrome. Am J Cardiol, 40: 514-520.

146. Sung RJ, Castellanos A, Mallon SM, Bloom MG, Gelband H, and Myerburg RJ (Sep). Mechanisms of spontaneous alternation between reciprocating tachycardia and atrial flutter-fibrillation in the Wolff-Parkinson-White syndrome. Circulation 1977, 56: 409-416.

147. Fujimura O, Klein GJ, Yee R, and Sharma AD (1990). Mode of onset of atrial fibrillation in the Wolff-Parkinson-White syndrome: how important is the accessory pathway? JACC, 15: 1082-1086.

148. Roark SF, McCarthy EA, Lee KL, and Pritchett EL (1901). Observations on the occurrence of atrial fibrillation in paroxysmal supraventricular tachycardia. American Journal of Cardiology 1986 Mar, 57: 571-575.

149. Sharma AD, Klein GJ, Guiraudon GM, and Milstein S (1985). Atrial fibrillation in patients with Wolff-Parkinson-White syndrome: incidence after surgical ablation of the accessory pathway. Circulation, 72: 161-169.

150. Wellens HJ (1994). Atrial fibrillation--the last big hurdle in treating supraventricular tachycardia [editorial; comment]. N Engl J Med, 331: 944-945.

151. Wathen M, Natale A, Wolfe K, Yee R, and Klein G (1993). Initiation of atrial fibrillation in the Wolff-Parkinson-White syndrome: the importance of the accessory pathway. Am Heart J, 125: 753-759.

152. Sung RJ (1983). Incessant supraventricular tachycardia. PACE, 6: 1306-1326.

153. Coumel P, Cabrol C, Fabiato A, Gourgon R, and Slama R (1967). Tachycardie permanent part rhythme reciproque. I. Preuves du diagnostic par stimulation auriculaire et ventriculaire. Arc Mal Coeur Vaiss, 60: 1830-1864.

154. Scheinman MM, Basu D, and Hollenberg M (1974). Electrophysiologic studies in patients with persistent atrial tachycardia. Circulation, 50: 266-273.

155. Gallagher JJ and Sealy WC (1978). The permanent form of junctional reciprocating tachycardia: Further elucidation of the underlying mechanism. Eur J Cardiol, 8: 413-430.

156. Ward DE and Camm AJ (1982). Ventriculo-atrial conduction over accessory pathways exhibiting decremental properties. Eur Heart J, 3: 267-275.

157. Okumura K, Henthorn RW, Epstein AE, Plumb JV, and Waldo AL (1986). "Incessant" atrioventricular (AV) reciprocating tachycardia utilizing left lateral AV bypass pathway with a long retrograde conduction time. PACE, 9: 332-342.

158. Critelli G, Gallagher JJ, Monda V, Coltorti F, Scherillo M, and Rossi L (1984). Anatomic and electrophysiologic substrate of the permanent form of junctional reciprocating tachycardia. JACC, 4: 610-610.

159. Lown B, Ganong SA, and Levine SA (1952). The syndrome of short P-R interval, normal QRS complex and paroxysmal rapid heart action. Circulation, 5: 693.

160. James TN (1961). Morphology of the human atrioventricular node with remarks pertinent to its electrophysiology. Am Heart J, 62: 756.

161. Denes P, Wu D, Amat-y-Leon F, Dhingra R, Wyndham CR, and Rosen KM (1977). The determinants of atrioventricular nodal re-entrance with premature atrial stimulation in patients with dual A-V nodal pathways. Circulation, 56: 253-259.

162. Benditt DG, Pritchett LC, Smith WM, Wallace AG, and Gallagher JJ (1978). Characteristics of atrioventricular conduction and the spectrum of arrhythmias in Lown-Ganong-Levine syndrome. Circulation, 57: 454-465.

163. Bauernfeind RA, Swiryn S, Strasberg B, Palileo E, Wyndham C, Duffy CE, and Rosen KM (1982). Analysis of anterograde and retrograde fast pathway properties in patients with dual atrioventricular nodal pathways: observations regarding the pathophysiology of the Lown-Ganong-Levine syndrome. Am J Cardiol, 49: 283-290.

164. Klein GJ, Guiraudon G, Guiraudon C, and Yee R (1994). The nodoventricular Mahaim pathway: an endangered concept? [editorial; comment]. [Review]. Circulation, 90: 636-638.

165. Wellens HJJ (1971). The preexcitation syndrome. In: Wellens HJJ (ed). Electrical Stimulation of the Heart. Baltimore, MD: University Park Press, pp. 97-109.

166. Gillette PC, Garson A Jr, Cooley DA, and McNamara DG (1982). Prolonged and decremental antegrade conduction properties in right anterior accessory connections: Wide QRS antidromic tachycardia of left bundle branch block pattern without Wolff-Parkinson-White configuration in sinus rhythm. Am Heart J, 103: 66-74.

167. Klein GJ, Guiraudon GM, Kerr CR, Sharma AD, Yee R, Szabo T, and Wah JA (1988). "Nodoventricular" accessory pathway: evidence for a distinct accessory atrioventricular pathway with atrioventricular node-like properties. JACC, 11: 1035-1040.

168. McClelland JH, Wang X, Beckman KJ, Hazlitt HA, Prior MI, Nakagawa H, Lazzara R, and Jackman WM (1994). Radiofrequency catheter ablation of right atriofascicular (Mahaim) accessory pathways guided by accessory pathway activation potentials. Circulation, 89: 2655-2666.

169. Cappato R, Schluter M, Mont L, and Kuck KH (1994). Anatomic, electrical, and mechanical factors affecting bipolar endocardial electrograms. Impact on catheter ablation of manifest left free-wall accessory pathways. Circulation, 90: 884-894.

170. Grogin HR, Lee RJ, Kwasman M, Epstein LM, Schamp DJ, Lesh MD, and Scheinman MM (1994). Radiofrequency catheter ablation of atriofascicular and nodoventricular Mahaim tracts [see comments]. Circulation, 90: 272-281.

171. Li HG, Klein GJ, Thakur RK, and Yee R (1994). Radiofrequency ablation of decremental accessory pathways mimicking "nodoventricular" conduction. Am J Cardiol, 74: 829-833.

172. Ursell PC, Gardner PI, Albala A, Fenoglio JJJ, and Wit AL (1985). Structural and electrophysiological changes in the epicardial border zone of canine myocardial infarcts during infarct healing. Circ Res, 56: 436-451.

173. Dillon SM, Allessie MA, Ursell PC, and Wit AL (1988). Influences of anisotropic tissue structure on reentrant circuits in the epicardial border zone of subacute canine infarcts. Circ Res, 63: 182-206.

174. Cardinal R, Vermuelen M, Shenasa M, Roberge F, Page P, Helie F, and Savard P (1988). Anisotropic conduction and functional dissociation of ischemic tissue during reentrant ventricular tachycardia in canine myocardial infarction. Circulation, 77: 1162-1176.

175. El-Sherif N, Smith RA, and Evans K (1981). Canine ventricular arrhythmias in the late myocardial infarction period. 8. Epicardial mapping of reentrant circuits. Circ Res, 49: 255-265.

176. Kramer JB, Saffitz JE, and Witkowski FX (1985). Intramural reentry as a mechanism of ventricular tachycardia during evolving canine myocardial infarction. Circ Res, 56: 736-754.

177. DiMarco JP, Lerman BB, Kron IL, and Sellers TD (1985). Sustained ventricular tachyarrhythmias within 2 months of acute myocardial infarction: results of medical and surgical therapy in patients resuscitated from the initial episode. JACC, 6: 759-768.

178. Wellens HJ, Duren DR, and Lie KI (1976). Observations on mechanisms of ventricular tachycardia in man. Circulation, 54: 237-244.

179. Josephson ME, Horowitz LN, Farshidi A, and Kastor JA (1978). Recurrent sustained ventricular tachycardia. 1. Mechanisms. Circulation, 57: 431-440.

180. Fisher JD, Cohen HL, Mehra R, Altschuler H, Excher DJ, and Furman S (1977). Cardiac pacing and pacemakers. II. Serial electrophysiologic testing for control of recurrent tachyarrhythmias. Am Heart J, 93: 658-668.
181. Cohen M, Wiener I, Pichard A, Holt J, Smith H Jr, and Gorlin R (1983). Determinants of ventricular tachycardia in patients with coronary artery disease and ventricular aneurysm. Am J Cardiol, 51: 61-64.
182. Wilensky RL, Yudelman P, Cohen AI, Fletcher RD, Atkinson J, Virmani R, and Roberts WC (1988). Serial electrocardiographic changes in idiopathic dilated cardiomyopathy confirmed at necropsy. Am J Cardiol, 62: 276-283.
183. Huang SK, Messer JV, and Denes P (1983). Significance of ventricular tachycardia in idiopathic dilated cardiomyopathy. Observations in 35 patients. Am J Cardiol, 51: 507-512.
184. Meinertz T, Hofmann T, Kasper W, Treese N, Bechtold H, Stienen U, Pop T, Leitner ER, Andresen D, and Meyer J (1984). Significance of ventricular arrhythmias in idiopathic dilated cardiomyopathy. Am J Cardiol, 53: 902-907.
185. Brigden W (1987). Hypertrophic cardiomyopathy. Brit Heart J, 58: 299-302.
186. McKenna WJ, Franklin RC, Nihoyannopoulos P, Robinson KC, and Deanfield JE (1988). Arrhythmia and prognosis in infants, children and adolescents with hypertrophic cardiomyopathy. JACC, 11: 147-153.
187. Fananapazir L, Tracy CM, Leon MB, Winkler JB, Cannon RO 3d, Bonow RO, Maron BJ, and Epstein SE (1989). Electrophysiologic abnormalities in patients with hyperrophic cardiomyopathy. A consecutive analysis in 155 patients. Circulation, 80: 1259-1268.
188. Spirito P, Chiarella F, Carratino L, Berisso MZ, Bellotti P, and Vecchio C (1989). Clinical course and prognosis of hypertrophic cardiomyopathy in an outpatient population. N Engl J Med, 320: 749-755.
189. Maron BJ, Bonow RO, Cannon RO, Leon MB, and Epstein SE (1987). Hypertrophic cardiomyopathy: Interrelations of clinical manifestations, pathophysiology and therapy (Part 1). N Engl J Med, 316: 780-789.
190. Maron BJ, Bonow RO, Cannon RO, Leon MB, and Epstein SE (1987). Hypertrophic cardiomyopathy: Interrelations of clinical manifestations, pathophysiology and therapy (Part 2). N Engl J Med, 316: 844-852.
191. Shakespeare CF, Keeling PJ, Slade AK, and McKenna WJ (1992). Arrhythmia and hypertrophic cardiomyopathy. Archives des Maladies du Coeur et des Vaisseaux, 85 Spec No 4: 31-36.
192. Kuck KH, Kunze KP, Schluter M, Nienaber CA, and Costard A (1988). Programmed electrical stimulation in hypertrophic cardiomyopathy. Results in patients with and without cardiac arrest or syncope. [Review]. Eur Heart J, 9: 177-185.
193. Kuck KH, Kunze KP, Geiger M, Costard A, and Schluter M (1987). Programmed electrical stimulation in patients with hypertrophic cardiomyopathy. Zeitschrift fur Kardiologie, 76: 131-136.

194. Kowey PR, Eisenberg R, and Engel TR (1984). Sustained arrhythmias in hypertrophic obstructive cardiomyopathy. N Engl J Med, 310: 1566-1569.
195. Lloyd EA, Zipes DP, Heger JJ, and Prystowsky EN (1982). Sustained ventricular tachycardia due to bundle branch reentry. Am Heart J, 104: 1095-1097.
196. Caceres J, Jazayeri M, McKinnie J, Avitall B, Denker ST, Tchou P, and Akhtar M (1989). Sustained bundle branch reentry as a mechanism of clinical tachycardia. Circulation, 79: 256-270.
197. Brooks R and Burgess JH (1988). Idiopathic ventricular tachycardia. Medicine, 67: 271-294.
198. Parkinson J and Papp C (1942). Repetitive paroxysmal tachycardia. Br Heart J, 10: 241-262.
199. Buxton AE, Waxman LH, Marchlinski FE, Simson MB, Cassidy D, and Josephson ME (1983). Right ventricular tachycardia: Clinical and electrophysiologic characteristics. Circulation, 5: 917-927.
200. Coumel P, Leclerq JP, and Slama R (1985). Repetitive monomorphic idiopathic ventricular tachycardia. In: Zipes DP and Jalife J (eds). Cardiac Electrophysiology and Arrhythmias. Orlando, FL: Grune and Stratton, pp. 455-466.
201. Kinoshita O, Fontaine G, Rosas F, Elias J, Iwa T, Tonet J, Lascault G, and Frank R (1995). Time- and frequency-domain analyses of the signal-averaged ECG in patients with arrhythmogenic right ventricular dysplasia. Circulation, 91: 715-721.
202. Ritchie AH, Kerr CR, Qi A, and Yeung-Lai-Wah JA (1989). Nonsustained ventricular tachycardia arising from the right ventricular outflow tract. Am J Cardiol, 63: 594-598.
203. Mont L, Sexas T, Brugada P, Simonis F, Kriek E, Smeets JL, and Wellens HJ (1992). The electrocardiographic, clinical and electrophysiologic spectrium of idiopathic monomorphic ventricular tachycardia. Am Heart J, 124: 746-753.
204. Lerman BB, Belardinelli L, West GA, Berne RM, and DiMarco JP (1986). Adenosine-sensitive ventricular tachycardia: evidence suggesting cyclic AMP-mediated triggered activity. Circulation, 74: 270-280.
205. Zipes DP, Foster PR, Troup PJ, and Pederson DH (1979). Atrial induction of ventricular tachycardia: Reentry versus triggered activity. Am J Cardiol, 44: 1-8.
206. Belhassen B, Rotmensch HH, and Laniado S (1981). Response of recurrent sustained ventricular tachycardia to verapamil. Br Heart J, 46: 679-682.
207. Okumura K, Matsuyama K, Miyagi H, Tsuchiya T, and Yasue H (1988). Entrainment of idiopathic ventricular tachycardia of left ventricular origin with evidence for reentry with an area of slow conduction and effect of verapamil. Am J Cardiol, 62: 727-732.
208. Ward DE, Nathan AW, and Camm AJ (1984). Fascicular tachycardia sensitive to calcium antagonists. Eur Heart J, 5: 896-905.
209. Touboul P, Saoudi N, Atallah G, and Kirkorian G (1989). Electrophysiologic basis of catheter ablation in atrial flutter. Am J Cardiol, 64: 79J-85J.

210. Olshansky B, Okumura K, Hess PG, and Waldo AL (1990). Demonstration of an area of slow conduction in human atrial flutter. JACC, 16: 1639-1648.
211. Cosio FG, Lopez GM, Goicolea A, and Arribas F (1992). Electrophysiologic studies in atrial flutter. Clin Cardiol, 61: 667-673.
212. Feld G, Fleck RP, Chen PS, Boyce K, Bahnson T, Stein JB, Calisi CM, and Ibarra M (1992). Radiofrequency catheter ablation for the treatment of human type I atrial flutter. Identification of a critical zone in the reentrant circuit by endocardial mapping techniques. Circulation, 86: 1233-1240.
213. Kirkorian G, Moncada E, Chevalier P, Canu G, Claudel JP, Bellon C, Lyon L, and Touboul P (1994). Radiofrequency ablation of atrial flutter. Efficacy of an anatomically guided approach. Circulation, 90: 2804-2814.
214. Poty H, Saoudi N, Abdel Aziz A, Nair M, and Letac B (1995). Radiofrequency catheter ablation of type 1 atrial flutter. Prediction of late success by electrophysiological criteria. Circulation, 92: 1389-1392.
215. Cauchemez B, Haissaguerre M, Fischer B, Thomas O, Clementy J, and Coumel P (1996). Electrophysiologic effects of catheter ablation of inferior vena cava-tricuspid annulus isthmus in common atrial flutter. Circulation, 93: 284-294.
216. Nath S, Mounsey JP, Haines DE, and DiMarco JP (1995). Predictors of acute and long-term success after radiofrequency catheter ablation of type 1 atrial flutter. Am J Cardiol, 76: 604-606.
217. Steinberg JS, Prasher S, Zelenkofske S, and Ehlert FA (1995). Radiofrequency catheter ablation of atrial flutter: procedural success and long-term outcome. Am Heart J, 130: 85-92.
218. Fischer B, Haissaguerre M, Garrigues S, Poquet F, Gencel L, Clementy J, and Marcus FI (1995). Radiofrequency catheter ablation of common atrial flutter in 80 patients. JACC, 25: 1365-1372.
219. Chen SA, Chiang CE, Wu TJ, Tai CT, Lee SH, Cheng CC, Chiou CW, Ueng KC, Wen ZC, and Chang MS (1996). Radiofrequency catheter ablation of common atrial flutter: Comparision of electrophysiologically guided focal ablation technique and linear ablation technique. JACC, 27: 860-868.
220. Ferguson TB Jr and Cox JL (1995). Surgery for atrial fibrillation. In: Zipes DP and Jalife J (eds). Cardiac Electrophysiology: From Cell to Bedside (ed 2nd). Philadelphia: W.B. Saunders Company, p. 1567.
221. Leitch JW, Klein G, Yee R, and Guiraudon G (1991). Sinus node-atrioventricular node isolation: Long term results with the "corridor" operation for atrial fibrillation. JACC, 17: 970-975.
222. van Hemel NM, Defauw JJ, Kingma JH, Jaarsma W, Vermeulen FE, de Bakker JM, and Guiraudon GM (1994). Long-term results of the corridor operation for atrial fibrillation [see comments]. Brit Heart J, 71: 170-176.
223. Cox JL (1993). Evolving applications of the maze procedure for atrial fibrillation. Ann Thorac Surg, 55: 578-580.

224. Cox JL, Boineau JP, Schuessler RB, Kater KM, and Lappas DG (1993). Five Year experience with the maze procedure for atrial fibrillation. Ann Thorac Surg, 56: 814-823.

225. Kosakai Y, Kawaguchi AT, Isobe F, Sasako Y, Nakano K, Eishi K, Kito Y, and Kawashima Y (1993). Modified maze procedures for patients with atrial fibrillation undergoing simultaneous open heart surgery. Circulation, 92: II-359-364.

226. Sandoval N, Velasco VM, Orjuela H, Caicedo V, Santos H, Rosas F, Carrea JR, Melgarejo I, and Morillo CA (1996). Concomitant mitral valve or atrial septal defect surgery and the modified Cox-maze procedure. Am J Cardiol, 77: 591-596.

227. Swartz JF, Lellersels G, Silvers J, et al. (1994). A catheter-based curative approach to atrial fibrillation in humans. Circulation, 90: I-335.

228. Haissaguerre M, Gencel L, Fischer B, Le Metayer P, Poquet F, Marcus FI, and Clementy J (1994). Successful catheter ablation of atrial fibrillation. J Cardiovas Electrophys, 5: 1045-1052.

229. Kim YH, O'Nunain S, Ruskin JN, and Garan H (1993). Nonpharmacologic therapies in patients with ventricular tachyarrhythmias. Catheter ablation and ventricular tachycardia surgery. [Review]. Cardiology Clinics, 11: 85-96.

230. Josephson ME (1993). Clinical Cardiac Electrophysiology: Techniques and Interpretations(ed 2nd). Philadelphia, Lea & Febiger.

231. D'Avila A, Nellens P, Andries E, and Brugada P (1994). Catheter ablation of ventricular tachycardia occurring late after myocardial infarction: a point-of-view. [Review]. Pace - Pacing & Clinical Electrophysiology, 17: 532-541.

232. Prystowsky EN and Klein GJ (1994). Cardiac Arrhythmias: An Integrated Approach for the Clinician. New York, McGraw-Hill,Inc.

233. Borggrefe M, Chen X, Hindricks G, Haverkamp W, Willems S, Kottkamp H, Rotman B, Martinez-Rubio A, Shenasa M, Block M, and Breithardt G (1995). Catheter ablation of ventricular tachycardia in patients with coronary heart disease. In: Zipes DP and Jalife J (eds). Cardiac Electrophysiology: From Cell to Bedside (ed 2nd). Philadelphia: W. B. Saunders Company, pp. 1502-1517.

234. Fitzgerald DM, Friday KJ, Wah JA, Lazzara R, and Jackman WM (1988). Electrogram patterns predicting successful catheter ablation of ventricular tachycardia. Circulation, 77: 806-814.

235. Garan H and Ruskin JN (1988). Reproducible termination of ventricular tachycardia by a single extrastimulus within the reentry circuit during the ventricular effective refractory period. Am Heart J, 116: 546-550.

236. Morady F, Frank R, Kou WH, Tonet JL, Nelson SD, Kounde S, De Buitleir M, and Fontaine G (1988). Identification and catheter ablation of a zone of slow conduction in the reentrant circuit of ventricular tachycardia in humans. JACC, 11: 775-782.

237. Stevenson WG, Khan H, Sager P, Saxon LA, Middlekauff HR, Natterson PD, and Wiener I (1993). Identification of reentry circuit sites during catheter mapping and radiofrequency ablation of ventricular tachycardia. Circulation, 88: 1647-1670.

238. Stevenson WG, Sager PT, Natterson PD, Saxon LA, Middlekauff HR, and Wiener I (1995). Relation of pace mapping QRS configuration and conduction delay to ventricular tachycardia reentry circuits in human infarct scars. JACC, 26: 481-488.

239. Josephson ME, Waxman HL, Cain ME, Gardner MJ, and Buxton AE (1982). Ventricular activation during ventricular endocardial pacing. II: role of pace-mapping to localize origin of ventricular tachycardia. Am J Cardiol, 50: 11-20.

240. Kuchar DL, Ruskin JN, and Garan H (1989). Electrocardiographic localization of the site of origin of ventricular tachycardia in patients with prior myocardial infarction. JACC, 13: 893-903.

241. Evans GT, Scheinman MM, and Zipes DP (1986). The percutaneous cardiac mapping and ablation registry: summary of results. Pace - Pacing & Clinical Electrophysiology, 9: 923-926.

242. Gonska BD, Cao K, Schaumann A, Dorszewski A, von zur Muhlen F, and Kreuzer H (1994). Catheter ablation of ventricular tachycardia in 136 patients with coronary artery disease: results and long-term follow-up. JACC, 24: 1506-1514.

243. Gonska BD, Cao K, Schaumann A, Dorszewski A, von zur Muhlen F, and Kreuzer H (1994). Management of patients after catheter ablation of ventricular tachycardia. [Review]. Pace - Pacing & Clinical Electrophysiology, 17: 542-549.

244. Tchou P, Jazayeri M, Denker S, Dongas J, Caceres J, and Akhtar M (1988). Transcatheter electrical ablation of right bundle branch. A method of treating macroreentrant ventricular tachycardia attributed to bundle branch reentry. Circulation, 78: 246-257.

245. Wilber DJ, Baerman J, Olshansky B, Kall J, and Kopp D (1993). Adenosine sensitive ventricular tachycardia: Clinical characteristics and response to catheter ablation. Circulation, 87: 126-134.

246. Nakagawa H, Beckman KJ, McClelland JH, Wang X, Arruda M, Santoro I, Hazlitt HA, Abdalla I, Singh A, Gossinger H, et al. (1993). Radiofrequency catheter ablation of idiopathic left ventricular tachycardia guided by a Purkinje potential. Circulation, 88: 2607-2617.

247. Klein LS, Miles WM, Hackett FK, and Zipes DP (1992). Catheter ablation of ventricular tachycardia using radiofrequency techniques in patients without structural heart disease. Herz, 17: 179-189.

248. Wen MS, Yeh SJ, Wang CC, Lin FC, Chen IC, and Wu D (1994). Radiofrequency ablation therapy in idiopathic left ventricular tachycardia with no obvious structural heart disease. Circulation, 89: 1690-1696.

249. Kottkamp H, Kindricks G, Chen X, Brunn J, Willems S, Haverkamp W, Block M, Breithardt G, and Borggrefe M (1995). Radiofrequency catheter ablation of sustained ventricular tachycardia in idiopathic dilated cardiomyopathy. Circulation, 92: 1159-1168.
250. Lawrie GM and Pacifico A (1995). Surgery for ventricular tachycardia. In: Zipes DP and Jalife J (eds). Cardiac Electrophysiology: From Cell to Bedside (ed 2nd). Philadelphia: W. B. Saunders, pp. 1547-1552.

Index